Alcohol:
No Ordinary Commodity

Alcohol:
No Ordinary
Commodity
Research and
public policy

SECOND EDITION

Thomas Babor

Raul Caetano

Sally Casswell

Griffith Edwards

Norman Giesbrecht

Kathryn Graham

Joel Grube

Linda Hill

Harold Holder

Ross Homel

Michael Livingston

Esa Österberg

Jürgen Rehm

Robin Room

Ingeborg Rossow

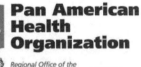

Pan American
Health
Organization

Regional Office of the
World Health Organization

OXFORD
UNIVERSITY PRESS

OXFORD
UNIVERSITY PRESS

Great Clarendon Street, Oxford ox2 6DP

Oxford University Press is a department of the University of Oxford.
It furthers the University's objective of excellence in research, scholarship,
and education by publishing worldwide in

Oxford New York

Auckland Cape Town Dar es Salaam Hong Kong Karachi
Kuala Lumpur Madrid Melbourne Mexico City Nairobi
New Delhi Shanghai Taipei Toronto

With offices in

Argentina Austria Brazil Chile Czech Republic France Greece
Guatemala Hungary Italy Japan Poland Portugal Singapore
South Korea Switzerland Thailand Turkey Ukraine Vietnam

Oxford is a registered trade mark of Oxford University Press
in the UK and in certain other countries

Published in the United States
by Oxford University Press Inc., New York

First published 2003

Second Edition 2010

British Library Cataloguing in Publication Data
Data available

Library of Congress Cataloging in Publication Data

Data available

Typeset in Minion by Glyph International, Bangalore, India
Printed in Great Britain on acid-free paper by Clays

ISBN 978-0-19-955114-9

3

Foreword

Alcohol is a source of pleasure for many consumers but it is also associated with a host of problems that afflict individuals and society at large. In recent years a strong body of evidence has emerged showing that these problems have increased in many parts of the world. The link between heavy alcohol consumption and some non-communicable diseases and injury is hardly contestable, and what was for some time a tenuous link with infectious disease is today being confirmed by studies that show the negative impact of alcohol on the outcomes of diseases like tuberculosis and HIV/AIDS (Rehm *et al.* 2009).

Much of what we know today about the impact of alcohol on health and social welfare is, primarily, from studies conducted in western industrialized societies, but our knowledge of alcohol problems in developing countries is increasing (Room *et al.* 2002). In these societies most adults are abstainers, women drink much less than men, and the pattern of consumption is characterized by drinking to intoxication. Through the work of the World Health Organization, and as reported in this book, we know that this pattern of consumption is a significant risk factor for burden of disease (WHO 2002; 2008). And yet, this knowledge has not been matched by appropriate policy responses to what is obviously a global public health menace.

It was not clear at the time, but the publication of the first edition of *Alcohol: No ordinary commodity* in 2003 was a landmark event in the history of alcohol control policies. Though it is difficult to measure the influence of a book, the world of alcohol policy has not been the same since its publication. There is more widespread knowledge among professionals and policy makers about the role that alcohol plays in society. The book made it clear to us that alcohol problems respond to sound public health measures; that because a measure is popular does not mean it is effective; and that policy should be guided by the best available evidence. In practical terms the book has served as the main resource material in alcohol policy training workshops and policy development in a variety of countries. I have heard it described as the "alcohol policy bible" by admirers, and its detractors have not been able to undercut its influence.

This second edition of *Alcohol: No ordinary commodity* looks very much like the first, except that all chapters have been updated, a new chapter has been added on the alcohol industry, and the rating table of alcohol control measures has been revised. You will find new information on the globalization of the alcohol industry, the potential impact of the industry's expansion into the emerging markets of the developing countries, including the industry's role in the policymaking process in these countries. Like the first edition, it does not pretend to have all the answers and popular strategies that have historically not lived up to expectation are not dismissed offhandedly. In this careful and painstaking analysis of a contentious issue in contemporary public health, the authors do not claim that every effective strategy will produce similar results in every country; but whether the problem is illicit production and trade, or what to do about heavy episodic ("binge") drinking, there is no better guide than this book. I have no doubt that this book will help to further strengthen our belief in evidence-based alcohol policies.

In a future edition one hopes that the evidence base will be further strengthened with more data and experiences from developing countries. It is to the interest of the global alcohol research and policy community that the research and monitoring capacity in these countries is enhanced. My hope is that the publication of this second edition of *Alcohol: No ordinary commodity* will finally render the argument about alcohol's contribution to economic development untenable (if it ever was), in the face of clear evidence that alcohol does not drive but hurts development. With such a knowledge base as provided by this book, there is indeed no excuse for any country or municipality for not applying the lessons learned. The time is past for uninformed arguments about what works and what does not. Instead, it is time to act in concert with the global community and under the leadership of the World Health Organization to develop and implement effective national strategies to reduce the harm associated with the consumption of this unusual commodity.

References

Rehm J., Anderson P., Kanteres F., Parry C.D, Samokhvalov A.V, **and** Patra J. (2009) *Alcohol, social development and infectious disease.* Stockholm: European Union.

Room R., Jernigan D., Carlini-Marlatt B., *et al.* 2002) *Alcohol in developing societies: A public health approach.* Geneva: WHO.

World Health Organization (2002) *The world health report 2002: Reducing risks, promoting healthy life.* Geneva: WHO.

World Health Organization (2008) *The global burden of disease: 2004 updates.* Geneva: WHO.

Isidore S. Obot, PhD, MPH
Professor and Head
Department of Psychology
University of Uyo
and
Director
Centre for Research and
Information on Substance
Abuse (CRISA)
Uyo, NIGERIA

Authors' preface to the second edition

From a public health perspective, alcohol consumption plays a major role in the causation of disability, disease, and death on a global scale. It also contributes substantially to family dysfunction, violence, and psychiatric disorder. With the increasing globalization of alcohol production, trade, and marketing, it is becoming apparent that alcohol control policy needs to be understood not only from a national but also from a global perspective.

In the past 50 years considerable progress has been made in the scientific understanding of the relationship between alcohol and health. Ideally, the cumulative research evidence should provide a scientific basis for public debate and governmental policymaking. However, much of the scientific evidence reported in academic publications has little apparent relevance to prevention strategy or treatment policy. To address this need for a policy-relevant translation of the alcohol research literature, a small group of experts under the leadership of Professor Griffith Edwards established in 1992 the Alcohol and Public Policy Project (APPP). The group recruited an international team of research scientists, consulted with experts throughout the world, and in the course of fewer than two years critically evaluated the accumulated knowledge on how to deal with alcohol problems in the public policy arena. The outcome of this work was *Alcohol Policy and the Public Good* (Edwards *et al.* 1994) and *Alcohol and Public Policy: Evidence and Issues* (Holder and Edwards 1995).

At a 1998 alcohol policy conference in Chicago, IL, USA, a small group of the APPP authors agreed to begin plans for work on another volume, based on the increasing knowledge base, the changing climate of alcohol policy, and international trends in drinking problems. The text of that volume, *Alcohol: No Ordinary Commodity—Research and Public Policy* (Babor *et al.* 2003) evolved through the development of background papers, the discussion of this material at five plenary meetings held in different parts of the world, and many stages of drafting. Like the previous books in this series, *No Ordinary Commodity* is a written rather than an edited volume, built on the joint input of all those involved, and speaking with one voice to the reader. Sponsored by the World Health Organization and the UK Society for the Study of Addiction, the major purpose of this volume was not only to show why alcohol is indeed no ordinary commodity, but also to direct attention to the emerging arsenal of evidence-informed policy options available to policymakers at the local, national, and international levels.

Although alcohol has been recognized since time immemorial as a special product requiring special controls on its production and availability, it was only since the 19th century that academics took an active interest in the effects of alcohol policies on individuals and populations. Building on this tradition, the modern era of alcohol policy research can be traced to the landmark publication of *Alcohol Control Policies in Public Health Perspective* (Bruun *et al.* 1975a), which showed how alcohol policy could be informed by an emerging corpus of epidemiological, theoretical, and intervention research. Continuing in that vein, the first edition of *Alcohol: No Ordinary Commodity* attempted to synthesize what was new and relevant to alcohol policy on an international level. We are pleased that the book was recognized by the British Medical Association as worthy of first prize in the public health category of its 2004 medical book competition, and has been cited repeatedly by the World Health Organization as an authoritative source in its plans to develop a Global Strategy on Alcohol.

The present volume was conceived out of a recognition that the scientific evidence for effective alcohol policy is expanding rapidly in many areas, and is therefore periodically in need of updating and expansion into new areas of knowledge. The policy needs of communities and nations change with each new generation and each new epidemic of alcohol-related problems, especially in less-resourced countries where policy-relevant research is desperately needed. Those parts of the world, particularly in Asia, Africa, and Latin America, which have traditionally had weak alcohol controls and relatively low aggregate levels of alcohol consumption, are being threatened by an expansion of commercial production and advanced marketing by the alcohol industry. These developments are likely to increase their susceptibility to alcohol-related problems.

This situation led the authors to re-examine the epidemiological data underpinning our original thesis that alcohol is no ordinary commodity, and to provide a critical evaluation of what had previously been ignored in the alcohol control debate: the role of the alcohol industry. Combined with new studies on the effectiveness of alcohol taxes and availability restrictions, new information about the impacts of alcohol marketing, and an expanding array of other evidence-based policies, the authors felt there was more than enough reason for a second edition. We therefore offer this volume as our contribution to the debate over how best to formulate, implement, and sustain a Global Strategy on Alcohol, which the World Health Organization has been charged with presenting to the World Health Assembly in 2010.

As we noted in our preface to the first edition, the purpose of this book is to describe recent advances in alcohol research that have direct relevance to the development of alcohol policy on the local, national and international levels. That focus has not changed, nor has our interest in providing updated evaluations of the effectiveness, generalizability, and cost of alcohol control strategies. We hope that by expanding our purview and updating the science base, this edition of *No ordinary commodity* will continue to inform the policy debate, empower the policymaker, and demonstrate how research can contribute to the advancement of a public policy response that reduces the social and personal harms related to alcohol consumption.

The Authors

A note on terminology and technical terms

Key terms that have technical or linguistic meanings that would not be familiar to the general reader are defined in the Glossary at the end of the book. These terms are indicated in bold when they are first used in a given chapter. Most often the terms refer to words or concepts used in epidemiology, alcohol research, addiction medicine, or popular culture in different parts of the world.

Preface

The harmful use of alcohol is among the leading risk factors for the burden of disease in the Region of the Americas, contributing to violence, injuries, suicides, chronic noncommunicable diseases, and mental health disorders besides alcohol dependence. It disproportionally affects individuals, families and societies in low and middle income countries of the Region and contributes to worsening inequities in health. Alcohol consumption is increasing particularly among young people and it is also starting at earlier ages, despite the scientific evidence of the risk of early alcohol use and the later development of alcohol dependence.

The Pan American Health Organization (PAHO) has increased technical cooperation to countries in the Region to respond to alcohol related problems in a more comprehensive way. In 2005, PAHO organized with the support of the government of Brazil the *First Pan American Conference on Alcohol Public Policies*, with participants from 26 countries of the Region, who signed the Brasilia Declaration. PAHO has also coordinated research on alcohol and domestic violence and is supporting training of health professionals in primary health care to screen and provide a brief intervention for those at risk of developing alcohol problems.

PAHO has contributed to the development of the World Health Organization (WHO) strategy to reduce harmful use of alcohol, by organizing a regional consultation meeting in 2009 and by contributing technical expertise to various documents, expert meetings and policy discussions with Member States.

In response to the need for evidence on the effectiveness, costs and generalizability of various alcohol policies and the relative role of various stakeholders, including the alcohol industry, I am pleased to introduce this book, which is an updated and expanded second edition of the landmark book published in 2003 by Oxford University Press and WHO. PAHO will support the publication of the Spanish version as well, aimed at reaching out to a much broader audience in the Americas Region.

I hope this publication will not only contribute to the discussions at global level but also provide support for effective country responses to the harmful consumption of alcohol.

Mirta Roses Periago
Director, PAHO

Acknowledgements

The authors are grateful to the World Health Organization (Copenhagen regional office and Geneva headquarters), which provided support for the first edition on which much of this volume builds, and to the UK Society for the Study of Addiction, which provided funding to cover the logistical costs of the project. No fees were paid for any of the writing, consulting work, or background papers connected with the project. All authors provided WHO Conflict of Interest assurances, which are available from the first author upon request. Most of the support for travel costs and manuscript preparation came from the participants' own centres and universities, as well as time donated by them to the project. Although the lead author of this volume was responsible for the overall coordination of the project, it should be noted that the authors' names are listed in alphabetical order to indicate that equal contributions were made by all to the substantive work behind the revisions. The authors wish to recognize Dr Robert Mann, of the Centre for Addiction and Mental Health, Toronto, Canada, for his important contributions to Chapter 11. Honey Bloomberg's contributions in collecting, organizing, and synthesizing resource documents for Chapter 13 are also appreciated. The authors are particularly grateful to Jean O'Reilly, PhD, who served as the chief editorial assistant to the project.

The following organizations and funding sources are acknowledged because of the institutional support they provided to the authors in the form of salaries and travel funds.

Thomas Babor's participation in this project was supported in part by the University of Connecticut PHS Endowed Chair in Community Medicine and Public Health, as well as by a grant from the US National Institute on Alcohol Abuse and Alcoholism (P60 AA03510).

Sally Casswell was supported in part by the Centre for Social and Health Outcomes Research and Evaluation, Massey University, New Zealand.

Kathryn Graham and Norman Giesbrecht were supported in part by the Centre for Addiction and Mental Health, Toronto, Ontario, Canada.

Linda Hill's work monitoring global alcohol corporations was supported initially by the Institute of Alcohol Studies, UK, for the Global Alcohol Policy Alliance, and then by the Centre for Health Outcomes Research and Evaluation (SHORE), Massey University, New Zealand.

Michael Livingston was supported by funding from the Alcohol Education and Rehabilitation Foundation of Australia.

Esa Österberg's participation in this project was supported by the national Research and Development Centre for Welfare and Health (until 2008) and by the National Institute for Health and Welfare (from the beginning of 2009).

Jürgen Rehm's participation was enabled by the Ontario Centre for Addiction and Mental Health and the Swiss Research Institute for Public Health and Addiction (until 2008). In addition, his underlying work was supported by the World Health Organization, the Swiss National Science Foundation, and the Global Burden of Disease and Injury Study.

Robin Room's professorship at the University of Melbourne was primarily funded by the Department of Health, State of Victoria, Australia.

Ingeborg Rossow's participation was enabled by the Norwegian Institute for Alcohol and Drug Research.

Contents

Contributors

Thomas Babor, PhD, MPH
Professor and Chairman
Department of Community Medicine
and Health Care
University of Connecticut School of
Medicine
Farmington, Connecticut, USA

Raul Caetano, MD, MPH, PhD
Professor of Epidemiology and
Regional Dean
University of Texas School of Public
Health, Dallas Regional Campus
Dallas, Texas, USA
Professor of Health Care Sciences and
Psychiatry
Dean, Southwestern School of Health
Professions
University of Texas Southwestern
Medical Center
Dallas, Texas, USA

Sally Casswell, PhD
Professor of Social and Health Research
Director, Centre for Social and Health
Outcomes Research and Evaluation
Massey University, Auckland,
New Zealand

Griffith Edwards, DM
Emeritus Professor of Addiction
Behaviour
National Addiction Centre, London, UK

Norman Giesbrecht, PhD
Senior Scientist, Section Public Health
and Regulatory Policies
Social, Prevention and Health Policy
Research Department
Centre for Addiction and Mental
Health, Toronto, Ontario, Canada

Kathryn Graham, PhD
Senior Scientist and Head, Social and
Community Prevention Research
Centre for Addiction and Mental Health
Adjunct Research Professor, Department
of Psychology
University of Western Ontario, London,
Ontario, Canada;
Professor (Adjunct), National Drug
Research Institute
Curtin University of Technology, Perth,
Western Australia

Joel Grube, PhD
Director and Senior Research Scientist,
Prevention Research Center
Pacific Institute for Research and
Evaluation
Berkeley, California, USA

Linda Hill, PhD
Senior Researcher
Centre for Social and Health Outcomes
Research and Evaluation
Massey University, Auckland,
New Zealand

Harold Holder, PhD
Senior Research Scientist, Prevention
Research Center
Pacific Institute for Research and
Evaluation
Berkeley, California, USA

Ross Homel, PhD, AO
Foundation Professor of
Criminology and Criminal Justice
Director
Griffith Institute for Social and
Behavioural Research Griffith University
Queensland, Australia

Michael Livingston, BA
Research Fellow, AER Centre for
Alcohol Policy Research
Turning Point Alcohol and Drug
Centre, Fitzroy, Australia

Esa Österberg, MSc
Senior Researcher, Department of
Alcohol, Drugs and Addiction
National Institute for Health and
Welfare, Helsinki, Finland

Jürgen Rehm, PhD
Senior Scientist and Co-Head, Section
Public Health and Regulatory Policies
Centre for Addiction and Mental
Health, Toronto, Canada;
Professor and Chair, Addiction Policy,
Dalla Lana School of Public Health
University of Toronto, Toronto,
Canada;
Head, Epidemiological Research Unit,
Technische Universität Dresden,
Klinische Psychologie & Psychotherapie,
Dresden, Germany

Robin Room, PhD
Professor, School of Population Health
University of Melbourne, Melbourne,
Australia;
Director, AER Centre for Alcohol Policy
Research
Turning Point Alcohol and Drug
Centre, Fitzroy, Australia;
Professor, Centre for Social Research on
Alcohol and Drugs
Stockholm University, Stockholm,
Sweden

Ingeborg Rossow, PhD
Research Director, Norwegian Institute
for Alcohol and Drug Research
Oslo, Norway

Chapter 1

Setting the policy agenda

1.1 **Introduction**

In Pitkäranta, Russia, Anatoly Iverianov, a 45-year-old log cutter, attributed the two heart attacks he suffered in 1998 to the fact that 'I've been drinking and smoking a lot.' Indeed, after a third heart attack ended his life soon after his news interview (Wines 2000), the autopsy results listed chronic alcoholism as the probable cause of death. As in other parts of Russia, violence, suicide, and cardiovascular disease play major roles in the precipitous decline in life expectancy observed here over the past decade. Alcohol control policies instituted in 1985 led to a reduction in drinking and an increase in life expectancy, but those policies were soon reversed.

In neighbouring Finland, just across the Russian border in North Karelia, epidemiological studies showed that people working in the timber industry once drank and smoked just as heavily as their Russian neighbours, and both regions shared the distinction of having the highest rates of cardiovascular disease in the world. Finland's response was to implement the North Karelia Project (Wines 2000), a five-year effort designed to change people's diet, exercise, smoking, and drinking habits through a combination of health promotion, disease prevention, and economic incentives. Twenty-five years after the policies were implemented, the rate of heart disease among working-age residents was significantly lower, in part because of the reduction in risk factors (Vartiainen *et al.* 2000).

In Kenya's capital of Nairobi, a homemade alcohol product fortified with methanol killed 121 people in November 2000, leaving 495 hospitalized, 20 of whom suffered blindness (Nordwall 2000). The toll was particularly pronounced in the urban slums surrounding the city, where unlicensed cafés serve illegal brews to the rural migrants seeking employment in the city. Policies restricting illicit alcohol distillation and the unlicensed sale of alcoholic beverages have been difficult to enforce.

In Tokyo, the headline of a newspaper article reads: 'Year-Ending Parties Pour Drunks onto Trains of Japan,' referring to the *bonenkai* New Year's holiday season. Railway officials estimated that at least 60% of the passengers were intoxicated during this period. In response, two policies were instituted. Extra security guards were hired to minimize injuries, and 'women only' railway cars were introduced to prevent sexual assaults. The article made no mention of whether the policies had their intended effects (Zielenziger 2000).

In Tennant Creek, Australia, aboriginal groups successfully pressed restrictions on Thursday trading (payday for social security checks), sales of four-litre cask wine, and hours of takeaway sale. The 'Thirsty Thursday'policy was associated with a reduction in alcohol-related police incidents, hospital admissions, and women's shelter presentations. During the same period, alcohol consumption decreased by 19% (Brady 2000).

What do these vignettes have in common? They all speak to the effects of alcohol consumption on individuals and populations, and draw attention to the search for policies that protect health, prevent disability, and address the social problems associated with the misuse of beverage alcohol. This book is at its core a scientific treatise on alcohol policy: what alcohol policy is, why it is needed, which interventions are effective, how policy is made, and how scientific evidence can inform the policymaking process.

1.2 Alcohol policy: a brief history

The control of alcohol production, distribution, and consumption was first exercised by local authorities in the emerging urban areas of ancient Greece, Mesopotamia, Egypt, and Rome (Ghalioungui 1979). Greek statesmen of the sixth century bce introduced supervised festivities to provide an alternative to the Dionysian revelries that promoted drunkenness. In 594, Solon prescribed the death penalty for drunken magistrates and required that all wine be diluted with water before being sold. For more than 2000 years, ingenious strategies like these were devised by monarchs, governments, and the clergy to prevent alcohol-related problems. But it was not until the rise of modern medicine and the emergence of the world temperance movement in the nineteenth century that alcohol policy gained greater potential as an instrument of public health (Babor and Rosenkranz 1991).

Measures affecting alcohol consumption are now a common feature of legal and regulatory systems throughout the world. All governments have to deal with alcohol or alcoholic beverages as consumer goods in one way or another. However, public policy that regards alcohol as a special social or health problem, or as a subject for comprehensive regulation, has been less common. In earlier times, alcoholic beverages were recognized as special commodities. This was done, for example, by giving a company monopoly control to trade in alcoholic beverages in a certain area or by using alcoholic beverages as a tax base for the state (Österberg 1985; Room 1993). In the nineteenth century, the temperance movement gave rise to national, regional, and local alcohol policies, especially in the Anglo-Saxon and Nordic countries. Between 1914 and 1921, laws prohibiting the manufacture and sale of all or most forms of beverage alcohol were adopted in Canada, Finland, Iceland, Norway, Russia, and the USA (Paulson 1973). Most of these laws were repealed during the 1920s and 1930s, to be replaced by laws and policies that allowed but regulated the manufacture and sale of alcohol. To view alcohol policies through the narrowly focused perspective of prohibition, however, is to ignore the fact that most policymaking during the past century has been incremental, deliberate, and respectful of people's right to drink in moderation. However, total alcohol prohibition still remains a crucial part of some government policies, mostly in Islamic countries and states of India.

In Europe, the last 50 years have seen a convergence in alcohol policies. In the early 1950s, alcohol policy in the Nordic countries was based on social policy and public health considerations, and included high excise duties on alcoholic beverages, comprehensive state alcohol monopoly systems for production and trade, and strict controls on alcohol availability (Karlsson and Österberg 2001). In the Mediterranean wine-producing countries there were very few alcohol control measures in force in the early 1950s, and most of them were motivated by industrial or commercial interests. Some countries between the Nordic and Mediterranean areas, like Ireland and the UK, developed a strict licensing system, especially for on-premises sales of alcoholic beverages. Other countries, like Belgium and The Netherlands, still have in force leftovers of former alcohol control systems.

The convergence of alcohol policies in the present European Union (EU) member states during the second half of the twentieth century can be best understood by looking separately at different areas of alcohol controls. On the one hand, the control of alcohol production, distribution, and sales has decreased in the EU member states (see Box 1.1). On the other hand, measures targeted at alcohol demand and the drinker, like alcohol education and drink-driving countermeasures, have become more prevalent and harsher during the last fifty years. In the present EU member states there have also been converging trends with regard to taxing alcoholic beverages, although the convergence has been rather weak.

In North America there has been a gradual decline in alcohol control in most jurisdictions in recent decades, with more dramatic changes such as full privatization of alcohol retail sales in several US states and one Canadian province, and an erosion of government-run systems in several other jurisdictions. In the last two decades, divergent trends were evident with regard to alcohol prices: in Canada, alcohol prices tended to parallel changes in the Consumer Price Index, whereas in the USA a general decline in real prices was evident in many jurisdictions. Alcohol taxes have not been raised to match inflation. Both countries have lax controls on alcohol advertising, especially in the USA. By contrast, there are extensive education and law enforcement efforts to control drink-driving.

Similar developments have taken place in other parts of the world. For instance, the collapse of the communist system in the former Soviet Union (see Box 1.2) and many

Box 1.1 Public policies are not always public health policies

In the Nordic countries, the influence of the commercial policies of the EU has undermined previously strong national alcohol policies (Holder *et al.* 1998; Sulkunen *et al.* 2000). As a consequence, there is now much greater interest in the local arena for handling alcohol-related problems (Larsson and Hanson 1999). For example, in Sweden, the Alcohol Act of 1995 not only disestablished the state monopoly for import, export, distribution, and production of alcohol, but also shifted responsibility for the licensing of on-premises sales and control of licensed establishments to a more local level, from the 25 counties to the 272 municipalities (Romelsjö and Andersson 1999). Similarly, in a number of North American contexts there has been a move toward full or partial privatization of government retail monopolies (Her *et al.* 1999), and increasing emphasis by government-run monopolies on commercial issues at the expense of control mandates.

Box 1.2 Alcohol policies in transition

A large vacuum in alcohol policy was created by the break-up of the Soviet Union, after which public administration and political authority became less unified within each of the countries in transition. Whereas it was possible to talk of a national policy before the break-up of the Soviet Union, after 1991 it was more appropriate to describe the situation in the Russian Federation as a national framework within which an assortment of local alcohol policies existed (Nemtsov and Krasovsky 1996; Reitan 2000). Furthermore, the weakness of the central governments in Eastern Europe following the fall of communism was a serious obstacle for preventive alcohol policies (Simpura 1995). The limited capacity of public authorities to control the alcohol trade and the opposition of the alcohol industry to state measures made it very difficult to bring public control and order to the alcohol trade.

Eastern European countries has meant that alcohol control, especially the control of alcohol availability, has lost much of its effect in these countries (Moskalewicz 2000; Reitan 2000). On the other hand, in the 1990s, under the impetus of the European Alcohol Action Plan, many Eastern European countries have adopted national alcohol programmes or participated in projects aimed at strengthening local alcohol control.

In many developed countries, general alcohol policies affecting the whole population and oriented to the collective good have been under sustained attack. Policies remaining from the past have been gradually eroded (e.g. privatization of monopolies, erosion of taxes by inflation, extension of opening hours). At the same time, however, popular concern about alcohol-related problems has risen, although it has only fitfully found political expression, for example, in concerns about drink-driving, or about public intoxication at football matches. The rise in public concern partly reflects an increase in the rates of alcohol-related problems. Public health advocacy, as well as scientific documentation of the hidden ways in which social and health harms often result from drinking, have also contributed to this growing concern.

In general, there has been a decline in alcohol control policies on several fronts, including those interventions that have the greatest and broadest potential for curtailing alcohol-related harms. Ironically, many of the studies that have documented the effectiveness of such interventions have only been possible because the strategies were being weakened or dismantled.

Trends in the developing world have been less well documented (Room *et al.* 2002). In some parts of the world, such as Papua New Guinea, prohibitions imposed by colonial powers lasted until the 1960s, provoking an association of drinking and western-style beverages with autonomy and prestige. Some forms of alcohol control, such as municipally owned beer halls in southern Africa, have in many places been weakened or dismantled, often under pressure from the 'structural adjustment' programmes of international development agencies. The control of alcohol advertising, **alcohol education**, and driving under the influence of alcohol have also become issues in developing countries. In many countries there has been an increase in educational programmes despite research on their lack of effect, along with some interventions to curtail drink-driving.

1.3 **Alcohol policy science**

If alcohol policy has a long history, then the scientific study of alcohol policy as a public health strategy has a much more abbreviated past. The growing interest in alcohol policy represented by this book is part of a maturation process in the study of alcohol problems that dates back to the 1960s (e.g. Seeley 1960) and in particular to the publication of a seminal monograph entitled *Alcohol Control Policies in Public Health Perspective* (Bruun *et al.* 1975a). Sponsored by the **World Health Organization** (WHO), the monograph drew attention to the preventable nature of alcohol problems, and to the role of national governments and international agencies in the formulation of rational and effective alcohol policies. *Alcohol Control Policies* stimulated a heated debate not just among academics, but also among policymakers and medical practitioners (Edwards *et al.* 1995). The most significant aspect of the book was its main thesis: the higher the average amount of alcohol consumed in a society, the greater the incidence of problems experienced by that society. Consequently, one way to prevent alcohol problems is through policies directed at the reduction of average alcohol consumption, particularly policies that limit the availability of alcohol.

In the early 1990s, a new project was commissioned by the WHO to review the development of the world literature pertaining to alcohol policy. The new study produced *Alcohol Policy and the Public Good* (Edwards *et al.* 1994), a book that elaborated key themes of its predecessor (Bruun *et al.* 1975a), summarizing the evidence on new topics and proposing a public health agenda for alcohol control policy (Edwards *et al.* 1994). The book concluded that public health policies on alcohol had come of age because of the strong evidential underpinnings derived from the scientific research that had grown in breadth and sophistication since 1975. After reviewing the evidence on taxation of alcohol, restrictions on alcohol availability, drink-driving countermeasures, school-based education, community action programmes, and treatment interventions, it was concluded that:

- ◆ The research establishes beyond doubt that public health measures of proven effectiveness are available to serve the public good by reducing the widespread costs and pain related to alcohol use.

- ◆ To that end, it is appropriate to deploy responses that influence both the total amount of alcohol consumed by a population and the high-risk contexts and drinking behaviours that are so often associated with alcohol-related problems. To conceive of these intrinsically complementary approaches as contradictory alternatives would be a mistake.

Building on the tradition of collaboration between the WHO and international alcohol researchers, preparation of the first edition of the present volume was undertaken for three reasons. First, new epidemiological research on the global burden of disease had implicated alcohol as one of the leading risk factors for death and disability in many regions of the world. Second, because of the rapidly changing trends in alcohol problems, there had been a growing international interest in the application of health policies, including prevention programmes and treatment services, as an important responsibility of national and local governments. Third, major improvements in the way that alcohol problems are studied had provided a growing body of scientific evidence to inform alcohol policies. That evidence base clearly established that alcohol is indeed no ordinary commodity, and for this reason a variety of different policies, aimed at both individuals and populations, targeting **aggregate** consumption as well as high-risk drinkers, were necessary to manage the threat alcohol poses to public health and social well-being.

This revised edition was undertaken for several reasons. First, however compelling that conclusion has been to policymakers and the public health community, it soon became apparent that if alcohol is no ordinary commodity, the public health response needs to focus on the entire production chain that brings alcoholic beverages to the consumer. Until recently, little attention had been devoted to the alcohol industry from a public health perspective, and even less to the role of the alcohol industry in the policymaking process. The present volume attempts to correct that deficiency, update the rapidly expanding policy and prevention literature, and at the same time strengthen the main thesis of the first edition, that alcohol is no ordinary commodity.

1.4 **Alcohol policy defined**

Bruun *et al.* (1975a) defined alcohol control policies as all relevant strategies employed by governments to influence alcohol availability, leaving health education, attitude change, and informal social control as beyond the scope of a public health approach. In 1994, Edwards *et al.* provided a broader view of alcohol policy, considering it as a public health response dictated in part by national and historical concerns. Though there was not an explicit definition of the nature of alcohol policy, its meaning could be inferred from the wealth of policy responses that were considered: alcohol taxation, legislative controls on alcohol availability, age restrictions on purchasing alcohol, media information campaigns, and school-based education, to name a few.

This book borrows from its predecessors in its definition of alcohol policy, but also expands the concept in keeping with nationally and internationally evolving views of public health. Public policies are authoritative decisions made by governments through laws, rules, and regulations (Longest 1998). The word 'authoritative' indicates that the decisions come from the legitimate purview of legislators and other public interest group officials, not from private industry or related advocacy groups.

When public policies pertain to the relation between alcohol, health, and social welfare, they are considered alcohol policies. Thus, drink-driving laws that are designed to prevent alcohol-related accidents, rather than those merely intended to punish offenders, are considered alcohol policies. Generally, alcohol policies affect populations (such as underage drinkers) or organizations (such as programmes and services within health systems). Based on their nature and purpose, alcohol policies can be classified into two categories: allocative and regulatory (Longest 1998). Allocative policies are intended to provide funding and other resources to a distinct group or type of organization in order to achieve some public objective. Subsidies that support alcohol education in schools, the training of waiters and waitresses in **responsible**

beverage service, and the provision of treatment for alcohol-dependent persons, are examples of policies that seek to reduce the harm caused by alcohol or to increase access to services for certain population groups. In contrast to allocative policies, regulatory policies seek to influence the actions, behaviours, and decisions of others through direct control of individuals or organizations. Economic regulation through price controls and taxation is often applied to alcoholic beverages to reduce demand and to generate tax revenues. Laws that impose a minimum purchasing age and limit hours of sale have long been used to restrict access to alcohol for reasons of health and safety. Federal and local laws pertaining to the potency, purity, and marketing of alcoholic beverages, and the times and places where they can be served or purchased, are examples of other regulatory policies.

From the perspective of this book, the central purpose of alcohol policies is to serve the interests of public health and social well-being through their impact on health and social determinants, such as **drinking patterns**, the drinking environment, and the health services available to treat problem drinkers. As discussed in Chapter 2, drinking patterns that lead to rapidly elevated blood alcohol levels result in problems associated with acute intoxication, such as accidents, injuries, and violence. Similarly, drinking patterns that involve frequent and heavy alcohol consumption are associated with chronic health problems such as liver cirrhosis, cardiovascular disease, and depression.

The environmental determinants of alcohol-related harm include the physical availability of the product, the social norms that define the appropriate uses of alcohol (e.g. as a beverage, as an intoxicant, as a medicine) and behaviour when drinking, and the economic incentives that promote its use. As noted in Chapter 5, the alcohol industry has been identified as an important environmental influence that may contribute to alcohol-related problems through its promotional activities and product design. Health and social policies that influence the availability of alcohol, the social circumstances of its use, and its retail price are likely to reduce the harm caused by alcohol in a society.

Another important determinant of health in relation to alcohol is the availability of and access to health services, particularly those designed to deal with **alcohol dependence** and alcohol-related disabilities. Alcohol-related health services can be preventive, acute, and rehabilitative, and can be either voluntary or coercive. Allocative health policies have a major impact on the alcohol treatment and preventive services available to people within a country through health care financing and the organization of the health care system.

1.5 Public health and the public good

The definition of alcohol policy proposed in this book relies heavily on concepts derived from public heath, a specialized field of knowledge and action that is not always understood by either the general public or the health professions. Public health is concerned with the management and prevention of diseases and injuries in human populations. Unlike clinical medicine, which focuses on the care and cure of disease in individual cases, public health deals with groups of individuals, called populations. The value of population thinking in alcohol policy lies in its ability to identify health risks and suggest appropriate interventions that are most likely to benefit the greatest number of people. The concept of 'population' is based on the assumption that groups of individuals exhibit certain commonalities by virtue of their shared characteristics (e.g. gender), shared environment (e.g. village, city, nation), or shared occupations (e.g. alcoholic beverage service workers) that increase their risk of disease and disability, including alcohol-related problems (Fos and Fine 2000). Because populations defined by geographic boundaries are often not homogeneous, it is sometimes fruitful to focus on subpopulations rather than total populations. This is a major difference between the present volume and the 1975 monograph, *Alcohol Policies in Public Health Perspective* (Bruun *et al.* 1975a), which restricted its analysis of alcohol control policies to their impact on total populations.

Why are public health concepts important to the discussion of alcohol policy? During the twentieth century public health measures have had a remarkable effect on the health of populations throughout the world. Life expectancy has increased dramatically worldwide during this period, thanks to the application of public health measures designed to improve sanitation, reduce environmental pollution, and prevent communicable and infectious diseases (WHO 1998). But even as epidemics of infectious and communicable diseases have receded, health risks associated with life-style behaviours and chronic diseases have increased in importance as major causes of mortality and morbidity. When population approaches are used instead of, or in conjunction with, individual level medical approaches, the effects on health and disease are much greater. As this book will show, public health concepts provide an important vehicle by which to manage the health of populations in relation to the use and misuse of alcohol. Whereas medical approaches oriented toward individual patients can be effective in treating alcohol dependence and alcohol-related disabilities (Chapter 14), population-based approaches deal with groups, communities, and nation states to improve the allocation of human and material resources to preventative and curative services. They also provide epidemiological data to monitor trends, design better interventions, and evaluate programmes and services.

In this context, the 'public good' served by effective alcohol policy refers to those things that are beneficial for all (or most) members of a given society. One such public good would be the prevention or effective management of alcohol-related harm by means of effective interventions, just as the eradication of malaria or prevention of human immunodeficiency virus (HIV) infection have been considered 'global public goods' because of their international dimensions (Smith *et al.* 2003). In this book it is argued that when alcohol policy is informed by public health considerations, it is more likely to achieve its goal of providing a public good. Not all policies, however, serve the public good. Some are ineffective; others are counterproductive. Thus our purpose in writing this book is to determine which policies serve the public good, and which do not.

1.6 **Alcohol, health, and public policy**

By locating alcohol policy within the realm of public health and social policy, rather than economics, criminal justice, or social welfare, this book draws attention to the growing tendency for governments, both national and local, to approach alcohol as a major determinant of ill-health. The pursuit of health, as one of modern society's most highly cherished values, accounts for the growing interest in alcohol policy. But it also creates a special challenge because public health often competes with other social values such as free trade, open markets, and individual freedom. In this book, health is viewed not only as the absence of disease and injury, but also as a state in which the biological, psychological, and social functioning of a person are maximized in everyday life (Brook and McGlynn 1991). The way in which health is defined and valued within a society has important implications for alcohol policy. If it is defined narrowly as the absence of disease, then the focus is often placed on the treatment of alcohol dependence and the clinical management of alcohol-related disabilities, such as cirrhosis of the liver and traumatic injuries. If health is defined more broadly, then alcohol policy can be directed at proactive interventions that help many more people attain more optimal levels of health.

1.7 Structure of this book

Following this Introduction, Chapter 2 explains why alcohol cannot be considered an ordinary commodity from a public health perspective. Not only is alcohol a toxic substance when taken in large amounts and over an extended period of time, it also affects the health of the drinker through the mechanisms of acute intoxication and alcohol dependence. The next two chapters deal with the epidemiology of alcohol use and misuse. Epidemiology is the scientific study of the occurrence and causes of diseases and other health-related conditions (e.g. injuries) in human populations, and the application of this information to the control of health problems. Health is influenced by a variety of factors, including the physical, social, and economic environments that people live in, and by their genetic make-up, their personal lifestyles, and the health services to which they have access. As Chapters 3 and 4 will show, alcohol-related health and social problems are influenced by the same factors. It follows that alcohol policies, to be effective instruments of public health and social welfare, must take into account, if not operate in, all of these domains, rather than be limited to a more circumscribed focus on either alcohol, the agent, or alcohol dependence, the result of chronic drinking.

Following this global overview of alcohol epidemiology, Chapters 5 and 6 deal with the alcohol industry and the international context of alcohol trade that has become so important in the marketing of alcohol as a global commodity.

Chapters 7 through 14 constitute the core of the book, to the extent that they systematically review the evidence supporting seven major approaches to alcohol policy: pricing and taxation measures, regulating the physical availability of alcohol, controlling the drinking environment, drink-driving countermeasures, regulating alcohol promotion, primary prevention programmes, and treatment and early intervention.

Chapter 15 provides a comprehensive framework to understand the alcohol policy-making process and how it can serve the interests of public health and social welfare. In the final chapter of the book, an attempt is made to synthesize what is known about evidence-based interventions that can be translated into policy. By comparing different intervention strategies in terms of their effectiveness, scientific support, generalisability, and cost, it becomes possible to evaluate the relative appropriateness of different strategies, both alone and in combination, to present problems and future needs. As the scientific basis for alcohol policy begins to take shape, it is becoming apparent that there is no single definitive, much less politically acceptable, approach to the prevention of alcohol problems; a combination of strategies and policies is needed. If this realization is sobering, so too is the conviction, argued in the pages of this book, that alcohol policy is an ever-changing process that needs constantly to adapt to the times if it is to serve the interests of public health.

1.8 Extraordinary measures

Whether it is holiday revelry in Tokyo, Japan, payday binging in Tennant Creek, Australia, or drinking to obliterate the Perestroika blues in Pitkäranta, Russia, alcohol is a product that enters into many aspects of social life in practically every part of the world. But as the pages of this book will show, alcohol is no ordinary commodity. For this reason, the public health response to the prevention of alcohol-related problems requires extraordinary measures, some of them relatively painless for a society to implement, others more demanding in terms of resources, ingenuity, and public support.

Chapter 2

Alcohol: no ordinary commodity

2.1 Introduction

Beer, wine, and distilled spirits are alcohol-based commodities that are bought and sold in the marketplace. And alcohol is a drug with toxic effects and other intrinsic dangers such as intoxication and dependence. This chapter examines these different aspects of alcoholic beverages, paying special attention to the contrast between alcohol's dual role as a commodity and as a drug.

An understanding of this contrast is essential to the book's central purpose. In recent years, public discussion of alcohol policies has too often ignored or downplayed the need to understand both the nature of the agent and its harmful properties, with an implicit acceptance of the idea that alcohol is only an ordinary commodity like any other marketable product. The validity of this assumption is questioned by evidence showing that alcohol intoxication, alcohol dependence, and the toxic effects of alcohol on various organ systems are key mechanisms linking alcohol consumption to a wide range of adverse consequences.

2.2 Alcohol's cultural and symbolic meanings

The history of alcoholic beverages shows that drinking has served many purposes for the individual and society. As Heath (1984) has noted, alcohol can be at the same time a food, a drug, and a highly elaborated cultural artefact with important symbolic meanings. Nowadays, alcohol products are mainly used as beverages to serve with meals, as thirst quenchers, as a means of socialization and enjoyment, as instruments of hospitality, and as intoxicants.

In earlier times, alcoholic beverages were frequently used as medicine (Edwards 2000). Presently, the best example of a medicinal use of alcohol is when it is consumed to protect against heart disease. Light regular consumption of alcohol (as little as a drink every second day) is associated with a reduction in heart disease, probably through its ability to increase levels of high-density cholesterol (HDL) and its anti-clotting effect (Suh *et al.* 1992; Corrao *et al.* 2000). As will be seen in Chapter 4, this protective effect is seen primarily for men 45 years of age and older and appears not to be reflected in terms of health benefit at the population level (Ramstedt 2006).

Until the advent of clean water supplies in Europe and America in the late nineteenth century, alcoholic beverages were considered to be a healthy alternative to polluted drinking water (Mäkelä 1983). Alcoholic beverages are used in many cultures in a variety of social situations, both public and private. They are frequently used to commemorate births, baptisms, and weddings. In a religious context, the consumption of alcohol may be limited by ritual expectations, as in the Catholic mass and the Jewish

Seder, where only very light drinking is condoned. In other cases, higher levels of consumption, including intoxication, are accepted. For example, alcohol is used to induce trance-like states in African-Brazilian religious rituals. Alcohol is frequently used as a relaxant and as a social lubricant. In some communities, the provision of an abundance of alcohol in social situations is almost mandatory, and is seen as a sign of wealth and power by those who provide it.

Alcohol's meanings change as individuals go through different stages of life, and as societies' norms about appropriate or acceptable drinking change accordingly (Fillmore *et al.* 1991b). Drinking can be a sign of rebellion or independence during adolescence, but societies across the world are concerned with the harmful consequences of drinking on youth. Epidemiological evidence reviewed in Chapters 3 and 4 indicates that there are good reasons for this concern. In a study of 26 developed countries, for instance, deaths from motor vehicle crashes peaked at ages 20–24 years for males and 15–19 years for females (Heuveline and Slap 2002). Thus, most societies, even those with very liberal policies toward alcohol consumption, agree that alcohol should not be made readily available to children and adolescents. Drinking during early adulthood is usually more frequent and heavier than in later life, although in some societies this can be modified by cultural factors and the demographic characteristics of the drinker (Fillmore *et al.* 1991b).

There are also important differences in the cultural meaning of drinking for men and women. In some societies, drinking has been almost exclusively a province of men (Roizen 1981), and this remains true, for instance, in India (Room *et al.* 2002). Though the percentage of abstainers is generally higher among adult women everywhere, in many countries of Europe the gender difference is not great (Simpura and Karlsson 2001). Nowadays, women consume one-fifth to one-third of the alcohol in most industrialized countries (see Chapter 3), and in a few countries there has been even greater convergence between the sexes (Bloomfield *et al.* 2001).

Societies' normative expectations regarding the use of alcohol vary across age groups. In many societies, abstention rates increase in the later stages of life for both men and women (Demers *et al.* 2001; Taylor *et al.* 2007). Besides ill-health, this often reflects societal norms; older people are not supposed to engage in the intoxicated partying that may be more or less accepted among the young. However, as individuals in industrialized countries live longer and healthier lives, these cultural views about the propriety of drinking by older individuals may change.

Alcohol is thus a drug used widely in many social situations. Throughout the life cycle from youth to old age it is associated with many positive aspects of life. It is used in traditional social rituals in many places. In some rituals, even intoxication is seen as an acceptable and pleasurable pursuit. However, these situations can rapidly change from being 'alcohol-safe' to being 'alcohol-dangerous' when party guests who have been drinking become belligerent or leave to drive their cars back home.

2.3 Alcohol as a commodity

Alcoholic beverages are produced and distributed in four ways (Jernigan 2000b; Room *et al.* 2002). First, there is home brewing and craft production, both of distilled spirits and traditional fermented beverages. Second, there is industrial production and distribution of commercial versions of these indigenous beverages, such as *chibuku* in southern Africa, *soju* in South Korea, and *pulque* in Mexico. Third, there is local industrial production of 'international' beverages, such as domestic whiskey in India and lager beer like Corona in Mexico. Fourth, there is the production of branded international beverages, which are increasingly marketed on a global scale. These structural issues are discussed in more detail in Chapter 5.

In many countries, the production and sale of alcoholic beverages is an important economic activity. It generates profits for the producers, advertisers, and investors, provides employment opportunities, brings in foreign currency for exported beverages, and generates tax revenues for the government. Alcohol is a major source of sales and profits for the travel and hospitality industries, including hotels and restaurants. For these reasons, there are many vested interests that support the continuation and growth of alcohol production and sales. It may take only a few hundred employees to operate a modern, large-scale brewery. But when beer is sold in grocery stores or restaurants, it becomes a significant source of retail sales, which bring profits to small business owners and employment to service and sales workers. However, as Room and Jernigan (2000) indicate, the increased industrialization brought by the alcohol industry to developing societies does not really lead to a clear increase in employment or expansion of the tax base.

Alcoholic beverages, particularly wine and beer, are considered agricultural products in many developed countries. Wine plays an especially important role in the agricultural economies of countries like France, Italy, and Spain. It is estimated than in Italy, alcohol production, mostly in the form of viniculture, provides employment for 1.5–2.0 million people. While beer and distilled spirits also have clear connections to agriculture, in many countries these activities come under the jurisdiction of the ministry of industry. In contrast to wine production, in developed countries beer and especially distilled spirits are mostly produced in large plants by large industrial enterprises.

Consumer spending on alcoholic beverages usually generates taxes, which make these products a popular source of income for local, state, and national governments. In many countries, taxes on alcohol are imposed under several headings and at several different administrative levels. Estimating the total amount of taxes collected from alcohol production and sales can therefore be difficult. In 2006, beverage alcohol's total contribution to state and local revenues in the USA was US $37 billion. Of that amount, $19 billion came from indirect revenues such as corporate, personal income, property, and other taxes generated by the alcohol industry (Distilled Spirits Council of the United States 2007).

In summary, alcohol is an important commodity with a complex supply chain and a considerable employment base. Its products must be manufactured, packaged, labelled, stored, distributed, sold, marketed, and advertised. It generates profits for the primary producers and for all sorts of middlemen and ancillary actors involved in the alcohol trade. Alcohol is a commodity that is demanded, purchased, and consumed globally. Taxation of alcoholic beverages brings in revenue in larger or smaller quantities to state budgets. Alcoholic beverages are, by any reckoning, an important, economically embedded commodity. But as we shall see in the remainder of this chapter, the benefits connected with the production, sale, and use of this commodity come at an enormous cost to society. Public health specialists and policymakers who forget the double nature of alcohol as a profitable commodity and as a source of harm do so only at their peril (Edwards and Holder 2000).

2.4 Mechanisms of harm: intoxication, toxicity and dependence

Looking back at the last 30 years, especially the past decade, it can be said that remarkable progress has been made in the scientific understanding of alcohol's harmful effects, as scientists continue to uncover biological, chemical, and psychological explanations for humans' propensity to consume what has been called 'the ambiguous molecule' (Edwards 2000). This knowledge is fundamental to an understanding of alcohol's capacity for physical toxicity, intoxication, and dependence. The remainder of this chapter will focus on recent scientific advances in the understanding of these important **mediators** of the relation between drinking and the different kinds of harm it produces.

Figure 2.1 shows the relationships among alcohol consumption, intoxication, and dependence as mediating factors, and various types of harm. **Drinking patterns** are characterized not only by the frequency of drinking and the quantity per occasion, but also by the variation between one occasion and another. The pattern represents the way in which drinkers consume a certain volume of alcohol in a given timeframe. The total volume of alcohol consumed and the pattern of drinking are related to one another. For instance, the ingestion of a very high volume of alcohol will almost inevitably lead to intoxication, a high-risk pattern of drinking. Different patterns can

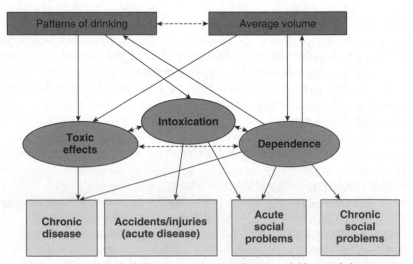

Fig. 2.1 Relations among alcohol consumption, mediating variables, and short-term as well as long-term consequences.

lead to different types of problems. Sustained heavy drinking, of the type that has been common in wine-drinking countries, may not lead to much evident intoxication, but can cause tissue damage and **dependence**. Daily drinking of even moderate amounts of wine per occasion over a long period of time can lead to cirrhosis because of the cumulative effects of alcohol on the liver. By contrast, a relatively low frequency of drinking together with consumption of a high number of drinks per occasion can lead, through the mechanism of acute intoxication, to a variety of medical and social problems, such as accidents, injuries, interpersonal violence, and certain types of acute tissue damage. Finally, sustained drinking may result in alcohol dependence. Once dependence is present, it can feed back to increase or sustain both the overall volume of drinking and the drinking pattern. Dependence can then lead to chronic medical problems as well as acute and chronic social problems.

2.5 **Alcohol as a toxic substance**

Alcohol is a toxic substance in terms of its direct and indirect effects on a wide range of body organs and organ systems. Some of alcohol's adverse health impacts can result from acute intoxication or **binge drinking**, even in a person who does not have a longstanding or persistent drinking problem. Alcohol poisoning (Poikolainen 2002), acute pancreatitis (Imrie 1997), and acute cardiac arrhythmias (Peters 1998) represent dangers of that kind. On occasion, some of these conditions may have fatal outcomes. Another category of harm can be designated as 'acute and chronic'. For example, a drinking binge in a chronic heavy drinker may turn liver impairment into liver failure, or cause the acute onset of brain damage.

A third category of harm is chronic disease resulting from long-term exposure to high doses of alcohol, with cancers and cirrhosis being prime examples. As discussed in more detail in Chapter 4, there is clear evidence for a causal role of alcohol in various cancers, including cancer of the mouth, oesophagus (gullet), larynx, and pharynx. Cirrhosis of the liver is also closely associated with alcohol consumption, with research showing that the direct toxic effect of alcohol is the main cause of the condition (Lieber 1988), as well as hepatitis and fatty liver (Sherman and Williams 1994). Other conditions that can be associated with tissue damage by alcohol are diseases of the heart muscle and cardiac arrhythmias (Peters 1998), pancreatitis (Searles *et al.* 1996), hypertension with consequent risk of stroke (Peters 1998), wasting of the limb muscles (Urbano-Márquez and Fernández-Solà 1996), peripheral neuritis, and brain damage of various kinds (Lishman 1998).

Heavy drinking by pregnant women can result in a range of damages to the foetus (Clarren and Smith 1978; Astley and Clarren 2000). The term 'fetal alcohol spectrum disorders' (FASD) describes a continuum of permanent birth defects, which, in their extreme form called 'fetal alcohol syndrome', are characterized by hearing disabilities, retarded growth, and heart disorders, together with certain characteristic facial abnormalities. There is still uncertainty as to the intensity and timing of the alcohol exposure needed to produce any type or degree of fetal impairment.

In summary, alcoholic beverages are items of consumption with many customary uses, and are also commodities important to many people's livelihood. But social customs and economic interests should not blind us to the fact that alcohol is a toxic substance. It has the potential to affect adversely nearly every organ and system of the body. No other commodity sold for ingestion, not even tobacco, has such wide-ranging adverse physical effects. Taking account of alcohol's potential for toxicity is therefore an important task for public health policy.

2.6 Alcohol intoxication

There is a popular tendency to view all problems related to drinking as a part of, or due to, **alcoholism**. Studies of drinking practices and problems in the general population question this assumption, showing a universe of drinking problems that lie outside the bounds of alcoholism (Cahalan and Room 1974). In the mid-1970s, partly based on evidence from general population studies, a population-based vision of the broad range of problems that alcohol sets for society began to emerge (Bruun *et al.* 1975a). This new approach cast off the constraints of the narrow view that made alcoholism the only salient issue. Given that alcohol-related social problems, interpersonal problems, and acute health problems are widely distributed throughout the population, the **prevention paradox** (Kreitman 1986) was put forward to draw attention to the broad range of alcohol-related problems in the drinking population at large. One of the main causes of alcohol-related harm in the general population is alcohol intoxication.

The term **alcohol intoxication** is defined here as a more or less short-term state of functional impairment in psychological and psychomotor performance induced by the presence of alcohol in the body. The major types of impairments (other than acute toxicity) that occur with alcohol intoxication are described in Box 2.1. The impairments produced by alcohol are mostly dose-related, are often complex, and involve multiple body functions. Some (such as slurred speech) are evident and easily recognized, while others, such as impaired driving ability, may be subtle and detected only via laboratory testing. Some of these effects stem directly and almost inevitably from a given blood alcohol concentration, while others depend on personal characteristics, the individual's previous experience with alcohol, and the setting and expectation of effect. Other psychoactive drugs, especially central nervous system depressants, may exacerbate the effects of alcohol when taken concomitantly.

As Box 2.1 underlines, intoxication and accompanying changes in behaviour are a matter of cultural and personal expectations and understandings as well as of the concentration of alcohol in the blood. The anthropological literature has long recognized that there are striking differences between cultures in drunken comportment (MacAndrew and Edgerton 1969; Room 2001). Even within a given culture, the meaning of 'drunk' can change over time. In 1979, when alcohol consumption in the USA was achieving record levels for the twentieth century, adult males reported that it would take an average of 9.8 drinks (about 118 g ethanol) for them to feel drunk, and 5.4 drinks to feel the effects of drinking. In 1995, after US consumption levels fell by 21%, men reported that it would take an average of 7.4 drinks to feel drunk and 4.6 to feel the effects (Midanik 1999). The amounts also fell for women, from 5.7 to 4.7 drinks to feel drunk and from 3.7 to 3.2 drinks to feel the effects. More recent analyses

Box 2.1 Types of impairments that occur with alcohol intoxication

♦ *Psychomotor impairment.* Alcohol can impair balance and movement in a way that increases the risk of many types of accidents.

♦ *Lengthened reaction time.* This classic dose-related impairment is of particular concern because of its causal role in traffic accidents.

♦ *Impairment of judgement.* Impaired judgement can result in dangerous risk-taking, such as getting into a car and then driving in a risky and aggressive way when intoxicated.

♦ *Emotional changes and decreased responsiveness to social expectations.* The factors involved in alcohol-related changes in mood, emotional state, and social responsiveness are complex and are likely to involve interaction of alcohol's physiological effects with psychological and social factors. In part because of these changes, intoxication can contribute to the risk of violence to others and intentional self-harm.

(Kerr *et al.* 2006) show a further decrease in the number of drinks US survey respondents think they need to feel drunk. In 2000, males reported they needed 6.6 drinks to feel drunk, while females reported 4.1 drinks. This reduction from 1995 to 2000 occurred at a time when US per-capita consumption was fairly stable at 2.15 (1995) and 2.18 (2000) gallons of ethanol for the population aged ≥14 years (Lakins *et al.* 2007).

Intoxication, occasional or regular, is a key risk factor for the adverse consequences of drinking, which in some cases might also involve dependence. However, just as behavioural changes associated with intoxication are influenced by social and cultural expectations, so too is the link between intoxication and adverse harms, especially social harms. These types of harms have been defined as a failure to fulfil major social obligations associated with family, job, and public demeanour (Room 2000b). Social reactions to intoxication are a key part of the mechanism by which social harms (public drunkenness, drink-driving, job-related problems such as absenteeism and loss of job, family problems such as separation and divorce) are recognized by society. In places where drinking is a daily or almost daily activity of many, and even heavier drinking is accepted in special circumstances (e.g. weddings, carnival), reactions to intoxication may take some time to develop, and so will related social harms. In other places, such as 'dry' cultures where most people do not drink and rules against intoxication are strict, reactions to small behavioural changes associated with drunkenness may be swift and severe, leading to social harms for intoxicated drinkers and those around them.

Social harms arise not only from the general environment in which drinking takes place but are also from the characteristics of the drinker. One will only have an alcohol-related problem with a spouse if one is married. Job problems will arise in relation to the extent to which the work being done is closely supervised by others. The drinking problems of a salesman who works alone outside the office may go undetected for quite some time, which would not happen with someone who works regular hours in an office environment side-by-side with others. Social harms also affect the drinker's immediate social network of co-workers, relatives, and friends. Social harms can also have a collective effect on society as a whole. Lost productivity in the workplace has such a general effect. Public intoxication, violence, and driving after drinking require responses by the police and the legal system, all of which come with considerable budget expenditures. These behaviours also affect a community's general sense of security and safety. As will be seen in Chapter 4, the link between intoxication and adverse social consequences is clear and strong for social harms such as violence (Room and Rossow 2001), traffic casualties (Hurst *et al.* 1994), and other injuries.

The following conclusions stem from these analyses:

1) Alcohol is a psychoactive substance that can impair motor skills and judgement. The impairment from intoxication is biological, but its manifestations are affected by expectancies and cultural norms.

2) Occasional drinking to the point of intoxication is quite common among drinkers. Intoxication, even when it occurs infrequently, can result in substantial social harm and injury. In fact, the chances of harm from a single intoxication event seem to be higher for those who drink infrequently than for those drinking more frequently (Hurst *et al.* 1994; Room *et al.* 1995a).

3) Prevention of alcohol intoxication is a potentially powerful strategy for preventing much of the harm from alcohol.

4) Since the link between intoxication and harm is very much affected by the social and physical context, harm can also potentially be averted by insulating the drinking behaviour. This insulation from harm can take many forms, e.g. physical (making the place of drinking safer) or temporal (separating the drinking from activities requiring vigilance).

5) The variety and complexity of social harms, their inherent interactional nature (Room 2000b), their effects on individuals, and the collective effect on society call for prevention policies that are also varied in nature and environmentally and contextually based.

2.7 **Alcohol dependence**

In 1976, Edwards and Gross (1976) put forward the concept of the **alcohol dependence syndrome**. Together with this new conceptualization of a core set of indicators, it was also noted that alcohol-related problems could occur without dependence, but that dependence was likely to carry with it many problems. The overall formulation was intrinsically two-dimensional. One dimension is represented by the syndrome concept, which refers to a cluster of inter-related physiological and psychological symptoms in which alcohol use takes on a much higher priority than other behaviours. The second dimension, alcohol-related problems, refers to harm resulting from drinking, regardless of whether the person is alcohol dependent.

The syndrome concept has been officially recognized in the *Diagnostic and Statistical Manual of Mental Disorders*, 4th edn (DSM-IV) of the American Psychiatric Association

Box 2.2 ICD-10 diagnostic criteria for dependence[a]

1. Evidence of tolerance to the effects of alcohol, such that there is a need for markedly increased amounts to achieve intoxication or desired effect, or that there is a markedly diminished effect with continued use of the same amount of alcohol.

2. A physiological withdrawal state when alcohol use is reduced or ceased, as evidenced by the characteristic withdrawal syndrome for the substance, or use of the same (or closely related) substance with the intention of relieving or avoiding withdrawal symptoms.

3. Persisting with alcohol use despite clear signs of harmful consequences as evidenced by continued use when the person was actually aware of, or could be expected to have been aware of, the nature and extent of harm.

4. Preoccupation with alcohol use, as manifested by important alternative pleasures or interests being given up or reduced because of alcohol use, or a great deal of time being spent in activities necessary to obtain alcohol, consume it, or recover from its effects.

5. Impaired capacity to control drinking behaviour in terms of its onset, termination, or level of use, as evidenced by alcohol being often taken in larger amounts or over a longer period than intended, or any unsuccessful effort or persistent desire to cut down or control alcohol use.

6. A strong desire or sense of compulsion to use alcohol.

[a] Adapted from World Health Organization (1992b).

(1994), and in the *International Statistical Classification of Diseases and Related Health Problems*, 10th edn (ICD-10; WHO 1992b). The criteria for a diagnosis of alcohol dependence in this latter classification are shown in Box 2.2. Three of the six criteria must have been present in the past 12 months for a positive diagnosis of alcohol dependence.

Two factors contributing to the development of alcohol dependence are reinforcement (negative and positive) and neuroadaptation (Roberts and Koob 1997). Reinforcement occurs when a stimulus (e.g. alcohol-induced euphoria or stimulation) increases the probability of a certain response (e.g. continued drinking to maintain a rising blood alcohol level). Neuroadaptation refers to biological processes by which initial drug effects are either enhanced or attenuated by repeated drug use. Acute drug reinforcement occurs because addictive drugs interact with neurotransmitter systems, which are part of the brain reward circuitry. Alterations in this system persist after acute withdrawal and may increase vulnerability to relapse. The mesolimbic dopamine system of the brain is important in the establishment of dependence to psychomotor stimulants such as cocaine or amphetamine, and also plays a role in dependence to alcohol. Opioid endogenous systems (morphine-like neurotransmitters) play an important role in positive reinforcement of opiates, alcohol, and nicotine. Thus, opiate antagonists such as naltrexone reduce alcohol reinforcement in both animals and humans. Serotonin systems are also important in regulating alcohol consumption. Finally, GABA (gamma-aminobutyric acid) systems are the primary inhibitory systems in the brain. Alcohol and other sedative-hypnotic drugs (benzodiazepines) modulate receptors in this system. Changes in these neurotransmitter systems may lead to sensitization (increase in positive reinforcing effects) and counter-adaptation (increase in negative reinforcing effects), according to Roberts and Koob (1997). The remarkable advances in neurobiological research point to alcohol's psychoactive properties as a critical feature in the development of alcohol dependence.

The prevalence rate of alcohol dependence varies according to the level of drinking in the general population. Patterns of drinking and a variety of social, psychological, and biological characteristics of the population may also affect dependence rates. In the US adult population, the overall 12-month prevalence rate of alcohol dependence based on diagnostic criteria in DSM-IV is 3.81% (Grant et al. 2004). These rates are higher among males than females and higher among those in the 18–29-year age group than in any other group. Alcohol dependence rates for various regions of the world are discussed in Chapter 3.

A number of studies have examined the relationship between drinking patterns and alcohol dependence. Independent of how drinking is measured (Dawson and Archer 1993; Hall et al. 1993), the more a population engages in sustained or recurrent heavy alcohol consumption, the higher the rate of alcohol dependence (Rehm and Eschmann 2002). Both average volume of drinking and the pattern of drinking larger amounts on occasion are related to the prevalence of dependence (Caetano et al. 1997), and the risk of dependence increases linearly with increased drinking. The nature and the direction of causality, however, are not clear. Dependence may perpetuate heavy drinking, or heavy drinking may contribute to the development of dependence, or these two mechanisms may operate simultaneously. As suggested in Figure 2.1, alcohol dependence is likely to have both direct and indirect effects on alcohol-related problems.

The fact that alcohol has self-reinforcing potential is of fundamental importance to understanding the dynamics of the relationship between a population and its drinking. Alcohol is not a run-of-the-mill consumer substance, but a drug with dependence potential.

The alcohol dependence syndrome concept was originally developed as a clinical construct that applies primarily to persons in treatment. But recent evidence strongly suggests that milder degrees of dependence are widely distributed in the population and are associated with increased experience of problems. This may be especially the case in younger populations. Dependence is a matter of continuities and variations with broader expression than the extreme seen in the clinic. Mild dependence is associated with a significant public health burden because it is common, and severe dependence, although less common, is likely to be associated with an intense clustering of problems.

Alcohol dependence has many different contributory causes, including genetic vulnerability, but it is a condition that is contracted by exposure to alcohol. The heavier the drinking, the greater the risk. The challenge to public health is to identify policies that make it less likely that drinkers will contract dependence, and the consequent relative chronicity in behaviour patterns damaging to the individual and costly to society. The fact that alcohol dependence, once established, can become a rather chronic influence on drinking behaviour (one likely to generate more and more problems over the individual's drinking career) gives added cogency to the need for population-based strategies.

2.8 **Conclusion**

The major public health implications of the evidence reviewed in this chapter may be summarized as follows:

- ◆ the dangers in alcohol are multiple and varied in kind and degree;
- ◆ some but not all are dose-related;
- ◆ they may result directly from the effect of alcohol or through interaction with other factors;
- ◆ intoxication is often an important mediator of harm;
- ◆ dependence can significantly exacerbate the hazards and cause protracted exposure to danger.

Public health responses must be matched to this complex vision of the dangers in alcohol as they seek to respond better to the population-level harm. Population-level policies (universal interventions) should be considered together with those directed at high-risk drinkers (selected interventions) and those targeting individuals who have already developed problems (targeted interventions) (Institute of Medicine 1989). The context for those responses should be an improved understanding of the nature of an agent that is far from being an ordinary kind of commodity.

Chapter 3

Alcohol consumption trends and patterns of drinking

3.1 Introduction

This chapter describes alcohol consumption trends and **patterns of drinking** in a global perspective. The typical frequency of drinking and the amount of alcohol consumed per occasion vary enormously, not only among world regions and countries, but also over time and among different population groups. As will be shown in this chapter, variations in these 'patterns' of drinking affect rates of alcohol-related problems, and have implications for the choice of alcohol policy measures.

Two aspects of alcohol consumption are of particular importance for comparisons across populations and across time. First, total alcohol consumption in a population is an important indicator of the number of individuals who are exposed to high amounts of alcohol. Adult per-capita alcohol consumption is, to a considerable extent, related to the prevalence of heavy use, which in turn is associated with the occurrence of negative effects. Second, the relationship between total alcohol consumption and harm is modified by the number of drinkers in a population and by the way in which alcohol is consumed.

Surveys have been invaluable in furthering our understanding of the drinking cultures of countries and their different subgroups. However, surveys are not without errors and biases. Overall, they tend to underestimate alcohol consumption for a country as compared with sales and production data. Unfortunately, underestimation may vary between 30% and 70%, which is one reason why comparisons between countries are often difficult to make with confidence.

3.2 Proportions of drinkers and levels of alcohol consumption

3.2.1 Methods of estimating and reporting alcohol consumption

The level of alcohol consumption in a population is usually expressed in litres of ethanol (100% alcohol or pure alcohol) per capita. An alternative procedure is to report litres of ethanol for each person aged ≥15 years. The age of 15 years is chosen as a lower limit to reflect the fact that children do not drink alcoholic beverages in most countries, and that most drinkers in many countries, especially established market economies, typically initiate drinking within a few years of this age.

Yet another way of expressing the level of consumption is in terms of litres of ethanol per drinker, excluding from the calculation those who abstain from alcohol. This
requires an estimate of the proportion of abstainers in the population, typically defined
in terms of having consumed no alcoholic beverages in the last 12 months, and usually derived from interview responses to population survey questions. Expressing per-
capita consumption in litres per drinker permits a comparison of levels of drinking
among drinkers in different nations, even if there are disparities in the proportion of
the population that drinks at all.

Rates of abstention vary greatly between different societies. In most European countries, drinking is common in the adult population, and 80–95% currently drink at
least occasionally (WHO 2004a). The proportion of drinkers varies significantly more
among countries in the Americas. Estimates for Argentina (84%) and Canada (78%)
are close to the European countries, whereas they are lower in the USA (66%), Mexico
(58%), Brazil (49%) and Jamaica (42%) (WHO 2004a). Surveys from 20 African countries show that the proportion of drinkers is generally less than 50% and in some—
mainly Muslim—countries the proportion of drinkers is close to 0% (Clausen *et al.*
2009). Data from surveys in Thailand, India, and Sri Lanka show that the proportion of drinkers in these countries tends to be around 20–30%, while the proportion
is higher in China (51%) and Japan (86%) (WHO 2004a). In the Western Pacific
region, the proportion of drinkers varies considerably, from more than 80% in New
Zealand and Australia to 45% in Papua New Guinea (WHO 2004a). Survey data from
the Eastern Mediterranean Crescent and other regions with Muslim societies generally show that the proportion of drinkers is low, some at 0–10% (WHO 2004a).
Consequently, when we compare the consumption per adult drinker, rather than
among all adults, we find that the consumption per drinker is slightly higher in the
USA than in Denmark, although the per-capita consumption is 40% higher in
Denmark than in the USA. We also find that the consumption per drinker is almost
40% higher in China than in Peru, whereas per-capita consumption is at the same
level. As noted by Room *et al.* (2002), a recalculation of per-capita consumption in
India gives approximately nine litres of pure alcohol per male drinker per year, which
corresponds to the average annual intake per drinker in many European countries.

In many developed societies, estimates of the annual amount of alcohol consumption are derived from statistics related to production and trade or sales. In addition to
this 'recorded consumption', in most countries there is also 'unrecorded consumption', which may include alcoholic beverages from a variety of sources (e.g. home brewing, informal or illegal production, travellers' imports), as well as consumption by the
country's residents outside the country. In most established market economies, unrecorded consumption amounts to less than 25% of total consumption (Leifman 2002).
But elsewhere, a much higher proportion of consumption is unrecorded. Estimates
from several former Soviet Union republics, Turkey, and the Indian subcontinent indicate proportions of up to two-thirds (Rehm *et al.* 2003a), and estimates for East Africa
are around 90% (Willis 2001). In such countries, estimates of overall alcohol consumption must go beyond conventional taxation and trade statistics, drawing on estimates
from agricultural sources and field studies (Rehm and Eschmann 2002; WHO 2004a).

3.2.2 Regional estimates of drinkers and drinking around the world

Our primary focus in this chapter will be on fifteen regional groupings of countries, covering the entire world. These regions, described in Appendix 3.1, have been defined as part of the WHO's effort to estimate the global burden of disease (Murray and Lopez 1996b) in Africa, the Americas, the Middle East, Europe (including all successor states to the former Soviet Union), South East Asia, and the Western Pacific. Within each general geographic area, countries are grouped in terms of adult and infant mortality (see WHO 2000). Estimates for drinkers and drinking in each of the 15 regional groupings are derived from a population-weighted averaging of country estimates. In regions like Western Europe or North America, the figures are mostly derived from country-level empirical data, but elsewhere the figures include a substantial element of extrapolation and expert judgement. The picture we are presenting is thus approximate rather than exact, but it does provide a framework to evaluate alcohol consumption on a global basis.

Table 3.1 shows the most salient characteristics of alcohol consumption in these different regions of the world, beginning with the predominant beverage type. The third column in Table 3.1 shows the figures for recorded alcohol consumption per resident aged ≥15 years in the fifteen regional groupings. Clearly, recorded alcohol consumption is highest in the economically developed regions of the world (e.g. Americans A, Europe A). By contrast, recorded consumption is generally lower in Latin America, Africa and parts of Asia, and particularly low in historically Muslim states and the Indian subcontinent (e.g. Americas D, Africa D, Africa E, Middle East B and D, South East Asia D).

Adding in estimates of unrecorded consumption changes the picture somewhat. The fourth column in Table 3.1 shows the estimated level of total alcohol consumption per resident aged ≥15 years in the fifteen regions. Western Europe, Russia and other non-Muslim parts of the former Soviet Union (e.g. Europe A, B and C) now show the highest per-capita consumption levels, but Latin American (Americas B) levels are not far behind. In proportional terms, it is in Africa and the Indian subcontinent that unrecorded consumption makes the greatest contribution. In terms of estimated total consumption per resident aged ≥15 years, there is a more than 13-fold difference between the region with the highest estimated consumption (Europe C) and the region with the lowest (Middle East D).

In all regions, men are much more likely than women to be drinkers. The fifth and sixth columns in Table 3.1 show the estimated proportions of drinkers among males and females for each region. As noted above, most adults in Western and Eastern Europe and in the region including Japan and Australasia are drinkers. In the Americas, a majority of adults are drinkers, but around one-third abstain. In the rest of the world, only a minority of adults are drinkers. Women are particularly unlikely to be drinkers in the Indian subcontinent and Indonesia, and in the Middle East. Differences between men and women in the proportion of drinkers are particularly marked in China and South East Asia.

The seventh column in Table 3.1 shows the total consumption per drinker for each of the fifteen regions; the abstainers are excluded from the population base on which alcohol consumption is calculated. On this basis, the range of variation among world

Table 3.1 Characteristics of alcohol consumption in different regions of the world (population weighted averages) in 2003 (consumption data underlying Rehm et al. 2009)

(1) WHO region (see definitions below)	(2) Predominant beverage type	(3) Recorded consumption[a]	(4) Total consumption[b]	(5) % drinkers among males[c]	(6) % drinkers among females[d]	(7) Consumption per drinker[e]	(8) Average drinking pattern[f]	(9) % alcohol dependent[g]
Africa D (e.g. Nigeria, Algeria)	Mainly fermented beverages	5.0	7.3	41.0	31.0	20.3	2.8	0.7
Africa E (e.g. Ethiopia, South Africa)	Mainly other fermented beverages and beer	4.0	6.7	45.0	27.0	18.8	3.1	1.6
Americas A (Canada, Cuba, USA)	>50% beer, ~25% spirits	8.3	9.4	68.0	48.0	16.4	2.0	5.1
Americas B (e.g. Brazil, Mexico)	Beer, followed by spirits	5.7	8.1	81.0	61.0	11.4	3.1	3.5
Americas D (e.g. Bolivia, Peru)	Spirits, followed by beer	3.6	7.5	68.0	49.0	12.8	3.1	3.2
Middle East B (e.g. Iran, Saudi Arabia)	Spirits and beer	0.3	1.0	12.0	5.0	12.0	2.6	0.0
Middle East D (e.g. Afghanistan, Pakistan)	Spirits and beer	0.1	0.6	9.0	1.0	11.6	2.6	0.0
Europe A (e.g. Germany, France, UK)	Wine and beer	10.7	12.0	88.0	76.0	14.7	1.5	3.4
Europe B 1 (e.g. Bulgaria, Poland, Turkey)	Spirits	5.3	8.3	61.0	36.0	17.1	2.9	0.8

Region	Predominant beverage	[a]	[b]	[c]	[d]	[e]	[f]	[g]
Europe B 2 (e.g. Armenia, Azerbaijan, Tajikistan)	Spirits and wine	2.1	4.1	67.0	39.0	7.9	2.9	0.2
Europe C (e.g. Russian Federation, Ukraine)	Spirits	9.0	15.1	87.0	73.0	19.0	3.9	4.8
South East Asia B (e.g. Indonesia, Thailand)	Spirits	1.3	2.3	22.0	3.0	18.4	3.0	0.4
South East Asia D (e.g. Bangladesh, India)	Spirits	0.3	1.9	21.0	2.0	16.6	3.0	0.8
Western Pacific A (e.g. Australia, NZ, Japan)	Beer and spirits	7.7	9.4	87.0	71.0	11.9	2.0	2.1
Western Pacific B (e.g. China, Philippines, Vietnam)	Spirits	4.9	6.0	74.0	37.0	10.9	2.2	0.9

[a] Recorded alcohol consumption (in litres of absolute alcohol) per resident aged ≥15 years.

[b] Estimated alcohol consumption per resident aged ≥15 years.

[c] Estimated proportion of male drinkers aged ≥15 years.

[d] Estimated proportion of female drinkers aged ≥15 years.

[e] Estimated total alcohol consumption (in litres of absolute alcohol) per adult drinker.

[f] Estimated hazardous drinking score (1 = low level of risk; 4 = high level of risk associated with a country's predominant pattern of drinking).

[g] Estimated rate of alcohol dependence, among those aged ≥15 years.

Source: Based on estimates (Rehm et al. 2001b,d, 2009) from the WHO Comparative Risk Analysis within the Global Burden of Disease study (2000). Recorded consumption is derived from official or industry figures; unrecorded consumption is estimated from a variety of sources. The percentages of drinkers (drinking at all in the last 12 months) among males and females are derived from population surveys, where possible. Where figures for a country were otherwise unavailable, they were extrapolated from nearby countries on the basis of similarity of alcohol culture. Hazardous drinking pattern is an estimate derived from survey data and expert judgements at the country level. Estimates of the total population alcohol dependent are derived from population surveys, especially the World Mental Health (WMH2000) Surveys (see WHO 2002a).

regions is much diminished, with the groupings that include Russia, South Africa, and Western Europe now being much more similar to the groupings that include China, Bolivia, and Pakistan. This means that, in a global perspective, a country's abstention rate has a very important influence on per-adult consumption levels.

3.3 Trends and dramatic shifts in per-capita alcohol consumption

3.3.1 Trends in per-capita alcohol consumption

International comparisons of changes in levels of consumption over time can only be made on the basis of recorded consumption. These comparisons thus do not pick up the results of any changes in levels of unrecorded consumption. Looking at trends in per-capita alcohol consumption worldwide, there seems to have been a decline in drinking in many of the high alcohol consumption countries from the early 1970s to the early 2000. Figure 3.1 shows that this is particularly the case in the traditional wine-producing countries in Europe, such as France, where the decrease is mostly due to reductions in wine consumption (Gual and Colom 1997; World Advertising Research Center 2005). Similar trends are also seen in the wine-producing countries in South America such as Argentina and Chile. In other developed countries with relatively high per-capita alcohol consumption, a smaller but still significant decrease has been observed over more than a decade, for instance in Canada and the USA— although consumption levels have increased since the mid-1990s. Some developed countries have countered this trend, particularly countries with a traditionally low- or medium-level consumption, such as Cyprus, Ireland, and Japan (World Advertising Research Center 2005).

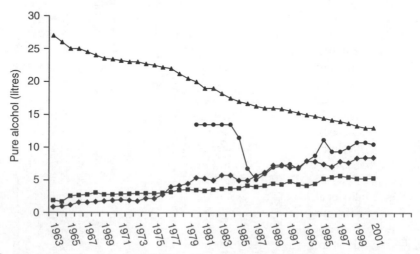

Fig. 3.1 Recorded consumption in litres of pure alcohol per inhabitant aged ≥15 years in Brazil (■), France (▲), Russia (●), and Thailand (◆).
Source: WHO 2004a.

By contrast with the general trends in developed countries, increases in recorded per-capita consumption have been noted for many developing countries (WHO 2004a). However, to some extent these increases in recorded consumption, often due to increased industrial production and importation, may reflect a comparable decrease in unrecorded consumption. This implies a need to be especially cautious when making statements about global trends. Overall, there does appear to have been a convergence in consumption among the developed countries as well as between developed and developing countries over the past 30 years. This conclusion is supported by more systematic data compiled from the *Global Status Report: Alcohol Policy* (WHO 2004b).

Adult per-capita consumption in Europe A (e.g. France) and B seems to be driven by long-term downward trends (Mäkelä *et al.* 1981b; Simpura 1998). For Europe C, there has been more variation. The sharp decline at the end of the 1980s is due to a forceful intervention, the anti-alcohol campaign of the Gorbachev period (1985–1988) in the former Soviet Union (e.g. Russia) (White 1996), as illustrated in Figure 3.1. No trends are apparent for Eastern Mediterranean B and D, nor for Africa D.

For the Western Pacific region there was an upward trend that seems to have stopped at the end of the 1980s. For Western Pacific B and South East Asia B (e.g. Thailand), consumption has clearly increased.

For the Americas, there has been a long wave for Americas A of increasing then decreasing consumption and a recent increase. For Americas B, the wine-producing countries Chile and Argentina have had significant downward trends in consumption (parallel to France, for instance), whereas other countries (e.g. Brazil) have witnessed increasing trends in consumption (See Fig 3.1).

3.3.2 Remarkable changes in consumption

Some remarkable and sudden shifts in alcohol consumption have taken place in recent decades, changes that are of particular concern from a public health perspective. As already noted, a number of developing countries have witnessed marked increases in recorded per-capita consumption. Moreover, in several countries in transition sudden changes over shorter periods of time have been observed. In Poland, the recorded per-capita consumption decreased markedly from 1980 to 1981 (a drop of 24%, from 8.4 litres of pure alcohol to 6.4 litres per adult inhabitant), concurrent with the anti-alcohol campaign launched by the 'Solidarity' trade union movement and co-opted in the government's declaration of martial law and its institution of alcohol rationing (Moskalewicz 2000). In the former Soviet Union, a similar decrease was observed in the mid 1980s during the anti-alcohol campaign of the Gorbachev era (White 1996; Reitan 2000). The campaign was initiated in 1985 in response to the enormous health and social costs of drinking and comprised a series of measures to reduce production and availability of alcohol. Illicit production and loss of government revenues may explain why the campaign gradually lost its momentum from 1987 onwards. The recorded per-capita consumption of pure ethanol in the Soviet Union dropped from 8.4 litres in 1984 to 3.3 litres in 1987 (Ivanets and Lukomskaya 1990). Even when illicit production is taken into account, there seems to have been a large net reduction of some 25% during the anti-alcohol campaign (Shkolnikov and Nemtsov 1997). At the end of the campaign, alcohol consumption returned to former levels.

3.4 Impact of total alcohol consumption

3.4.1 Distribution of alcohol consumption in the population

Studies from a number of countries demonstrate that alcohol consumption is very unevenly distributed in a population and among drinkers; most of the alcohol in a society is drunk by a relatively small minority of drinkers. Lemmens (1991) estimated for The Netherlands in the mid 1980s that the top one-tenth of drinkers consumed more than one-third of the total alcohol, and that the top 30% of the drinkers accounted for up to three-quarters of all consumption. Greenfield and Rogers (1999) found even more extreme results with US data. They found that the top 20% drink almost 90% of all alcohol and that young adults (aged 18–29 years), comprising roughly one-quarter of the adult population, account for almost half of all adult consumption. A Canadian study estimated that 10% of the drinkers consumed 50% of the alcohol (Stockwell *et al.* 2009). In China, it has been estimated that the top 11% of the drinkers (or less than 7% of the total population) consume 55% of the total amount of alcohol (Hao *et al.* 2004).

Skog (1991b) compared the distribution of alcohol consumption of Norway, a relatively low-consumption country, with France, a high-consumption country. In Norway the upper 10% of the drinkers consumed 50% of the total alcohol, whereas in France the upper 10% of drinkers consumed 30% of the alcohol. Skog argued that this exemplifies a general pattern: consumption is likely to be more strongly concentrated in a small segment of the population in low-consumption countries, whereas the concentration is less pronounced where per-capita consumption is higher. The skewness of the distribution of consumption can also be illustrated in another way; a significant fraction (i.e. 10–15%) of the drinkers consumes more than twice the average of all drinkers in a population (Skog 1985).

Studies of the distribution of alcohol consumption have also shown a significant regularity in the relationship between the mean consumption among drinkers and the consumption level in various consumer groups. Thus, the higher the mean consumption in a population, the higher the consumption level for the most modest drinkers in that population (e.g. the 25th percentile) and for the somewhat heavier drinkers (i.e. the 50th and 75th percentiles) as well as for the heaviest drinkers (i.e. the 90th or 95th percentile) (Skog 1985; Lemmens 1991). This implies that there is a strong relationship between the total consumption of alcohol in a population and the prevalence of people who are heavy drinkers.

It should, however, also be noted that although studies on the distribution of alcohol consumption have been undertaken in many populations covering a wide spectrum of mean consumption, they have only covered a limited number of established market economies where alcohol consumption is widespread. Thus, it is quite possible that the distribution pattern may deviate significantly in other socio-cultural systems, such as those with stricter informal social control of consumption (Skog 1985).

3.4.2 Relationship between total alcohol consumption and prevalence of heavy drinkers

It follows from the observations on the distribution of consumption that when total alcohol consumption increases in a society, there tends to be an increase in the prevalence of heavy drinkers, defined in terms of a high annual alcohol intake. This is referred to as the total consumption model. Because heavy drinkers account for a significant proportion of total alcohol consumption, it would be difficult for the total consumption level to increase without an increase in their drinking. It is, however, not only the consumption among heavy drinkers that affects the total consumption. An increase in total consumption seems to imply an increase in consumption in all consumer groups.

In Finland, total alcohol consumption increased by 46% from 1968 to 1969 in the wake of substantial increases in alcohol availability, and the increase in consumption was influenced most by the addition of new heavy drinking occasions (Mäkelä 1970). An increase in consumption was observed in all consumer groups, but the increase was greater in heavier consumption groups (Mäkelä 2002). The connection between heavy drinkers and the level of total consumption in the population has also been explained by the social nature of most drinking. People tend to influence each other's drinking with their own drinking behaviour, which implies that heavier drinkers, along with other drinkers, tend to drink more when consumption increases (Bruun *et al.* 1975a; Skog 1985, 2001b).

3.5 **Drinking patterns**

The term 'drinking pattern' refers to regularities in the frequency, amount and type of alcohol consumed over a period of time, and whether or not it is consumed with food. Drinking patterns are important because they have a direct effect on the drinker's blood alcohol level and other aspects of a person's drinking that are likely to lead to harm.

3.5.1 **Type of beverage**

One aspect of the drinking pattern is the type of alcoholic beverage consumed. As noted in Chapter 2, there are many varieties of alcoholic beverages, with varying levels of alcohol content. In many places, one or two beverage types account for most of the alcohol consumption. Predominant beverage types tend to change relatively slowly in a culture, although there are historical exceptions. For example, in 1917 a major tax increase in Denmark on distilled spirits suddenly altered the predominant alcoholic beverage from spirits to beer. The excise duty rate for distilled spirits was increased 12-fold and that of beer two-fold. The consumption of distilled spirits decreased much more than that of beer, so the share of beer as a percent of total alcohol consumption increased (Thorsen 1990).

Historically, spirits drinking was often regarded as more problematic than drinking fermented beverages like wine or beer. From a medical perspective, the choice of beverage makes little difference in terms of most long-term health consequences, such as liver cirrhosis (Smart 1996a) and cancers of the mouth and upper digestive tract (Bofetta and Hashibe 2006); it is the total amount of pure alcohol consumed regardless of beverage type that accounts for the toxic effects. But spirits drinking does bring some special problems. Fatal alcohol poisoning and aggressive behaviour seem to be more strongly associated with spirits than with other types of alcoholic beverages (Mäkelä *et al.* 2007). And yet, the harmful effects of specific beverages are less important than the specific cultural associations of different alcoholic beverages, and the drinking patterns associated with them. In the USA and the UK, beer, rather than stronger beverages, is most often involved in hazardous drinking (Rogers and Greenfield 1999; Naimi *et al.* 2007), in part because of its cultural meaning as a recreational beverage. In Finland beer and cider constitute almost two-thirds of the total amount of alcohol consumed; however, the heavier the binge drinking episode, the greater the proportion of spirits (Mäkelä *et al.* 2007). In Norway spirits were most often consumed in heavy drinking occasions two to three decades ago, whereas nowadays beer and wine account for most of the heavy drinking occasions (Horverak and Bye 2007).

The second column of Table 3.1 lists the predominant beverage types in the fifteen world regions. On a global basis, grape wine is a relatively unimportant part of alcohol consumption, although it dominates in specific areas like southern Europe. Rice-based fermented beverages, traditionally called rice wines, are important beverages in some Asian countries like Japan, as are medium strength spirits (~25%) such as *shochu*. *Arrack* and other spirits tend to predominate in the lowest consumption areas, and spirits such as vodka predominate in the highest consumption area, Slavic Europe.

In Africa and Latin America, traditional fermented beverages such as *sorghum* beer, *pulque* (made from the maguey plant), and *chicha* (made from maize) play an important role, with much of their production now industrialized. But nearly everywhere in the developing world, European-style lager beer is the prestige commodity among everyday alcoholic beverages (Jernigan 2000a). This style of beer, typically promoted and produced by multinational firms or their partners, shows growth in consumption levels in most parts of the developing world.

3.5.2 Drinking context

The extent to which alcohol is consumed in public settings (i.e. pubs, bars, restaurants) rather than in private settings has implications for harmful consequences (particularly violence), as well as prevention strategies. Quantitative data on drinking contexts from surveys are fairly sparse (Single *et al.* 1997). Comparative survey data from six European countries show some variability in the proportion of drinking occasions that occurred in bars or restaurants, ranging from around 10% to 25% of the drinking occasions (Leifman 2002). On the other hand, estimates from data on recorded consumption (Brewers Association of Canada 1997) show that the proportion of alcohol being consumed in public venues varies considerably across countries, i.e. from around 20% in Denmark and Canada to around 75% in Ireland.

The association between drinking context and alcohol problems probably varies by culture and over time. For instance, Finnish drinkers consumed more alcohol per occasion at home than in public drinking places in the 1950s, but by the mid 1960s differences by location in amount consumed had diminished among Helsinki drinkers (Partanen 1975). Survey studies in several countries have found that drinking in public drinking venues is particularly associated with heavy drinking and intoxication (Cosper *et al.* 1987; Single *et al.* 1997; Mustonen and Mäkelä 1999; Horverak and Bye 2007), although this picture is not entirely consistent (Demers 1997; Kairouz *et al.* 2002).

3.5.3 Distribution of drinking occasions and intake per occasion

Total consumption can be regarded as a combination of two dimensions—drinking frequency and average quantity per occasion—each with its own distribution. Two equal distributions of total consumption may thus be composed of different combinations of drinking frequency and quantity. If regular drinking has different health effects than occasional heavy drinking, two apparently equal overall levels of drinking may lead to different outcomes.

Simply assessing total consumption may thus lead to erroneous conclusions. For example, Knupfer (1987) has noted that in several epidemiological studies on cardiovascular risk, consumption was presented as average number of drinks per day, which was subsequently misinterpreted as daily drinking of the particular amounts. She noted, however, that in US surveys 'daily light' drinkers are rare, and those who drink daily are mostly heavy drinkers. In line with this, Lemmens (1991) found drinking frequency to be positively associated with quantity per occasion. Similar findings are reported from Canada (Paradis *et al.* 2009) where only 6% of the drinkers reported a usual intake of one to two drinks per occasion and five to seven drinking occasions per week, and there was a positive correlation between drinking frequency and usual quantity per occasion. The prevalence of frequent light drinkers appears to be even smaller in other parts of the world such as India (Benegal *et al.* 2005), Mexico (Mendoza *et al.* 2005), and Sri Lanka (Hettige and Paranagama 2005), although somewhat higher rates are also reported in Brazil (Kerr-Correa *et al.* 2005) and Uganda (Tumwesigye and Kasirye 2005). Recent surveys from African countries where alcohol abstention is predominant have also showed that among drinkers the proportion of frequent light drinkers is low (Clausen *et al.* 2009).

3.5.4 Intoxication

As discussed in Chapter 2, intoxication is a major mechanism through which alcohol causes harm. Intoxication results from drinking a relatively large amount of alcohol on one particular occasion, although the term covers more than simply the amount of alcohol consumed. To understand the implications of total consumption, we must differentiate between drinkers whose amount of intake varies considerably from one occasion to another and drinkers who consistently drink about the same amount on each occasion. Risks will be quite different for a person who drinks three bottles of beer every evening and a person who drinks one bottle every day but fifteen bottles on a Saturday night, though their drinking frequency and average consumption will be the same.

Cultures vary in the extent to which drinking to intoxication is a characteristic of the drinking pattern. They also differ in how intoxicated people become, and how people behave while intoxicated (Room and Mäkelä 2000). It seems that drinking pattern and the extent to which people drink to intoxication in a population are fairly stable over time and less variable than the overall consumption (Horverak and Bye 2007). The eighth column in Table 3.1 shows the average drinking pattern score for each of the fifteen regions, compiled as a population-weighted average of the scores of the included nations. The score was derived from survey data, extrapolation, and expert judgement.

Nations were assigned a score from 1 to 4, indicating the level of hazard associated with the predominant pattern of drinking (Rehm *et al.* 2001b,d). Note that the score is independent of both the proportion of abstainers and the volume of alcohol consumption. In principle, it is intended to indicate the differential risk of problems associated with the dominant patterns of drinking in the country or region. It can be viewed as an indication of the extent to which intoxication is a characteristic mediator between alcohol consumption and social and casualty harms in that nation.

The two regions with the lowest average score for hazardous drinking pattern are Europe A and Western Pacific A. Europe A, especially, includes countries assigned a higher drinking pattern score than the average. For instance, the score assigned to Sweden, Norway and Finland is three, but the score for the region as a whole is brought down by more populous countries with lower hazardous drinking pattern scores.

The region including Russia and Ukraine (Europe C) has the highest drinking pattern score, but the scores are also high in Africa, Latin America, Eastern Europe, and India. The level of hazard thus has relatively little relationship to the per-adult level of consumption. A hazardous pattern can be associated with either high or low consumption levels in the population at large.

Intoxication is a particularly marked characteristic of drinking by teenagers and young adults in many cultures. As they are relative neophytes to drinking, their episodes of intoxication may be particularly prone to harmful consequences. A recent multinational study of drinking habits and drug use among school children provides a basis for comparisons among European countries as well as the USA (Hibell *et al.* 2009). The second column in Table 3.2 shows the average number of drinking events in the last year reported by 15–16-year-olds in a selection of mostly European countries in 2007. The third column presents the average number of intoxication occasions in the last year in the same samples. The fourth column is the ratio of intoxication occasions to drinking occasions. This ratio thus represents the proportion of drinking occasions that become occasions of drunkenness and gives an indication of the relative significance of drinking to intoxication in the various countries. The fifth, sixth and seventh columns present corresponding figures from adult sample populations in the same countries. As can be seen, the intoxication frequency:drinking frequency ratio varies significantly between countries and tends to fall into a north–south gradient across European countries. In southern European countries a smaller proportion of drinking occasions leads to a state of subjective intoxication compared with Northern European countries. Moreover, we also see that drinking to intoxication is more likely to occur in a drinking occasion among adolescents than among adults. The variation in the extent to which drinking occasions become occasions of intoxication is also illustrated in Figure 3.2.

3.5.5 Alcohol dependence

As discussed in Chapter 2, alcohol dependence may be viewed as a mediator between alcohol consumption and alcohol-related problems. That is, someone who has become alcohol dependent is more likely to continue to drink in ways that result in health or social harm. On the basis of advances in psychiatric epidemiology, it is now possible to estimate alcohol dependence rates from surveys conducted in the WHO global regions (last column of Table 3.1; Rehm and Eschmann 2002).

Table 3.2 Average numbers of drinking occasions (D) and intoxication occasions (I) and I:D ratio in adolescent and adult population samples by country

(1) Country	(2) Adolescents	(3)	(4)	(5) Adults	(6)	(7)
	D	I	I:D	D	I	I:D
Denmark	22.1	6.1	0.28	139	11	0.08
Finland	8.3	2.9	0.35	53	13	0.25
France	12.5	1.5	0.12	91	7	0.07
Germany	19.7	2.5	0.13	76	9	0.11
Italy	11.3	1.3	0.12	150	18	0.12
Norway	6.4	2.3	0.36	47	6	0.13
Russia	10.5	2.2	0.21	61	15	0.25
Sweden	7.3	2.2	0.30	31	8	0.27
Ukraine	10.7	1.8	0.17	53	16	0.30
UK	16.9	4.7	0.28	92	32	0.33
USA	5.9	3.0	0.51	103	12	0.12

Average numbers of drinking occasions and intoxication occasions in adolescent sample populations are calculated based on data from European School Project on Alcohol and Drugs (ESPAD) surveys in 2007 (reported in Hibell *et al.* 2009). Note that values for intoxication frequency and thus also I:D are not comparable to the values from previous ESPAD surveys presented in Babor *et al.* (2003) due to changes in measurement. Average numbers of drinking occasions and intoxication occasions (i.e. ≥5 or ≥6 drinks per occasion) in adult population samples are calculated based on data from Mäkelä *et al.* (1999; Denmark and Norway), Leifman (2002; Finland, France, Germany, Italy, Sweden, and the UK), Pomerleau *et al.* (2005; Russia and Ukraine), Dawson (2000; USA). Note that in Russia and Ukraine larger amounts of alcohol are consumed at intoxication occasions (Pomerleau *et al.* 2008).

In general, there is a strong relationship between the estimated per-adult total consumption in a global region and the estimated rate of alcohol dependence. Patterns of drinking reflected in high hazardous drinking scores may also lead to dependence. It is also likely that cultural differences in attributions and in the experience and recognition of affective states are related to dependence rates, as suggested by a WHO study of the cross-cultural comparability of the criteria for alcohol dependence (Room *et al.* 1996). Thus rates of dependence in the three American regions, in Europe C (primarily Russia), and in South East Asia A (primarily India) seem systematically higher than would be expected from per-adult total consumption rates.

3.6 Distribution of drinking across demographic subgroups and over the lifespan

3.6.1 Gender

A large research literature, based primarily on survey studies of drinking habits, has consistently shown that there are significant differences in drinking patterns between men and women, between younger and older people, and often among ethnic or religious groups. As Table 3.1 suggests, there are striking gender differences in whether a person drinks; men are more likely to be drinkers and women abstainers. Among drinkers, men drink on average significantly more than women do. There is variation among countries in the proportion of total alcohol consumed by men, but the range of variation in Europe and North America is not great: from less than 70% (in Denmark, Switzerland and the USA) to more than 80% (France and Russia) (Simpura *et al.* 1997, p. 102). In some developing countries, men's share of the overall consumption is much greater. For instance, survey data from China indicate that around 93% of alcohol is consumed by men (Hao *et al.* 2004), and a similar figure has been reported from the Seychelles (Perdrix *et al.* 1999). Some studies have shown that the gender difference in drinking has diminished over time in some countries, yet this has not been consistently reported from the relatively few affluent countries where this has been studied (Holmila and Raitasalo 2005).

Moreover, men drink heavily (i.e. to intoxication, or large quantities per occasion) much more often than women. This is consistently reported from a variety of countries (WHO 2004a; Wilsnack *et al.* 2005). Hence, there are more heavy drinkers and more heavy drinking occasions among men, and consequently harmful drinking is more likely to characterize men than women. Although the evidence is still sparse, it seems that this phenomenon may be even more distinctive in developing countries (Room *et al.* 2002).

3.6.2 Age groups and life cycle

Drinking habits in various age groups are difficult to compare across countries because different measures of drinking and age groupings have been used in population surveys. Moreover, most surveys that compare drinking in various age groups have been conducted in the established market economies of Europe and North America, so the findings may not necessarily apply to other regions of the world. Nevertheless, a common picture emerges from these studies: abstinence or infrequent drinking are more prevalent in older age groups, and intoxication or heavy drinking episodes are relatively more frequent among adolescents and young adults. This has been reported from the Nordic countries (Mäkelä *et al.* 1999), Canada (Demers 1997), the USA (Dawson 1998), and The Netherlands (San José *et al.* 2000) (see also Figure 3.2). On the other hand, studies from Germany (Bloomfield 1998), the USA (Weisner *et al.* 2000), the Nordic countries (Mäkelä *et al.* 1999), and the Seychelles (Perdrix *et al.* 1999) have found that the average consumption or the proportions of high-volume consumers do not vary much across age groups.

Of particular concern in many countries is hazardous drinking among youth. In most of the countries where alcohol consumption is widespread (e.g. most European and American countries, New Zealand and Australia), a large proportion of adolescents drink alcohol, at least from time to time (WHO 1999; Hibell *et al.* 2000). Data from the 2007 European School Survey Project on Alcohol and other Drugs (ESPAD: Hibell *et al.* 2009) showed that in 34 of the 36 participating countries a clear majority of the 15–16-year-old students reported drinking in the previous year. In three-fourths of the countries the majority of drinkers reported fewer than ten drinking occasions in

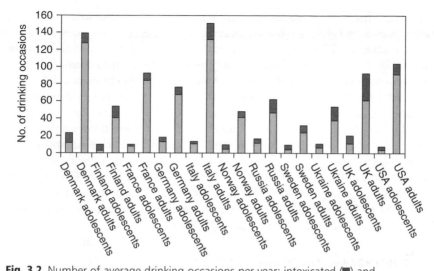

Fig. 3.2 Number of average drinking occasions per year; intoxicated (■) and non-intoxicated (▨) occasions by country and adolescent/adult population. Source: Our calculations, based on data presented in Table 3.2.

the preceding year. In more than half of the countries, the majority of the students had their first drink before the age of 14 years (Hibell *et al.* 2009). A number of studies from western industrialized countries have shown that young people consume alcohol in public drinking places (e.g. bars, cafes) more often than middle-aged and elderly people (Cosper *et al.* 1987; Single 1993; Demers 1997), and that a large proportion of young people's consumption tends to take place in bars and pubs (Engels *et al.* 1999).

The age gradient in drinking level and abstinence described in recent cross-sectional studies may be interpreted as an age effect (i.e. people tend to drink less heavily or become abstinent as they get older), a cohort effect (i.e. those who grew up in the second half of the twentieth century have learned or have been socialized into more drinking or heavy drinking than older cohorts), or a combination of both. Longitudinal studies have shown that middle-aged and elderly people are more likely than younger people to reduce their drinking or become abstinent, and much less likely than younger people to increase their drinking or take up heavy drinking (Fillmore *et al.* 1991a; Hajema *et al.* 1997; Mulder *et al.* 1998). In a study of drinking careers in a Native American (Navajo) population, Kunitz *et al.* (1994) found that young people who would have been classified as alcoholic tended to moderate or quit drinking as they became older. But there appear to be cultural differences in the extent and timing of reducing heavy drinking with increasing age. A cross-ethnic study by Caetano (1997) showed that the stability and incidence of problem drinking was higher among Hispanics and blacks than among whites in the US general population.

3.6.3 Indigenous minority groups

In developed countries, rates of abstention are often higher in indigenous minority groups than in the surrounding population (e.g. Hunter *et al.* 1992; Brady 2000).

Studies of indigenous populations in Australia and North America have shown that these groups often have a significantly higher alcohol intake than the general population (see Brady 2000 for a review), although there is considerable variation among groups (Heath 1983). In the 1980s, the per-capita consumption in Greenland (with a mainly Inuit population) was almost twice as high as in the rest of Denmark (National Institute for Alcohol and Drug Research 2001), whereas no differences in amount of consumption have been found, for instance, between the Saami population and the general population in Norway (Larsen and Saglie 1996). However, there is particular concern about the pattern of consumption among indigenous minority groups. Fewer indigenous people seem to drink daily and drinking tends to be more hazardous, with any drinking at all often implying drinking to intoxication (Dawson 1998; Brady 2000). Surveys from New Zealand showed that although Maori reported a lower drinking frequency they also reported a significantly larger intake on a typical drinking occasion compared to non-Maori (Bramley *et al.* 2003).

3.7 **Summary and implications**

Sales data from established market economies show a slight overall decrease in alcohol consumption in recent years, as well as converging trends in traditional high- and low-consumption countries. Of particular concern, however, is the increasing consumption in some of the emerging economies, given that the drinking appears to be concentrated in a smaller fraction of the population in these countries.

While levels of alcohol consumption vary greatly from one part of the world to another, it appears that much of this variation is attributable to differences in the proportions of adults who abstain from drinking altogether. On a base limited to drinkers, the consumption level of the highest-consuming region is less than three times that of the lowest-consuming region. This suggests that registered per-capita consumption will increase steeply if the proportion of abstainers declines, particularly in places where abstention is very common, as is true in much of the developing world.

It is not only the level of total alcohol consumption that is relevant to the health and social problems from drinking; the drinking pattern and societal reactions to drinking are also of considerable importance. Thus, the same amount of consumption may be associated with quite different problem levels in different societies. The large variation in total consumption and drinking patterns across population subgroups also implies that alcohol-related problems will be very unevenly distributed within a given country.

In terms of the mediators between alcohol consumption and social and health problems discussed in Chapter 2, there are large variations between one country and another in the extent to which drinking is concentrated into occasions of intoxication. We have presented data from a hazardous drinking pattern score for global regions, which gives an indication of the relative prominence of intoxication occasions in the drinking of the region. We have also presented estimates for the rates of alcohol dependence, a second mediator between levels of consumption and the occurrence of social and health problems. The global regions appear to cluster into two groups when the proportion of drinkers who report being alcohol dependent is compared with the consumption level per drinker. Some parts of the world, as noted—the Americas, Eastern Europe, and the Indian subcontinent—report higher rates of dependence than the consumption per drinker would suggest. Within each group of regions, however, there seems to be an association between the average consumption per drinker and rates of dependence.

The differences in amounts and patterns of drinking between different countries and global regions imply differences in the composition and mixture of social and health problems from drinking, the issue to which we turn in Chapter 4. The differences also imply that it may be necessary for the mixture of prevention and intervention strategies to vary from one society to another.

Appendix 3.1

The fifteen regional groupings below (which comprise the 191 United Nations Member States) have been defined by the World Health Organization on the basis of geographical location as well as high, medium, or low levels of adult and infant mortality. WHO's EUR B has been subdivided to separate out the relatively low-consumption southern republics of the former Soviet Union.

Africa	D	Algeria, Angola, Benin, Burkina Faso, Cameroon, Cape Verde, Chad, Comoros, Equatorial Guinea, Gabon, Gambia, Ghana, Guinea, Guinea-Bissau, Liberia, Madagascar, Mali, Mauritania, Mauritius, Niger, Nigeria, Sao Tome and Principe, Senegal, Seychelles, Sierra Leone, Togo
Africa	E	Botswana, Burundi, Central African Republic, Congo, Côte d'Ivoire, Democratic Republic of the Congo, Eritrea, Ethiopia, Kenya, Lesotho, Malawi, Mozambique, Namibia, Rwanda, South Africa, Swaziland, Uganda, United Republic of Tanzania, Zambia, Zimbabwe
America	A	Canada, Cuba, USA
America	B	Antigua and Barbuda, Argentina, Bahamas, Barbados, Belize, Brazil, Chile, Colombia, Costa Rica, Dominica, Dominican Republic, El Salvador, Grenada, Guyana, Honduras, Jamaica, Mexico, Panama, Paraguay, Saint Kitts and Nevis, Saint Lucia, Saint Vincent and the Grenadines, Suriname, Trinidad and Tobago, Uruguay, Venezuela
America	D	Bolivia, Ecuador, Guatemala, Haiti, Nicaragua, Peru
Eastern Mediterranean	B	Bahrain, Cyprus, Iran (Islamic Republic of), Jordan, Kuwait, Lebanon, Libyan Arab Jamahiriya, Oman, Qatar, Saudi Arabia, Syrian Arab Republic, Tunisia, United Arab Emirates
Eastern Mediterranean	D	Afghanistan, Djibouti, Egypt, Iraq, Morocco, Pakistan, Somalia, Sudan, Yemen
Europe	A	Andorra, Austria, Belgium, Croatia, Czech Republic, Denmark, Finland, France, Germany, Greece, Iceland, Ireland, Israel, Italy, Luxembourg, Malta, Monaco, Netherlands, Norway, Portugal, San Marino, Slovenia, Spain, Sweden, Switzerland, UK
Europe	B 1	Albania, Bosnia and Herzegovina, Bulgaria, Georgia, Poland, Romania, Slovakia, The Former Yugoslav Republic of Macedonia, Turkey, Yugoslavia
Europe	B 2	Armenia, Azerbaijan, Kyrgyzstan, Tajikistan, Turkmenistan, Uzbekistan
Europe	C	Belarus, Estonia, Hungary, Kazakhstan, Latvia, Lithuania, Republic of Moldova, Russian Federation, Ukraine
South East Asia	B	Indonesia, Sri Lanka, Thailand
South East Asia	D	Bangladesh, Bhutan, Democratic People's Republic of Korea, India, Maldives, Myanmar, Nepal

Western Pacific	A	Australia, Brunei, Darussalam, Japan, New Zealand, Singapore
Western Pacific	B	Cambodia, China, Cook Islands, Fiji, Kiribati, Lao People's Democratic Republic, Malaysia, Marshall Islands, Micronesia (Federated States of), Mongolia, Nauru, Niue, Palau, Papua New Guinea, Philippines, Republic of Korea, Samoa, Solomon Islands, Tonga, Tuvalu, Vanuatu, Vietnam

Chapter 4

The global burden of alcohol consumption

4.1 Introduction

This chapter describes the enormous range of alcohol-related consequences within two broad categories: alcohol's contribution to the burden of illness carried by individuals and societies, and alcohol's harmful effect on the social fabric of families, communities, and nations. It also discusses the potential health benefits of moderate alcohol use.

Establishing that alcohol consumption is a direct cause of specific social and health problems is a task with great significance for public health. If a social or health problem is at least in part attributable to drinking, the evidence generally helps to suggest specific measures to prevent or control the problem. Quantifying the strength of the relationship is an additional tool in making decisions about policy priorities, taking into account as well the prevalence of the particular problem. For instance, the invention of reliable instruments to measure blood alcohol concentration (BAC) opened the way for the scientific study of drink-driving behaviour. As a result it soon became clear that drinking was implicated in a much larger share of traffic fatalities than had been thought. This eventually led to substantial policy changes concerning drink-driving. We begin this chapter with a discussion of how epidemiologists establish causal relations between drinking and its consequences. We then consider the evidence on health consequences in three different frames:

1) The role of alcohol in the global burden of disease and disability.

2) Alcohol and all-cause mortality.

3) The relation of alcohol to specific causes of death and disease.

The relation of drinking to different types of social problems is then considered. A case study of the Russian experience during the anti-alcohol campaign of 1985–1987 is used to illustrate the potential changes in health and social problems that follow from reductions in alcohol consumption. Before turning to conclusions, the available evidence is considered on the relative magnitude of health and social problems from drinking.

4.2 Measurement and inferential issues

4.2.1 The nature of health and social problems

To varying degrees, different health and social problems have both an objective element and an element that is a matter of social definition. At one end of the continuum is the fact that death can be measured objectively and reliably. But when we want to divide deaths into different categories (or 'causes of death', as they are conventionally called), social definition becomes important. For both acute and chronic causes of death, recording and coding practices often vary from one country to another (e.g. Ramstedt 2002a). For health problems short of death, social definition plays an even larger part. The threshold at which a potential disability is socially noticeable, for instance, varies between cultures (Room *et al.* 2001). Despite these difficulties, there has been substantial progress in international efforts to employ standard codes for causes of death and disease that are cross-culturally applicable, such as the International Classification of Disease, Tenth Revision (ICD-10) (WHO 1992a). In addition, modern comparative statistics such as the Global Burden of Disease study correct for cultural differences in coding practices (Lopez *et al.* 2006). While these efforts have contributed to the advance of epidemiology and other health sciences (WHO 2001a), the apparent objectivity of the international classification system should not obscure the fact that an element of social definition is still present in the recognition of alcohol-related harms.

While internationally comparable statistics by causes of death have long been available, and there are similar data on hospitalizations by cause at least for established market economies, there are no cross-nationally comparable data on disabilities (Goerdt *et al.* 1996; Rehm and Gmel 2000a), since the revised system for classifying and recording disability has only recently been adopted by the WHO (2001a). The paucity of data on morbidity and especially disability is especially problematic for estimating alcohol's role, as there are indications that alcohol is more related to disability than to mortality (Murray and Lopez 1996a; Rehm *et al.* 2004).

For social problems, as the term itself implies, the element of social definition becomes more prominent. Child marriage and polygamy are accepted customs in some societies, but these would be defined as social problems and indeed crimes in others. Even within a given society, the existence of a social problem is itself often a matter of judgement and dispute—the partners in a couple may disagree about whether there is a marital problem at all. And often the way social matters are thought about in a given society changes over time. In English-speaking countries around 1900, for instance, divorce was commonly viewed as a social problem, and the then-difficult process of getting a divorce created legally defined categories of divorce, such as divorce due to the partner's 'inebriety' (i.e. drunkenness). The shift in many jurisdictions in recent decades to 'no-fault divorce' abolished these categories (Room 1996).

Scientific progress depends on objective definitions and measures. For this reason the role of alcohol as a causal factor in disease is presently more clearly understood scientifically than the role of alcohol in the causation of social harm. Nevertheless, reliable measurement and cross-national comparisons are not only possible for many social problems, but are also useful for public policy purposes.

4.2.2 Alcohol as a cause

As noted in Chapter 2, there are three main aspects of alcohol that contribute to harms from drinking. In the context of estimations of the global burden of alcohol consumption, which are primarily concerned with alcohol's role in ill-health and injury, these aspects play different roles. For many chronic diseases, the primary aspect considered is the toxic effect, primarily through the cumulative volume of drinking. Conversely, for injuries the primary focus is on drinking in a specific event, including intoxication. However, both aspects of alcohol can play a role in chronic disease, and also in injuries. In global burden estimates, **dependence** primarily appears as an outcome—as a mental disorder—rather than as a risk factor for other health harm. The effect of dependence on other health harms is primarily accounted for through the high volume and excessive patterns of consumption, to which dependence presumably contributes.

In classifications of disease and crime, some categories are alcohol-specific. For instance, the category of 'alcohol poisoning' in the ICD-10 specifies a causal role of alcohol in the death or injury. The 'attributable fraction' (the proportion of cases in the category assumed to be caused by drinking) is thus set at 1.0 or 100% for these conditions. But the causal attribution built into these categories is substantially influenced by social factors. The doctor or health worker making the attribution to alcohol may be oversensitive to a potential alcohol attribution. More commonly, however, alcohol's involvement in a death may be missed by those certifying the death, or may be deliberately not mentioned to protect the reputation of the deceased. Thus a landmark study of death-recording in twelve cities in ten countries found that the number of deaths assigned to the ICD-10 category 'liver cirrhosis with mention of alcoholism' rose by 135%, after taking into account additional information obtained from hospital records and interviews with attending physicians and family members. The majority of the new cases were previously coded in categories like cirrhosis without mention of alcoholism (Puffer and Griffith 1967).

For other categories of death, disease, disability, or crime, alcohol's involvement may be a matter of increased probability rather than certainty. Thus some of those who die in traffic accidents involving a driver who had been drinking would have died even if there had been no drinking (Reed 1981), for example, because the other driver might have been at fault. To take the proper measure of alcohol's role in this wider range of categories, it is necessary to draw on epidemiological studies to estimate relative risks (i.e. how much particular levels and patterns of drinking increase the risk of mortality or morbidity) for each of the disease categories where alcohol is potentially involved. For some causes of death—notably for casualties—the relative risk varies between cultures and countries. Combining information on the relative risk with prevalence data on the relevant levels and patterns of drinking, the attributable fraction can then be calculated for a particular society.

It should be noted that alcohol's causal role in social and health problems is usually contributory, being only one of several factors responsible for the problem. For example, hepatitis and malnutrition may be involved in a cirrhosis death, as well as heavy drinking. Ice on the road and poor street lighting may play a causal role in a traffic crash, along with drinking by a driver. The minimum kind of causation in which we are interested is based on the following question: Would the event or condition have occurred in the absence of the drinking? Box 4.1 provides further insights into current epidemiological thinking about causal attribution.

Box 4.1 How epidemiologists estimate alcohol's causal contribution to death, disease and social harm

Determination of causality may vary between classes of consequences and, implicitly, according to the causal logic of the underlying sciences (Rehm and Fischer 1997; see also Pernanen 2001). For health outcomes, the usual epidemiological definitions have been used, which stress not only consistent relations but also biological pathways (Rothman *et al.* 2008). Thus, the consistent relationship between alcohol and lung cancer found in many epidemiological studies (English *et al.* 1995) was not included here as an alcohol-attributable disease because no biological pathway has yet been identified, and because the higher incidence of lung cancer in drinkers is believed to be caused by smoking (Bandera *et al.* 2001).

This example is interesting from another perspective. One might argue that smoking, or the persistence of smoking, is part of a causal chain linked to alcohol (Rothman *et al.* 2008), and if such a causal relationship could be established, then some cases of lung cancer would be attributable to drinking. Despite the consistent relationship between alcohol and smoking, we have not included lung cancer in this overview, because the evidence of alcohol *causing* smoking was not judged sufficient. Current knowledge seems to indicate that both behaviours stem from common third causes (Little 2000). In this decision, as in other decisions underlying this chapter, care was taken not to overstate the impact of alcohol.

While the causal status of the relationship between alcohol and health outcomes often depends on the plausibility of potential biological pathways, the causal status of the relationships between alcohol and social harm cannot usually be determined this way. An exception is aggressive behaviour, for which a causal link between alcohol intoxication and aggression has been supported by epidemiological and experimental research, as well as by research indicating specific biological mechanisms linking alcohol to aggressive behaviour. Experimental studies suggest a causal relationship between alcohol and aggression (Bushman 1997; Bushman and Cooper 1990), although this relationship is clearly moderated by gender and personality as well as by situational and cultural factors (Lipsey *et al.* 1997; Graham *et al.* 1998). There is also evidence pointing to the biological pathways through which alcohol increases aggressive behaviour (Miczek *et al.* 1993, 1997; Pihl *et al.* 1993). Alcohol may also contribute to aggression by impairing cognitive functioning (Peterson *et al.* 1990), which can reduce problem-solving ability (Sayette *et al.* 1993).

For other social problems, the estimation of alcohol's causal contribution has no easy solution. For many social problems, there may be record-keeping attribution by a police officer, a social worker, or another professional dealing with the problem. Other possible sources of attribution, much used in population surveys, are the drinker's own attribution of causality to alcohol, and those of the drinker's family members, friends, bystanders, or victims. There is often considerable variation in attribution between observers of the same phenomenon, and this methodology has been criticized because survey respondents' attributions may not

> **Box 4.1** How epidemiologists estimate alcohol's causal contribution to death, disease and social harm *(continued)*
>
> be sufficient evidence of causality (see Gmel *et al.* 2000). But such attributions sometimes constitute the essence of the social problem and thus become part of the data: if someone considers that his or her spouse's drinking causes problems, then that in itself indicates that there is a marital problem connected to the drinking.
>
> In addition to the consistency of empirical evidence from all of these sources, theoretical underpinnings and methodology play an important role in making inferences about alcohol's contribution to social harm.

4.2.3 Role of average volume and drinking patterns

So far we have only spoken about relationships between alcohol and problems in general terms. Clearly, different dimensions of alcohol consumption have to be distinguished to arrive at a better understanding of such relationships. In this chapter, as in the previous one, we distinguish between two dimensions: average alcohol consumption and **drinking patterns** (for definitions see Chapter 3 and the Glossary, respectively). Drinking patterns include but are not limited to heavy drinking occasions. For instance, one study showed that all-cause mortality in light to moderate male drinkers (0–2 drinks a day) was about twice as high if they had occasional heavy drinking episodes (Rehm *et al.* 2001b). Heavy drinking episodes not only play a role in mortality, but also contribute to acute consequences, particularly accidents and injuries. Thus, any discussion of the relationship between alcohol consumption and consequences needs to take into account both the nature of the problem (health vs social), and the dimension of drinking involved (average volume vs pattern of drinking).

4.2.4 Evidence on alcohol's role: individual and population level research

Death, disability, and social problems happen to individuals, and there is thus an inherent interest in the following question: At the individual level, what is alcohol's causal role in harm or benefit? From a public health perspective, an equally important question is: At the population level, what happens if there is an increase or decrease in alcohol consumption, or a change in the drinking pattern? The answers to these two questions often point in the same direction, but not always (Skog 1996). Complicating this issue is the fact that each level of analysis has its own difficulties in measurement and in causal attribution. Establishing causality from **aggregate** changes is complicated because it is difficult to control for **confounding** factors (Morgenstern 1998).

To better understand these phenomena, epidemiologists have developed a variety of research methods that focus on medical samples as well as population-level analyses. With many of the health and social problems related to drinking, the causal role of alcohol cannot be discerned from an individual case. The establishment of cause depends in part on the degree of statistical association in a large sample of cases. Thus the focus of an aetiological study in medical epidemiology commonly involves summarizing and comparing the individual outcomes across a large sample of cases.

Nevertheless, in most such studies the sample does not represent the experience of a whole population. This experience is represented by another type of evidence, population-level analyses (e.g. data from a whole country), particularly **time-series analyses** looking at the covariation from one point in time to another between an alcohol variable and a potential outcome variable. In recent years, the number of time-series analyses has grown considerably in the alcohol field.

If the results from individual- and population-level studies point in the same direction, our confidence in the findings is increased substantially. Such is the case, for instance, for studies of the relation of drinking to homicide. But if the results do not point in the same direction, judgements must be made about the relative weight of evidence from the different studies. Despite the complexity involved in establishing causal relations between alcohol and problems, and the difficulties of estimating the strength of this relationship, the science of alcohol epidemiology has advanced to the point that alcohol's specific role in a variety of health and social problems is now much more clearly understood, as the remainder of this chapter will show.

4.3 Alcohol consumption and health consequences

To estimate the burden of disease attributable to alcohol-related health consequences, it is necessary to take into account both its deleterious and its beneficial effects. Deleterious effects stem from alcohol's contribution to many chronic and infectious disease conditions, as well as accidents, injuries, and acute toxic effects (see Rehm *et al.* 2004 for a complete listing except for infectious disease). Box 4.2 describes the major conditions associated with alcohol-related morbidity and mortality. In addition, some specific drinking patterns have been found to have beneficial effects on coronary heart disease and ischaemic stroke (see contributions in Chadwick and Goode 1998; Puddey *et al.* 1999). The relationship between alcohol consumption and diabetes is not clear, but there is suggestive evidence for a beneficial effect of light to moderate drinking, including plausible biological pathways (Ashley *et al.* 2000).

The following paragraphs (and in Boxes 4.3–4.7) review the evidence for some of the most important diseases and conditions related to alcohol: coronary heart disease, breast cancer, tuberculosis, motor vehicle accidents, and suicide. Each box summarizes the research evidence derived from individual-level studies and studies based on population (aggregate level) time-series analyses. Except for traffic accidents, the focus of this research is primarily on mortality. Evidence from **meta-analytic** reviews and key studies is summarized in terms of the effects of total volume of alcohol consumed, moderate drinking, drinking pattern, plausible biological mechanisms, and interactions with factors that mediate or moderate the relationship between alcohol and the condition.

4.3.1 Coronary heart disease (CHD)

Box 4.3 summarizes the evidence for coronary heart disease. In individual-level studies, which have been carried out mainly in developed societies, the relationship between

Box 4.2 Major alcohol-related health conditions contributing to morbidity and mortality[a]

- ◆ **Cancers**: head and neck cancers, liver cancer, colorectal cancers, female breast cancer

- ◆ **Neuropsychiatric conditions**: alcohol dependence syndrome, alcohol abuse, depression

- ◆ **Diabetes** (protective and adverse effects)

- ◆ **Cardiovascular conditions**: ischaemic heart disease, hypertensive disease, cerebrovascular disease (protective and adverse effects for all cardiovascular conditions)

- ◆ **Gastrointestinal conditions**: liver cirrhosis, pancreatitis

- ◆ **Infectious diseases**: tuberculosis, pneumonia

- ◆ **Maternal and perinatal conditions**: low birth weight, fetal alcohol syndrome

- ◆ **Acute toxic effects**: alcohol poisoning

- ◆ **Accidents**: road and other transport injuries, falls, drowning and burning injuries, occupational and machine injuries

- ◆ **Self-inflicted injuries**: suicide

- ◆ **Violent deaths**: assault injuries

[a] Conditions are listed only where a causal impact of alcohol on incidence has been established (see Rehm *et al.* 2004; Lönnroth *et al.* 2008; see text for detail on definition of causality). Effects are adverse except as noted. Alcohol also plays a causal role in many less common causes of illness and death. Many more conditions have associations with alcohol, such as most neuropsychiatric diseases, but causality has not been established according to standard criteria.

alcohol consumption and CHD is negative overall, indicating a cardioprotective effect. As noted above, this effect explains the lower death rate of light drinkers relative to abstainers. It has been found consistently in many studies, even after adjusting for potential confounders (e.g. diet: Rehm *et al.* 1997; social isolation: Murray *et al.* 1999), and after correcting for the **'sick-quitter' effect** (Shaper *et al.* 1988; Shaper 1990a,b). Although the evidence on the effect has recently been contested (Fillmore *et al.* 2006), our current conclusion is that the effect had been overestimated on poorly designed studies, but still persists at a lower level in well-designed studies. The evidence for biological mechanisms is strong but not fully conclusive for all mechanisms discussed (e.g. Zakhari 1997; Puddey *et al.* 1999; Rehm *et al.* 2003b). At least half of the effect seems to be short term (mainly by preventing blood clots), so there may be little benefit from sporadic drinking, the most common drinking pattern in developing countries.

With respect to heavy drinking, the results are less clear, but overall detrimental effects were mainly found, especially for females (e.g. Rehm *et al.* 1997; Corrao *et al.* 2000). Heavy binge drinking, as is common in Russia, is associated with increased deaths from CHD. Thus, deaths from circulatory disease, including CHD, dropped by

Box 4.3 Effects of alcohol on ischaemic heart disease (ICD-10: I20–I25)

Individual-level studies

Volume of alcohol	Moderate drinking	Patterns of drinking	Mechanisms	Interactions
All meta-analytic reviews found significant beneficial effects (e.g. Maclure 1993; English *et al.* 1995; Single *et al.* 1999; Corrao *et al.* 2000) for light to moderate consumption; there is indication of detrimental effects of heavy drinking (Rehm *et al.* 1997; Corrao *et al.* 2000). Recent methodological critiques (e.g. Fillmore *et al.* 2006) have not been persuasive that there is no beneficial effect, but that the effect may have been overestimated.	Significant beneficial effect in meta-analytic studies; effect seems to be confined to regular drinking without heavy drinking episodes.	Irregular heavy drinking episodes were detrimentally related to coronary heart disease (Puddey *et al.* 1999; Rehm *et al.* 2003b). A meta-analysis confirmed that the effect of volume is mediated by heavy drinking occasions (Bagnardi *et al.* 2008).	Sufficient evidence for some mechanisms (blood lipids, blood coagulation: Mukamal and Rimm 2001), and some evidence for others (e.g. inflammation: see Puddey *et al.* 1999; Rehm *et al.* 2003b).	No consistent interaction found; some beverages found to be more protective but this may only indicate that beverage preference is a marker for other protective factors (see also Rimm *et al.* 1996).

Aggregate-level studies

Mixed results: most analyses have found no effect or weak relationship (e.g. Hemström 2001 for EU countries). Leon *et al.* (1997) found a decrease in circulatory disease following a decrease in consumption during the Gorbachev reform, with a subsequent increase in this category when consumption increased again (see text, especially section 4.5). Rehm *et al.* (2004) showed that the relationship depended on patterns of drinking, with protective effects only in countries without high prevalence of heavy drinking occasions.

9% among males and 6% among females in Russia between 1995 and 1998, when total consumption dropped by an estimated 25% (Leon *et al.* 1997; Shkolnikov and Nemtsov 1997).

The small number of aggregate level studies show no significant effect beyond that expected from random variation (e.g. Hemström 2001). This result is consistent with the postulate that the effects of changes in the level of drinking in a population are spread through the whole population (Skog 1996), so that those whose hearts benefit from a rise in consumption are matched by those whose hearts are harmed by the rise. A multi-level analysis produced results consistent with individual level studies, i.e. beneficial effects for countries where drinking patterns are mainly regular (often with meals), and detrimental effects for countries with more irregular patterns and heavy drinking occasions (Rehm *et al.* 2004).

Overall, we conclude that there is good evidence for the cardioprotective effect of regular light and moderate alcohol consumption at the level of the individual drinker. This effect applies mainly to the age group of ≥45 years, where the overwhelming majority of CHD occurs (e.g. Lopez *et al.* 2006; for the relationship to alcohol by age, see Rehm and Sempos 1995a,b).

However, the public health implications of this conclusion are limited. Most aggregate-level studies suggest that there may be no net protective effect at the population level from an increase in the level of consumption, and little protective or even a detrimental effect in societies where drinking patterns are sporadic with heavy drinking occasions.

In considering the public health implications of the individual-level cardioprotective findings, attention must be paid to strategies that increase the number of light regular drinkers without significantly increasing the number of heavy drinkers. If a segment of the population could successfully be encouraged to have one drink every day or every second day, they would obtain most of the heart benefits (Criqui 1994, 1996; Di Castelnuove *et al.* 2006) without experiencing alcohol-related problems. But there is very little evidence for effective strategies to accomplish this goal (as discussed later in this book). If there is an increase in consumption in the light-drinking segment of the population, there tends to be an increase at the heavier-drinking segment as well. As noted above, this tendency is consistent with the finding of no significant effect in the aggregate-level CHD studies. Therefore, a safer strategy to maximize potential benefits would be to effect decreases in consumption to light–moderate levels among heavier drinkers in the population.

4.3.2 Breast cancer

As shown in Box 4.4, alcohol seems to have a small dose-dependent effect on breast cancer (e.g. Singletary and Gapstur 2001). There is a likely interaction with hormones, especially estrogen. With respect to drinking patterns, binge drinking may be related to higher risks, but the evidence is only suggestive. Some studies show differences among alcoholic beverages in the relationship to breast cancer, but beverage preference may be a marker for other factors. We conclude that there is a modest relationship of volume of drinking to breast cancer: the more alcohol is consumed on average, the higher the risk for breast cancer, with an increase in risk already demonstrated for one drink per day (Hamajima *et al.* 2002; Baan *et al.* 2007).

4.3.3 Tuberculosis

As early as 1785 the American physician Benjamin Rush listed tuberculosis (TB) and pneumonia as infectious sequelae of sustained heavy drinking (Rush 1785). Since then there have been numerous publications describing the associations between alcohol, alcohol use disorders (AUDs) and TB (e.g. Jacobson 1992; Szabo 1997a).

Box 4.4 Effects of alcohol on breast cancer and/or carcinoma in situ of breast (ICD-10: C50/D05)

Individual-level studies

Volume of alcohol	Moderate drinking	Patterns of drinking	Mechanisms	Interactions
All meta-analytic reviews after English *et al.* (1995) report significant detrimental effects (Smith-Warner *et al.* 1998; Corrao *et al.* 1999; Single *et al.* 1999; Gutjahr *et al.* 2001). In addition a pooled analysis of 53 individual-level studies with more than 50 000 cases found a clear dose–response relationship (Hamajima *et al.* 2002).	Significant detrimental effect in meta-analytic studies, even if tested not as a linear trend but categorically (Corrao *et al.* 1999; Hamajima *et al.* 2002). One drink per day on average was associated with increased risk (Hamajima *et al.* 2002).	Trend for binge drinking (Kohlmeier and Mendez 1997; Kinney *et al.* 2000).	Plausible hypotheses, not yet fully clarified (Baan *et al.* 2007). The International Agency for Research on Cancer found that there is sufficient evidence for a causal impact of alcohol on breast cancer (Baan *et al.* 2007).	Estrogen, estradiol (pre- vs post-menopausal women) in many studies (Ginsburg *et al.* 1996; Ginsburg 1999).

Aggregate-level studies

No studies available.

However, the causality of the relationship remained in doubt until new evidence from immunology research and better statistical methods to control for confounding allowed medical epidemiologists to settle this question. Overall, we can conclude that sufficient evidence exists in support of a role of alcohol in TB incidence (see Box 4.5; see also Parry *et al.* 2009). However, unlike breast cancer, the effect has only been observed for heavy drinking and for alcohol abuse or dependence. There is no evidence linking TB to light or moderate drinking.

In addition, alcohol consumption worsens the course of disease and is associated with less treatment success (e.g. Jakubowiak *et al.* 2007) by compromising the immune system and by reducing compliance in taking medication. Related to this, alcohol has been associated with the emergence of drug-resistant TB forms (Fleming *et al.* 2006).

4.3.4 Traffic injuries and deaths

Motor vehicle crashes are clearly linked to alcohol (Box 4.6). A dose–response relationship has been demonstrated with respect to level of consumption prior to

Box 4.5 Effects of alcohol on tuberculosis (TB; ICD-10: A15–A19, B90)

Individual-level studies

Volume of alcohol	Moderate drinking	Patterns of drinking	Mechanisms	Interactions
A meta-analysis on TB risk given alcohol abuse (as defined by ≥40 g alcohol per day, or by a clinical diagnosis of alcohol use disorder) yielded a pooled relative risk across all studies of >3 (Lönnroth et al. 2008).	Lönnroth et al. (2008) did not find an association between consumption of <40 g alcohol per day and risk of TB.	The effect of alcohol is for heavy drinking, and regularity of drinking as an additional factor, is not clarified yet.	Two plausible hypotheses: (1) effect of alcohol via the immune system (Szabo 1997a,b); (2) effect via social drift of alcoholics. A technical review concluded that there was a causal effect of alcohol on TB incidence (Parry et al. 2009).	Poverty, nutritional status and co-infections significantly mediate the effect of alcohol on TB.

Aggregate-level studies

No studies available

driving, with a threshold for negative consequences estimated at 40 mg% (.04%, Eckardt *et al.* 1998). Biological evidence supports this relationship. There is some indication of positive effects below this threshold for experienced drinkers, but the evidence is not extensive. There is a relationship between accidents and average volume, but it is not clear whether this relationship is independent of drinking patterns. At the population level, changes in the legal BAC limit have an effect on motor vehicle crash rates, especially single-vehicle night-time crashes associated with drink-driving (Mann *et al.* 2001). This strongly supports the findings from individual-level case–control studies of the important role of alcohol in motor vehicle accidents.

4.3.5 Suicide

The relationship between alcohol and suicide or attempted suicide is well established for heavy drinkers (Rossow 2000), both from individual and aggregate level studies (Box 4.7). The strength of the overall relationship seems to vary between cultures. Individual and aggregate level studies both suggest that more 'explosive'drinking patterns (e.g. irregular, heavy drinking occasions) are linked to a higher incidence of suicide.

Box 4.6 Effects of alcohol on injuries and deaths from motor vehicle crashes (ICD-10: V codes)

Individual-level studies

Volume of alcohol	Moderate drinking	Patterns of drinking	Mechanisms	Interactions
Volume of drinking is related to risk of traffic crashes (e.g. Midanik et al. 1996). It is not clear if this effect is independent of patterns of drinking (see Rehm and Gmel 2000b), e.g. if the relationship is only a reflection of the correlation between heavy drinking occasions and volume and between such occasions and crashes.	Threshold for negative effect of alcohol on subjective and psychomotor performance measures when blood alcohol concentrations (BAC) are ≥40 mg% (~0.4 g pure alcohol/kg). Subjective feelings of being 'intoxicated' occur as low as 0.25 g pure alcohol per kg or BACs from 10 to 30 mg% (Eckardt et al. 1998). There are indications of a J-shaped dose–response curve on subjective measures and psychomotor performance measures. The positive effects occur at very low levels of consumption, however.	As psychomotor performance is linked to acute intake of alcohol, there is a strong effect of patterns (e.g. Gruenewald et al. 1996; Eckardt et al. 1998; Rossow et al. 2001).	At the neuro-chemical level, ethanol affects the function of gamma-aminobutyric acid, glutamatergic, serotonergic, dopaminergic, cholinergic and opioid neuronal systems. Ethanol can affect these systems directly, and/or the interactions between and among these systems become important in the expression of ethanol's actions (Eckardt et al. 1998).	Some evidence for adaptation or learning, and that the adverse effect on performance is less in experienced drinkers (Cherpitel 1996; Rossow et al. 2001). Some evidence for differences between beverages, but beverages may just be proxies for other variables (e.g. Gruenewald and Ponicki 1995).

Aggregate-level studies

Fatal accident rates increase with increased per-capita consumption in many European countries (Skog 2001a). Numerous studies show that interventions such as reducing legal BAC limits are associated with reductions in traffic crashes (Mann et al. 2001).

Box 4.7 Effects of alcohol on suicide (ICD-10: X60–X84, Y870)

Individual-level studies

Volume of alcohol	Moderate drinking	Patterns of drinking	Theoretical underpinnings	Interactions
Some studies indicate a linear relationship between consumption level and risk of suicidal behaviour (e.g. Andréasson *et al.* 1988; Dawson 1997). Numerous studies show a significantly increased risk of suicide and attempted suicide among alcohol abusers and heavy drinkers (Rossow 2000; Rossow *et al.* 2001)	No protective effect of moderate drinking, but rather a slightly increased risk (e.g. Andréasson *et al.* 1988; Dawson 1997).	Some studies show increased risk of attempted suicide with increasing frequency of intoxication (Rossow and Wichstrøm 1994; Dawson 1997), and a stronger association with intoxication frequency than with consumption level (Dawson 1997).	Plausible hypotheses: social disintegration, social losses and mental illness suggested as intermediate factors (Skog 1991a; Murphy 2000).	Psychiatric comorbidity increases the risk of suicidal behaviour among alcohol abusers (Murphy 2000). The relationship also varies markedly according to cultural norms (see aggregate level studies).

Aggregate-level studies

Suicide rates are found to increase with increased per-capita consumption in a number of studies (Rossow 2000; Ramstedt 2001), yet the strength of the association varies considerably, tending to be higher in countries with an 'explosive'drinking pattern than in other countries, and remaining insignificant in some countries (Norström 1988; Gmel *et al.* 1998; Ramstedt 2001). The impact of drinking pattern is supported by cross-cultural comparisons of the aggregate-level associations; i.e. a stronger association occurs in drinking cultures where intoxication is a more prominent characteristic (Norström 1988, 1995; Ramstedt 2001).

4.3.6 Alcohol and all-cause mortality

All-cause mortality is one potential summary measure for combining different alcohol effects. Figure 4.1 shows the effects of alcohol on male adults aged <45 years (Rehm *et al.* 2001c). The relationship between average volume of alcohol consumed and all-cause mortality is almost linear in this age group, reflecting increased risk of death with increased level of alcohol consumption.

A slightly different pattern emerges for persons aged >45 years, however, where the beneficial effects of alcohol on mortality come into play. Figures 4.2 and 4.3 show the

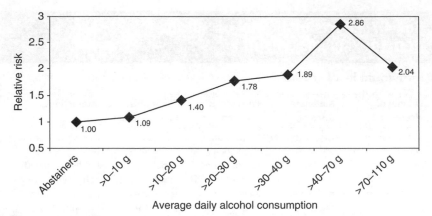

Fig. 4.1 Average daily alcohol consumption and risk of all-cause mortality (males aged <45 years).
Source: from Rehm *et al.* (2001a,c), with permission.

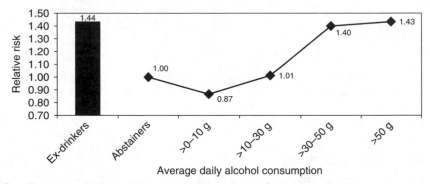

Fig. 4.2 Average daily alcohol consumption and risk of all-cause mortality (females aged ≥45 years).
Source: Rehm *et al.* (2001a,c), with permission.

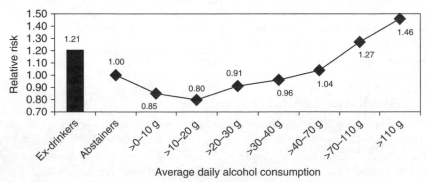

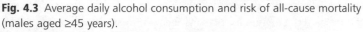

Fig. 4.3 Average daily alcohol consumption and risk of all-cause mortality (males aged ≥45 years).
Source: Rehm *et al.* (2001a,c), with permission.

relationship between average volume consumed and all-cause mortality for older age groups of men and women, respectively (Rehm *et al.* 2001c). For both genders, relationships are J-shaped, with the females experiencing deleterious effects at lower levels of alcohol consumption. These curves can be interpreted as reflecting the beneficial effects of moderate alcohol consumption on CHD (see Box 4.3) and ischaemic stroke, together with the detrimental effects of alcohol on many other chronic diseases.

Up to this point, we have considered only average volume. Based on recent research on drinking patterns and all-cause mortality, we can expect the beneficial effects of alcohol to be inversely related to the number and frequency of heavy drinking occasions (Rehm *et al.* 2001b). Sex, age, and different dimensions of alcohol consumption influence the effect of alcohol on all-cause mortality. In addition, the underlying mix of causes of death for all-cause mortality influences the exact shape of the risk curve (Rehm 2000; Rehm *et al.* 2001b).

4.3.7 **Alcohol and health consequences**

The results summarized thus far point to the following conclusions:

- Volume of drinking is linked to most disease outcomes through specific dose–response relationships. These relationships can be linear (as in the case of breast cancer or suicide), accelerating (as in the case of liver cirrhosis or motor vehicle accidents), or J-shaped (as in the case of heart disease or all-cause mortality). For some disease categories such as tuberculosis, there may be a threshold effect in that only heavy drinking or AUD seem to be associated with this disease.

- Patterns of drinking also play an important role in both the disease burden and the health benefits of drinking. Drinking patterns have been linked to CHD, motor vehicle accidents, and suicide, and are suspected to be linked to breast cancer.

- Moderate drinking has negative as well as positive health outcomes. Although it has some CHD benefits for some individuals, moderate drinking has also been linked to an increased risk of cancer and other disease conditions.

- Many disease conditions have interactions with other factors. These interactions make it difficult to estimate the contribution of alcohol to causation of disease.

- For some disease conditions, individual and population level analyses do not show consistent findings. This is the case for CHD, where individual level studies suggest a biologically plausible beneficial effect, whereas the limited evidence from population-level studies does not show this effect.

4.4 **Alcohol in the global burden of disease**

The preceding sections have described the relationship between alcohol consumption and some of the most important health conditions. However, alcohol affects morbidity and mortality through many other diseases as well. According to the Global Burden of Disease study sponsored by the World Health Organization and the World Bank

Box 4.8 Disability-adjusted life-years (DALYs)

The term 'DALYs' refers to a composite health summary measure used to estimate the burden of disease in a given country (Murray *et al.* 2000). It combines years of life lost to premature death with years of life lost due to disability. In this calculation, disability is indirectly calculated from morbidity, where time lived with disease is multiplied by a disease-specific weight. For example, major depression has a weight of 0.6, which means that an episode of depression in a single individual lasting 2 years would be counted as 1.2 DALYs (2×0.6). Disease-specific weights were derived from expert evaluations (for details see Murray and Lopez 1997) using standard methodologies (Drummond *et al.* 1997). When evaluating the results of the Global Burden of Disease study, one should keep in mind that these estimates have been based on conservative assumptions, and that infectious diseases are not included as categories impacted by alcohol.

(Murray and Lopez 1996; WHO 1999), in 1990 alcohol-related death and disability accounted for 3.5% of the total cost to life and longevity. More recent estimates (Rehm *et al.* 2009) indicate that during the last decade of the twentieth century alcohol's global health impact was 4.6%, as quantified in terms of **disability-adjusted life-years** (DALYs). This apparent increase is partly due to refinement of methods, but probably includes some real increase. Box 4.8 provides an explanation of this combined measure of death and disability.

Table 4.1 shows global alcohol-attributable DALYs for 2004 (Rehm *et al.* 2009). Alcohol-attributable DALYs are proportionally higher overall than either alcohol-attributable deaths or years of life lost because this summary measure includes years lived with a disability prior to death, and many alcohol-attributable diseases are not fatal. For DALYs, the burden of alcohol-attributable neuropsychiatric disorders now approximately equals that of all injury categories combined. DALYs for neuropsychiatric diseases are mainly due to AUD, and specifically to alcohol dependence.

Overall, neuropsychiatric diseases account for the largest portion of alcohol-attributable disease burden (36.4%) as measured in DALYs. A large part of this Figure is comprised of AUDs, particularly alcohol dependence and harmful use. Other neuropsychiatric disorders, such as depression, are often disabling but not lethal, and this is reflected in the markedly higher proportion of overall disease burden caused by this category, compared with alcohol-attributable mortality (34% of alcohol-attributable DALYs; 5.5% of alcohol-attributable deaths; see Rehm *et al.* 2006). The second largest category in alcohol-attributable disease burden is injuries (35.9%), with unintentional injuries by far outweighing intentional injuries. The next categories are about equal in size and each accounts for 9.5% of global disease burden: liver cirrhosis and cardiovascular diseases. Malignant neoplasms were responsible for 8.6% of global burden. Overall, the detrimental effects of alcohol on disease burden by far outweigh the beneficial effects.

As shown in Figure 4.4, males have far more alcohol-related disease burden than females (7.6% vs 1.4%, respectively), with a ratio of about 5.5:1. This ratio is much

Table 4.1 Global burden of disease (DALYs, in thousands) attributable to alcohol consumption by major disease categories in the world 2004[a]

Disease category	Men (M)[b]	Women (W)[b]	Total M + W	%M	%W	Total %M + %W
Maternal and perinatal conditions (low birth weight)	64	55	119	0.1	0.5	0.2
Cancer	4732	1536	6268	7.6	13.5	8.6
Diabetes mellitus	0	28	28	0	0.3	0.0
Neuropsychiatric disorders	23 265	3417	26 682	37.6	30.1	36.4
Cardiovascular diseases	5985	939	6924	9.7	8.3	9.5
Cirrhosis of the liver	5502	1443	6945	8.9	12.7	9.5
Unintentional injuries	15 694	2910	18 604	25.4	25.6	25.4
Intentional injuries	6639	1021	7660	10.7	9.0	10.5
Total alcohol-related burden 'caused' in DALYs	61 881	11 349	73 231	100.0	100.0	100.0
Diabetes mellitus	−238	−101	−340	22.2	8.1	14.6
Cardiovascular diseases	−837	−1145	−1981	77.8	91.9	85.4
Total alcohol-related burden 'prevented' in DALYs	−1075	−1246	−2321	100.0	100.0	100.0
All alcohol-related DALYs	60 806	10 104	70 910	100.0	100.0	100.0
All DALYs	799 536	730 631	1 530 168			
Percentage of all net DALYs attributable to alcohol	7.6%	1.4%	4.6%			
CRA 2000 (for comparison)	6.5%	1.3%	4.0%			

CRA, comparative risk assessment; DALYs, disability-adjusted life-years.

[a] See Rehm *et al.* 2009 for a description of the underlying study.

[b] Numbers are rounded to the nearest thousand. Zero indicates fewer than 500 alcohol-attributable DALYs in the disease category. Percentages refer to all DALYs either caused or prevented by alcohol.

larger in developing regions, as the vast majority of drinking is confined to males in most of these countries. Overall, there are also tremendous differences between regions, ranging from about 0.5% in the Eastern Mediterranean region to more than 11.6% in the European regions. Among the ten most populous countries, Russia shows the largest rate of alcohol-attributable burden (28.1%) for males, followed by Brazil (17.7%), China (12.9%) and Germany (12.8%). In general, poor populations and low-income countries have an even greater disease burden per unit of alcohol consumed than do high-income populations and countries.

Over the life course, 33.6% of the alcohol-related burden of disease occurs in the 15–29 year age group, followed by 31.3% for those aged 30–44 years and 22.0% for the

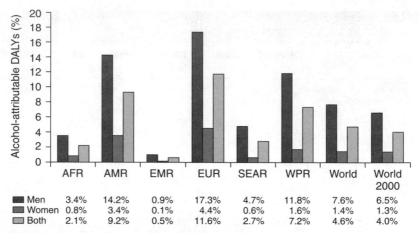

	AFR	AMR	EMR	EUR	SEAR	WPR	World	World 2000
■ Men	3.4%	14.2%	0.9%	17.3%	4.7%	11.8%	7.6%	6.5%
■ Women	0.8%	3.4%	0.1%	4.4%	0.6%	1.6%	1.4%	1.3%
□ Both	2.1%	9.2%	0.5%	11.6%	2.7%	7.2%	4.6%	4.0%

Fig. 4.4 Alcohol-attributable burden of disease in disability-adjusted life-years (DALYs) as a proportion of all DALYs by sex and WHO region.
AFR, African region; AMR, American region; EMR, eastern Mediterranean region; EUR, European region; SEAR, southeast Asian region; WPR, western Pacific region. Redrawn from Rehm *et al.* (2009), with permission.

45–59 year age group (Rehm *et al.* 2009). Although the effect of alcohol is most pronounced in early and middle adulthood, all phases of life are affected, from newborn babies (0.3%) to the elderly (3.7% of those aged ≥70 years).

Compared with traditional health risk factors such as tobacco, high cholesterol, and hypertension, in 2000 alcohol accounted for approximately the same amount of global burden of disease as tobacco (Ezzati *et al.* 2004). In developed countries, alcohol ranked as the third most detrimental risk factor whereas in emerging economies like China alcohol ranked first among the 26 examined.

4.5 Alcohol consumption and social harm

Although public discussion has often concentrated on alcohol-related problems connected with disease and other medical conditions, alcohol is also linked to consequences in the social realm, which have been called 'the forgotten dimension' (Klingemann and Gmel 2001). Box 4.9 describes the areas included within this dimension. It is worth noting that in contrast to the majority of the health-related impacts of alcohol, many of the social harms are borne by someone other than the drinker. Systematic examination of the significance of harms due to other people's drinking have yet to be undertaken, but clearly alcohol consumption has external consequences through alcohol-related crime (e.g. violence, domestic violence, property damage), family dysfunction, traffic accidents, problems in the workplace, and through the overall cost of alcohol-related harm to society.

The conceptual diversity of these social consequences makes it difficult to evaluate this field systematically. As suggested above, there is no common metric that would

Box 4.9 Categories of alcohol-related social harm

Violence[a]

Vandalism

Public disorder

Family problems: divorce/marital problems, child abuse

Other interpersonal problems

Financial problems

Work-related problems other than work accidents[b]

Educational difficulties

Social costs

[a] Injuries from violence are also part of accidents and injuries in the morbidity and mortality section.

[b] Work-related accidents are part of accidents and injuries in the morbidity and mortality section.

allow comparisons between social and medical outcomes, or even within social outcomes alone. Social cost studies have been suggested as such a metric, but these have often excluded social problems—for instance, family problems—for lack of data (Single *et al.* 1998). The overall Figures from the cost studies also depend heavily on indirect costs such as productivity losses, which are difficult to estimate (Gutjahr and Gmel 2001a,b).

A second possibility is to work from employment records, social welfare data, and law-court reports. Here, an attribution of the problem to drinking is often made by a third party, such as a social worker, police officer, or employer. But alcohol attributions in such records are usually not kept or not available. The main social records system that still routinely provides some data on social problems related to alcohol is police arrests and other criminal justice actions (Aarens *et al.* 1977). In the police records system, the crime may be alcohol specific, or there may be an attribution of it to drinking by the arresting officer, although this is often under-attributed. Victimization surveys supply an alternative method of estimating alcohol-related crimes, but these methods too raise questions about the validity of respondents' attributions.

Boxes 4.10–4.13 give some insight into the evidence for selected social consequences. Except for violence, the epidemiological evidence on the extent of alcohol's role in social problems is quite weak.

4.5.1 Violence

Individual as well as population-level studies (Box 4.10) indicate a causal relationship between alcohol consumption and violence (Room and Rossow 2001). The strength of the relationship seems to be culturally dependent. Patterns of drinking, especially drinking to intoxication, seem to play an important role in causing violence. Violence against intimate partners is strongly associated with the amount of alcohol consumed (Foran and O'Leary 2008).

Box 4.10 Effects of alcohol on violence

Individual-level studies

Volume of alcohol	Moderate drinking	Patterns of drinking	Theoretical underpinnings	Interactions
A number of studies indicate a linear relationship between consumption level and risk of involvement in violent incidents (Dawson 1997; Rossow 2000; Wells et al. 2000). A large number of studies have demonstrated a significantly increased risk of involvement in violence among alcohol abusers/ heavy drinkers (Pernanen 1991; Rossow et al. 2001). Several studies have also shown that heavy drinkers are more likely to be the victims of violence (Room and Rossow 2001; Rossow et al. 2001).	Survey studies indicate no protective effect of moderate drinking, but rather a slightly increased risk (Dawson 1997; Rossow 2000; Wells et al. 2000). However, experimental research suggests that alcohol does not have a reliable effect on aggression at very low blood alcohol concentrations (Graham et al. 1998).	Studies have demonstrated increased risk of violent events with increasing frequency of intoxication (Dawson 1997; Rossow et al. 1999; Wells et al. 2000), and an apparently stronger association with intoxication frequency than with consumption level (Dawson 1997; Wells et al. 2000).	Several underlying mechanisms are probable (see Pernanen 1991; Galanter 1997; Graham et al. 1998, 2000; Gustafson 1993).	A number of individual and environmental characteristics moderate the relationship between alcohol and violence (Gustafson 1993; Graham et al. 1996, 1998; Pernanen 1996).

Aggregate-level studies

Rates of reported (non-fatal) violence have been found to increase with increased per-capita consumption in a few studies (Skog and Bjørk 1988; Lenke 1990; Norström 1993, 1998), and homicide rates have also been found to increase with increased per-capita consumption. Again, the strength of the association varies, and tends to be higher in countries with 'explosive' drinking patterns than in other countries (Lenke 1990; Norström 1998; Parker and Cartmill 1998; Rossow 2001). The impact of drinking pattern is supported by cross-cultural comparisons of the aggregate-level magnitude of the association; i.e. a stronger association occurs in drinking cultures where intoxication is a more prominent characteristic (Lenke 1990; Rossow 2001).

4.5.2 Divorce and marital problems

The epidemiological evidence for any causal relationship between alcohol consumption and marital problems such as divorce is weak (Box 4.11). In many countries, a partner's heavy drinking was a common legal justification for divorce, when such justifications were needed, and subjective attributions are common (Rehm *et al.* 1999). The proposition that alcohol consumption is a cause of divorce lacks any evidence, either for or against, from well-controlled epidemiological studies.

4.5.3 Child abuse

The systematic empirical evidence for any causal relationship between alcohol consumption and child abuse is weak (Box 4.12; Rossow 2000). Only the effect of heavy drinking or abuse/dependence seems to be substantiated.

4.5.4 Work-related problems (other than work accidents)

Clearly, there is an association between alcohol consumption and different outcome variables at the workplace (Box 4.13). However, the direction and nature of causality are often unclear. Most findings suggest rather complex interactions with both individual characteristics and environmental factors, including work characteristics (Rehm and Rossow 2001). No protective effect of alcohol has been found at any level.

4.5.5 Alcohol and social problems: the overall findings

The situation with respect to social consequences of alcohol can be summarized as follows. Clearly, alcohol is related to many negative social outcomes. This is evidenced by the correlation between different alcohol variables (especially alcohol abuse/dependence) and different social outcomes. However, causal relationships to alcohol are not established for many of these outcomes. In many instances, weak research designs have been used, and longitudinal and experimental studies are scarce. The situation is complicated by the fact that alcohol seems to be part of a complex causal web (e.g. Murray and Lopez 1999; Rehm 2000) where its effects depend on or are modified by a multitude of other factors on different levels.

4.6 Problem rates in relation to changes in alcohol consumption: the Russian experience

Changes in mortality rates in Russia during the latter part of the twentieth century provide a striking example of how alcohol-related problems, especially CHD and violence, can affect mortality rates when there are significant changes in the volume of alcohol consumed in a society. The Russian experience is instructive for three reasons: (1) it shows how the pattern and amount of alcohol consumption can contribute to an epidemic of rising mortality in one of the largest countries in the world; (2) it demonstrates how advances in alcohol epidemiology can be used to explain these trends; and (3) it provides a case study of the political and economic forces that limit the effectiveness of alcohol policies in countries were popular support is lacking.

Box 4.11 Effects of alcohol on divorce and marital problems

Individual-level studies

Volume of alcohol	Moderate drinking	Patterns of drinking	Theoretical underpinnings	Interactions
A large number of cross-sectional studies have demonstrated a significant positive association between heavy drinking and divorce, but only a few well-designed studies have demonstrated a significantly increased risk of separation or divorce among married alcohol abusers/heavy drinkers compared with others (Leonard and Rothbard 1999). No studies of a dose–response relationship between volume of consumption and divorce risk was found. Fu and Goldman (2000) found no significant association between alcohol consumption and risk of divorce. A few longitudinal studies on alcohol consumption and marital aggression (see Quigley and Leonard 1999) have shown that husbands' heavy drinking is predictive of marital violence.	No systematic study on this relationship was found.	The impact of alcohol consumption on marital relation and divorce has been related to aspects of heavy drinking/alcohol abuse, but not to drinking patterns beyond that.	No systematic theory.	Effects probably mediated by marital satisfaction (marital functioning, marital aggression, etc.: Leonard 1990).

Aggregate-level studies

Divorce rates are found to increase with increased per-capita consumption in one study (Cases et al. 1999), and rates of domestic violence (mostly partner violence) are also found to increase with increased per-capita consumption (Norström 1993).

Box 4.12 Effects of alcohol on child abuse

Individual-level studies

Volume of alcohol	Moderate drinking	Patterns of drinking	Theoretical underpinnings	Interactions
A large number of studies have reported a variety of childhood adversities to be more prevalent among children of heavy drinkers than others, although many of these studies have been criticized for inadequate methodology (Barber and Gilbertson 1999; Rossow 2000). A few recent reports from well-designed studies have shown a higher risk of indicators of child abuse in families with heavy drinking caretakers (see Rossow 2000 for a review). There is little research to suggest any specific relationship between drinking level and risk of child abuse.	No systematic study on this relationship was found.	The impact of alcohol consumption on child abuse has been related to aspects of heavy drinking/alcohol abuse, but not to drinking patterns beyond that.	No systematic theory.	May probably interact with family resources and functioning (Windle 1996).

Aggregate-level studies

Norström (1993) analysed the association between per-capita consumption and physical abuse of children in a time-series analysis of Swedish data, and found a weak and positive but not statistically significant association.

Beginning in the 1960s, mortality rates in Russia and other parts of eastern Europe began to increase, while in Western Europe they were gradually declining. Then, in the period from 1985 to 1988, mortality in Russia and other parts of the Soviet Union took a sudden sharp turn for the better. The trend then reversed, and in the period from 1990 to 1994 mortality increased dramatically, to an extent never seen before in peacetime in industrialized societies. After 1995, the rates declined somewhat, returning by 1998 to approximately the level of 1984 (Shkolnikov *et al.* 2001). There was a new rise after 1998, reaching a peak in 2002–2004 close to the earlier peak in 1994 (Zaridze *et al.* 2009).

Box 4.13 Effects of alcohol on work-related problems other than work accidents

Individual-level studies

Volume of alcohol (the following effects have not always been clearly linked to volume, but to alcohol in general; see Rehm and Rossow 2001)	Moderate drinking	Patterns of drinking	Theoretical underpinnings	Interactions
◆ Absenteeism (including tardiness and leaving work early) due to illness, or disciplinary suspension, resulting in loss of productivity. ◆ Turnover due to premature death, disciplinary problems or low productivity from the use of alcohol. ◆ Inappropriate behaviour (such as behaviour resulting in disciplinary procedures). ◆ Theft and other crime. ◆ Poor co-worker relations and low company morale.	There is some indication that some negative effects are also related to moderate drinking (Mangione *et al.* 1999).	Intoxication and heavy drinking occasions are related to work problems even after control of volume (Rehm and Rossow 2001). Alcohol abuse and dependence have been linked to many work problems (Rehm and Rossow 2001).	Diverse, often weak, theoretical underpinnings. Often 'eclectic' theories like Ames and Janes (1992).	Many factors have been found to be interacting with alcohol in producing work problems. These can be broadly classified in the following headings: individual factors, environmental factors, and work-related factors (Rehm and Rossow 2001). Most of the effect of alcohol on work problems seems to be mediated by other variables.

Aggregate-level studies

No studies found.

The improving trend in mortality in the 1980s corresponds to the period of the anti-alcohol campaign of the Gorbachev era. The declining trend after that corresponds to the dissolution of the Soviet Union, and the state's subsequent loss of control of the alcohol market. Shkolnikov *et al.* (2001) attribute the rebound in the late 1990s to a reduction in drinking compared to the early 1990s. While many other changes were occurring in the period after 1990, recent analyses support the position that alcohol plays a primary role in the mortality crisis of the 1990s and early 2000s in Russia and neighbouring countries (Ramstedt 2009; Zaridze *et al.* 2009). Not only does alcohol account for most of the large fluctuations in Russian mortality, in recent years alcohol was a cause of more than half of all Russian deaths between ages 15 and 54 years (Zaridze *et al.* 2009).

Focusing on the effects of the anti-alcohol campaign in the 1980s, the changes in this period were remarkable (Table 4.2). Between 1984 and 1987, age-standardized death rates fell among males by 12% and among females by 7% (Leon *et al.* 1997). The causes of death accounting for these changes were quite specific. Deaths among males from alcohol-specific causes were most affected (Leon *et al.* 1997): they fell by 56%. Deaths from accidents and violence fell by 36%. Deaths from pneumonia (40%), other respiratory diseases (20%), and infectious diseases (25%) also fell. And deaths from circulatory diseases, which accounted for more than half of all deaths, fell among males by 9%. The trends were similar among females, but the changes were less marked. Cancer deaths did not follow the general trend; they actually rose slightly.

Estimates of the actual alcohol consumption (Shkolnikov and Nemtsov 1997) show total ethanol consumption, combining legal and illegal sources, to have declined from 14.2 litres per capita in 1984 to 10.7 litres per capita in 1987—much less than the decline in officially recorded sales, but still a decline of about 25%.

The experience of the Soviet Union in the latter half of the 1980s suggests that a substantial cut in the alcohol supply can produce beneficial effects on the population's health. For each litre of ethanol by which per-capita consumption fell in Russia, the age-standardized mortality fell by 2.7%. Thus, given appropriate circumstances, alcohol can have a much greater net impact on a population's health than findings from previous studies have suggested. The figure is considerably higher than the

Table 4.2 Age-standardized mortality rates per million for Russia by gender, comparing 1987–1984 and 1994–1987 (standardized to European population)[a]

Cause of death	1984 (rate/million)		Ratio, 1987/1984 rates		Ratio, 1994/1987 rates	
	Male	Female	Male	Female	Male	Female
All causes	21 293	11 606	0.88	0.93	1.37	1.2
Accidents and violence	2519	597	0.64	0.76	2.26	1.91
Alcohol-specific causes	455	123	0.44	0.48	4.29	3.9
Pneumonia	279	118	0.6	0.68	2.29	1.26
Other respiratory diseases	1531	523	0.8	0.78	1.16	0.94
Infectious and parasitic diseases	308	88	0.75	0.77	1.6	1.15
Circulatory diseases	11 798	8037	0.91	0.94	1.29	1.17
All neoplasms	5252	1488	1.04	1.03	1.04	1.05

[a] Source: recalculated from Leon *et al.* (1997).

estimated Western European experience showing a 1.3% net decrease in mortality from a one-litre fall in per-capita consumption (Her and Rehm 1998; see also Norström 1996). This discrepancy illustrates that the effects of a given volume of alcohol on health and disease can vary from one society to another. Among the factors that can have a major effect on this relationship are the dominant patterns of drinking in a society. In Russia and in a number of other newly independent states, there is a long-standing tradition of repeated heavy binge drinking, particularly among males. This pattern of drinking seems to be strongly implicated in the finding that a litre of ethanol has about twice as much effect on mortality in Russia as it does in Western Europe.

The second major lesson from this experience pertains to the relation between drinking and heart disease. The lesson is that the drinking pattern matters. Thus, deaths from heart disease actually declined in Russia during the anti-alcohol campaign of the 1980s, before rising rapidly again in the early 1990s (Ramstedt 2009). The medical epidemiological literature was so committed to the idea that alcohol had predominantly protective effects for the heart that at first this finding was interpreted as showing that alcohol could not be playing a role in the improvement in Soviet mortality in the late 1980s and the deterioration in the early 1990s. It has taken some time to come to a realization that, in cultural contexts like the former Soviet Union, alcohol is detrimental rather than beneficial for the mature heart.

4.7 Comparing health and social harm from drinking

Although at present there is no adequate comparative measure of the relative magnitude of social and health problems attributable to drinking, some comparisons can be made that are relevant to the issue, primarily in terms of estimates of the relative burden of alcohol problems in social and health services. Such estimates do not take into account private costs and problems, such as disruption of family life or work roles, except as they come to the attention of public agencies.

Cost-of-illness studies of the economic costs attributable to alcohol include estimates of the 'direct costs' of health and social services used by those with alcohol-related problems. Typically, the ongoing cost to the society for handling these cases is estimated to be larger in the social welfare and criminal justice sectors than in the health sector. For instance, a study of Scotland (CATALYST 2001) estimated alcohol-attributable health care costs of 95.6 million pounds, social work service costs of £85.9 million, and criminal justice and fire services costs of £267.9 million.

In a mixed urban, suburban and rural county in northern California, those reporting 'problem drinking' (defined in terms of having heavy drinking occasions, serious social consequence of drinking, or dependence symptoms) who came for services to one or another system were distributed as follows: 41.0% were seen by the criminal justice system, 8.0% by the social welfare system, 42.1% by the general health system (primary health clinics and emergency rooms), 3.1% by the public mental health system, and 5.9% by public alcohol or drug treatment agencies (Weisner 2001). It seems that in California the resources devoted to social problems related to drinking are at least as extensive as those devoted to health problems related to drinking.

A third way of estimating the relative burden of health and social harm is from survey research, where the attribution is by the drinker or those around the drinker.

A telephone survey, for instance, found that 7.2% of Canadians reported that they had been pushed, hit, or assaulted by someone who had been drinking, 6.2% had had friendships break up as a result of someone else's drinking, and 7.7% reported that they had had family problems or marriage difficulties due to someone else's drinking, all within the previous 12 months. In the same study, 2.3% reported that their own drinking had had a harmful effect on their home life or marriage in the past year, 3.7% said that it had harmed their friendships or social life, and 5.5% reported that it had harmed their physical health (recalculated from pp. 258, 274 of Eliany *et al.* 1992). Although questions have been raised about the accuracy of these kinds of survey data, particularly in terms of what respondents mean by 'health' problems (Greenfield 1995; Bondy and Lange 2000), a consistent finding from survey studies is that social problems due to someone's drinking extend more broadly in the population than health problems due to drinking.

4.8 Do the heaviest drinkers account for most of the harms—the 'prevention paradox'?

Although the heaviest drinkers have a much higher risk of various alcohol-related harms compared with other drinkers, it is not necessarily the heaviest drinkers who account for most of the alcohol burden. Particularly with respect to acute alcohol-related harms it is often found that most of the harms are not attributable to the heaviest drinkers, who constitute a distinct minority, but rather to the remaining majority of light or moderate drinkers (Jones *et al.* 1995; Leifman 1996; Stockwell *et al.* 1996; Skog 1999; Gmel *et al.* 2001; Rossow and Romelsjö 2006). For instance, Jones *et al.* (1995) found that the lower 90% of drinkers by volume accounted for 59% of alcohol-related work absenteeism. Poikolainen *et al.* (2007) reported that 70% of all self-reported problems, 70% of alcohol-related hospitalizations, 64% of all alcohol-related deaths, and 64% of the premature life-years lost before age 65 occurred among the lower 90% of Finnish men classifield by their drinking volume. Similarly, Rossow and Romelsjö (2006) found that the majority of acute alcohol problems occurred among the majority of drinkers with low or moderate risk (i.e. the lower 90%) by drinking volume. Drinkers who occasionally drink heavily but whose overall volume of drinking is low or moderate play a large part in these findings. On this basis it is often argued that prevention measures should be directed toward all drinkers (population strategies) rather than at the small group of very heavy drinkers (high-risk strategies). This is often referred to as the prevention paradox (Kreitman 1986; Rose 2001).

4.9 Conclusion

Alcohol accounts for a significant disease burden worldwide and is related to many negative social consequences. Although direct causality is not established unequivocally for some of these consequences on the social side, the conclusions for alcohol policy are the same, whether alcohol is the causal factor for a consequence, a causal factor among many others, or a factor mediating the influence of another causal factor. In all cases alcohol contributes to social burden, and public policy must strive to reduce this burden. While there may be some offsetting psychological benefits from drinking (Peele and Brodsky 2000), the best way to minimize the social harm from drinking is to lower the consumption.

Conclusions are more complicated for the health side. There is the beneficial effect on CHD at the individual level, with plausible biological pathways and some experimental evidence. This becomes an issue in public health policymaking, although the implications at the population level are debatable. The CHD protective effect also has to be balanced in policymaking against the detrimental consequences, even at low levels of drinking (e.g. the effects of alcohol on breast cancer and the risk of developing alcohol abuse or dependence).

Overall, the conclusion must be that the level of alcohol consumption matters for the health and social well-being of a population as a whole. In addition to this, the predominant pattern of drinking in a population can have a major influence on the extent of damage from extra alcohol consumption. Patterns that seem to add most to the damage are drinking to intoxication and recurrent binge drinking. In sum, the overall conclusion for alcohol policy is that alcohol contributes to both social and health burden, and that public policy must strive to reduce this burden.

Alcohol is a risk factor for a wide range of health conditions and social problems. It accounts for approximately 4% of deaths worldwide and 4.6% of the global burden of disease, placing it alongside tobacco as one of the leading preventable causes of death and disability.

Chapter 5

Global structure and strategies of the alcohol industry

5.1 Introduction

The context of decision-making about policies to reduce alcohol-related harm includes the role, strategies and influence of the alcohol industry. With the growth of modern industrial production, the proliferation of new product designs and the development of sophisticated marketing techniques, the alcohol industry represents an important if understudied part of the environment in which drinking patterns are learned and practised. For these reasons it is instructive to consider not only the global structure of the alcohol industry, but also its role in the promotion of alcohol consumption.

At the national level, the industry comprises large and small beer, wine or spirits producers or importers, as well as bars, restaurants and bottle stores and often food stores which sell alcohol to the public. These players, large and small, have diverging interests as well as interests in common in regard to policy frameworks. This chapter sets the scene for several later chapters by examining in particular the recent consolidation and globalization of alcohol production, distribution, and marketing in the hands of large alcohol corporations that increasingly dominate national, regional and global markets. The role of the alcohol industry in the policymaking process will be taken up in Chapter 15.

As the changes triggered by globalization have shifted western economies from a manufacturing base to greater reliance on the service sector, economic and social analysts have begun to describe society as a set of consumer markets, rather than as systems of production (Hayward and Hobbs 2007). The public health sector, responsible for treatment services and health promotion, tends also to focus on consumers' drinking patterns and resulting harms. From these perspectives, alcohol consumption and alcohol problems are seen as 'demand-driven', the result of good or poor decisions by individual drinkers. This focuses policy and action on reducing harm to young or vulnerable drinkers, and on how responsible management of drinking contexts can shape drinkers' behaviour in high-risk situations. Recently, however, the role of the industry that produces the alcohol has been attracting greater attention (see for example Grieshaber-Otto *et al.* 2000; Holder 2000; Jernigan 2000a, 2009; Anderson and Baumberg 2006b; Room 2006b; Anderson *et al.* 2009c; Babor 2009; Zeigler 2009). The producers and distributors of alcohol play important roles in sustaining consumption levels and consequent problems, not only through their obvious role in supply and marketing but also as political actors seeking to sustain and increase alcohol sales.

From a production perspective, the alcohol market is very far from the neoclassical ideal in which many players compete to respond to consumer preferences. A characteristic of the recent wave of globalizing industries is that they are 'marketing-driven'

(Klein 2000; Room *et al.* 2002). The alcohol market is now dominated by corporations whose huge expenditure on highly sophisticated marketing creates preferences and drives growth in emerging markets around the world, as well as maintaining sales in their countries of origin. They promote and sell a high-risk product which contributes directly and indirectly to disease, injury and social problems, as described in Chapters 3 and 4. Majnoui d'Intignano has described alcohol-related harm, like that of tobacco, as an 'industrial epidemic'—an epidemic caused not by a natural agent or force but by a commercial product. This epidemic is driven at least in part by the producer corporations and their allies in the retail, advertising and media industries (Jahiel and Babor 2007; Majnoni d'Intignano 1998).

In this chapter, our primary focus is on multinational corporations and global markets for alcohol, since this is the most rapidly expanding sector of the alcohol industry and the most politically powerful. However, more than half of the world's alcohol supply still falls outside the scope of the multinational producers, in the hands of 'informal' home producers, often of traditional beverages, and local producers of industrialized traditional beverages and 'international'-style beverages. Those sectors are also briefly discussed below, emphasizing relationships and common interests in the sale of alcohol as the alcohol industry consolidates on a global basis.

5.2 Unrecorded alcohol supply

Informal production is part of what is often referred to as 'unrecorded' consumption—that is, unrecorded by customs or tax officials as paying tariffs or taxes. This is alcohol from quite different sources. 'Informal' production includes home-made fermented or distilled beverages and small-scale village production of beverages traditional to a region, such as *chibuku* in southern Africa, *soju* in South Korea and *pulque* in Mexico. Unrecorded consumption also includes alcohol smuggled across borders and alcohol produced illegally within a country in order to avoid tariffs and taxes. Unrecorded alcohol is a relatively small proportion of total consumption in developed alcohol markets with large-scale commercial production and marketing, but in less developed markets it is estimated to be high.

There may be health risks associated with home brews and illegal production of spirits, although these are often overestimated (Lachenmeier and Rehm 2009). There may be health benefits in using regulation of production and tax policies to encourage drinkers to shift to a lower strength beverage type. Fermented beverages produced informally often are less strong than industrially produced products. The primary concerns for governments, however, are the loss of tax revenue and the low price of unrecorded alcohol that may contribute to heavy drinking. Smuggling (and some cross-border shopping situations) may undermine price and availability policies. Low prices and ready availability of informal or illegal alcohol are also of concern to tax-paying commercial producers and importers as it undercuts their products in the market.

In many countries, policy attention is being given to bringing informal production and types of illegal supply under systems of taxation and regulation. Global companies moving into emerging markets are in favour of such policy moves, which may suppress potential market competitors. They emphasize the quality of their production methods, offer technical advice, and support the regulation and taxation of alcohol from all sources (International Center for Alcohol Policy 2008). Some global companies have also moved into direct competition with informal beverage producers by marketing industrialized forms of traditional beverages. For example, SABMiller played a role in bringing village production and sale of traditional 'cloudy' beer made from sorghum under South Africa's licensing system (Parry 1998), and now makes sorghum beer as well as lager on an industrial scale. The Japanese alcohol giants Kirin and Asahi also produce and market potato-and-rice spirits **shochu** and other regional specialities alongside their international and imported beers and spirits.

5.3 **Alcohol retailers**

Alcohol is seen as an important contributor to business opportunities and jobs in the hospitality and retail sectors. In both high- and low-income countries, alcohol sales are a source of profit for the travel and tourism industries. Nightlife, specifically drinking in clubs, pubs, and bars, is playing an increasingly important economic role in many cities and towns. For example, a market research report on New York nightlife concluded that 'the nightlife industry generated an estimated $9.7 billion in economic activity, $2.6 billion in earnings (primarily wages) and 95,500 jobs in New York City' and 'contributed an estimated $391 million in tax revenues to New York City and an additional $321 million to New York State' (Audience Research and Analysis 2004). The impact on smaller communities may be relatively more important than that recorded for New York City, especially when entertainment districts serve to revitalize previously rundown city neighbourhoods. Hobbs *et al.* (2003) noted the key role of the night-time economy in revitalization of cities in the UK, reinforced by the conversion of inner city areas into residential neighbourhoods.

Although in many entertainment districts problems related to the number, density and size of nightclubs are recognized, local economic benefits from these establishments are often perceived as outweighing the costs. This may result in reluctance to impose and enforce effective regulations, and city governments' interests in stimulating a successful and vibrant night-time economy may run counter to the efforts of local communities to reduce harm by limiting or regulating alcohol outlets (Greater London Authority 2002; Hobbs *et al.* 2003; Roberts 2004; Hayward and Hobbs 2007).

Most alcohol laws regulate the retail sellers of alcohol to the public, with some measures related to the consumers themselves, such as minimum purchasing age and drink-driving laws. In many mature alcohol markets, the bars and retail outlets that sell alcohol to the public for drinking on or off the premises are regulated through licensing systems to control supply, ensure responsible management and reduce harm, most typically as a means of ensuring compliance with laws against selling to underage or intoxicated drinkers. Owners of bars and retail outlets are part of their local community and can be monitored at the local level (Ayres and Braithwaite 1992; Hauritz *et al.* 1998a). The hospitality industry profits from the sale of food, coffee and entertainment as well as alcoholic drinks and has an interest in managing intoxicated patrons on the premises. This offers opportunities to reduce local harms associated with drinking venues, as discussed in Chapters 9 and 10.

Retail outlets for take-away alcohol may be similarly licensed but the drinking and the risk occurs elsewhere, and prices are typically much lower than at drinking venues. In some countries, supermarket chains are now major retailers for beer and wine. They have begun advertising these products as cut-price 'loss leaders' to attract customers to shop with them. In Australia, the bulk-buying power of the two big supermarket chains means that 'specials' can cost less than the wholesale price to other alcohol retailers (Television New Zealand 2008).

Other retail outlets and bars advertise price specials and venue events, but overall retailers rely on their suppliers, the major producers, to promote the alcohol brands they sell. Retailers' interests are also linked to those of the major alcohol producers by supply agreements, financial loans or sometimes ownership.

In the UK, breweries were required by the national Monopolies Commission to relinquish ownership of pubs, most of which are now in the hands of large pub-owning companies ('pubcos') whose supply contracts based on price are mainly with the major breweries. By 2002 the top 10 pub operators owned close to 50% of all pubs, resulting in fewer opportunities for independent operators and similar establishments, normalizing a certain style of drinking at the expense of local diversity. Local concerns about economic benefits may advantage pub chains because these larger corporations are presumed to be safer investments (Chatterton and Hollands 2002; Davies and Mummery 2006).

In New Zealand, the breweries themselves chose to shift out of pub ownership when regulation of liquor licensing and broadcasting was liberalized. They then moved into owning or franchising liquor store chains, supported by brand advertising on television.

The complex relationships between producers, wholesalers and the retail level mean that the hospitality and alcohol retail industries have their own distinct perspectives on some regulatory issues but align with alcohol producers on others.

Not all alcohol is sold by private businesses. In sixteen countries around the world, including a number of US states, most Canadian jurisdictions, the Nordic countries and several Indian states, a large share of the distribution of alcohol is controlled through state monopoly ownership of retail outlets for take-away alcohol (Kortteinen 1989; WHO 2004b). This has been challenged under trade agreements as an inappropriate activity for government (see Chapter 6), although the status of the surviving monopolies is stable as of 2009. Government monopoly or partial monopoly of the retail market in alcohol often serves interests other than public health, including revenue generation and collection, protectionist interests and employment. But a public health interest has also been served, even when not stated explicitly, in that the number of outlets is kept down. In southern Africa, for example, municipally owned beer halls have been the main retail outlet for some alcoholic beverages. Privatization of municipally owned beer halls in Zimbabwe resulted very quickly in an increase in the number of outlets (Jernigan 1999). Government monopoly over an aspect of alcohol production or distribution also removes or mutes an important source of advocacy for greater alcohol availability.

5.4 **Alcohol producers**

In developed economies, the trend has been away from state controls over production levels and distribution. In Russia, the Commonwealth of Independent States, Estonia, and, most recently, Sweden, privatization of state alcohol production has provided opportunities for local and global companies. But in a few growing economies alcohol, particularly beer, is produced by state-owned enterprises or joint ventures, as in China. Large-scale industrial production, whether by the state or global corporations, has some advantages in terms of alcohol tax collection and safety of manufacture. In privatizing state production, Estonia licensed producers. One reason for retaining some state control over production was demonstrated in 2001 when 68 Estonians died from consuming illicitly produced spirits that contained methanol (Paasma *et al.* 2007).

Producers are the main advertisers of alcoholic beverages, yet governments that restrict alcohol advertising do so by laws regulating the media in which the advertising appears, rather than the producers directly. The major producers promote alcohol brands through advertisements, sponsorships, and direct marketing, including point of sale displays provided to retailers. It is the major alcohol corporations who drive market consumption through brand advertising and other promotions.

Most global alcohol-producing corporations are public companies answerable to shareholders, with a very different set of national and international interests from those of public health decision-makers. The size and profitability of these companies both arises from and drives global expansion to new markets that can ensure future growth. Industry consolidation nationally and internationally gives these large companies an increased capacity to influence policy (see Chapter 15) and a greatly increased capacity to promote alcohol brands and a drinking lifestyle.

5.5 **Global consolidation of alcohol ownership**

The global alcohol market is now dominated by a handful of large corporations. This consolidation has implications for public health because the resulting economies of scale and profit growth provide these companies with unprecedented resources for buying into new markets, for promoting alcohol brands and for influencing policy.

Most of the global companies trace their origins back a century or two to small local breweries or distilleries, and make much of this history in brand imagery. These companies grew through mergers or acquisitions in the 1960s and 1970s, began to operate internationally and consolidate regionally in the 1980s, then went global in the 1990s. One of the largest, SABMiller, reports that since 2000 the top 20 brewers have been involved in more than 280 mergers and acquisitions with a total transaction value of more than US $80 billion (SABMiller 2007).

A review of annual reports, company policies, media releases and websites of 24 large alcohol corporations showed a rapid consolidation of holdings since 2000, as part of rapid expansion into emerging markets around the world (Hill 2008). The major mergers are summarized below.

In 2003 the ten top distilling companies were producing 306 million 9-litre cases of spirits. By 2006 world production was dominated by just two companies, Diageo and

Table 5.1 Global beer manufacturers

Corporation (country of registration)	2006 revenues (US $ million)[a]	Ownership changes 2006 to mid-2008
1 SABMiller (South Africa)	15,744.0	
2 Inbev (Belgium)	15,448.6	
3 Heineken (Netherlands).	14,841.4	
4 Anheuser-Busch (USA)	12,386.4	Inbev
5 Asahi Breweries (Japan)	8,227.7	
6 Scottish & Newcastle (UK)	7,644.3	Heineken/Carlsberg
7 Carlsberg (Denmark)	6,902.4	
8 Molson Coors (Canada/USA)	5,845.0	SABMiller
9 FEMSA (Mexico)	3,261.3	Licensed to Anheuser-Busch in the USA
10 Sapporo Holdings (Japan)	2,805.8	

[a] Source: Datamonitor (2007).

Pernod Ricard, which also own much of the world's wine production. Diageo was the largest overall alcohol company with beers (notably Guinness) as well as leading spirits brands and wines. It resulted from a 1997 merger of Irish and British interests. In 2001 it bought 60% of Canadian distiller Seagram's, the remainder going to Allied Dolmecq, and it also owns a third of Moët Hennessy wines and cognacs. French distiller Pernod Ricard became the second largest wine and spirits company in 2004 when it bought the previous second runner Allied Dolmecq, passing some brands on to Fortune Brands, makers of Jim Beam. By 2006 half of Pernod Ricard's sales were in the Americas and Asia. In 2008 Pernod Ricard bought V&S Group, a Swedish state-owned company that marketed the globally successful Absolut vodka and other brands. Pernod Ricard expected its capital outlay of €5,626 million to pay off in about four years. This acquisition puts Pernod Ricard up alongside Diageo as co-leader of the global wine and spirits industry.

In 2005, 60% of the world's commercially brewed beer was produced by global companies, with 44% made by the largest four: Inbev, Anheuser-Busch, SABMiller, and Heineken. Inbev, with around 14% of the world beer market, was created through a 2004 merger of Ambev and Interbrew, amalgams of Latin American/Canadian and Belgium/European brewery interests. Anheuser-Busch, the largest brewer in the USA, makes Budweiser, now the largest single beer brand worldwide. In 2002, South African Breweries (SAB), which went global after the international apartheid boycott ended, purchased a controlling interest in Miller Brewing, second largest USA brewer with interests in Central America. SABMiller's experience in Africa has contributed to rapid success in other markets with limited infrastructure. In 2007, its US operations merged with Molson Coors, a 2004 merger of Canadian and US breweries. Heineken describes itself as the 'most international brewer', with 115 breweries and 170 brands in 65 countries. In 2008 Heineken and Carlsberg purchased Scottish & Newcastle, leading UK and sixth largest brewer, for £10,000 million and divided its regions between them. This gave Carlsberg full control of BBH, a major brewer in Eastern Europe and Russia, which it had jointly owned with Scottish & Newcastle. Then in mid-2008, Inbev bought Anheuser-Busch. This makes it the largest brewer in the US market as well as in the world.

Others among the top 24 reviewed have a large market share in particular regions, such as Fosters in Australia, the Pacific and South-east Asia, and Japanese companies Kirin and Asahi mainly in Asia. Still others have focused on one or two truly global brands, such as V&S Group (Absolut), Bacardi, and Forman Brown (Jack Daniels).

In addition to concentrating alcohol production in the hands of fewer companies, these multinational corporations have been consolidating their own global operations. Common strategies used by the top 24 global alcohol corporations are summarized in Box 5.1. Most have shed the business diversification of the 1990s to focus on their 'core business' of alcohol. Non-alcoholic drinks and bottling operations are the businesses most commonly retained. This may be strategic. For example, in Africa the commercial drinks industry is underdeveloped and SABMiller is now producing drink containers, lager, sorghum beer, and non-alcoholic drinks throughout the region. Most global companies now own a wide range of brands but have adopted a strategy of promoting a limited number of premium (i.e. higher-priced) global brands alongside key local brands.

In 2006–2007, the top companies reported organizational changes to rationalize and consolidate their production, distribution and back-office functions, following mergers and acquisitions. The stated purpose of this is to achieve considerable savings that will be 'invested behind brands'—that is, increased spending on advertising, sponsorships and other promotion of alcohol in established markets as well as new ones (Hill 2008).

Box 5.1 Common strategies among twenty-four global alcohol corporations

Identified from annual reports to shareholders, 2003–2007 (Hill 2008):

- Refocus on 'core business'of alcohol.
- Global marketing of a set of higher priced 'premium'brands.
- Target emerging markets for alcohol in growing or recovering economies.
- Buy or part-buy the largest local competitor, then run international and local brands together.
- Consolidate after mergers/acquisitions and put savings into increased brand marketing.
- Adopt corporate social responsibility policy.
- Support free trade agreements and challenges to barriers to trade and competition.

5.6 **Targeting new markets**

Economies of scale benefit companies with a global footprint (Mackay 2003; Jernigan 2009). With alcohol consumption stabilizing in industrialized countries, this has been achieved through a scramble for new markets in the deregulating countries of Eastern Europe and the growing economies of Latin America and Asia. Some economists consider that the global economy is meeting natural limits of overproduction and stagnation (Bello 2006), but outside their home territories the alcohol corporations are still on the upward swing. Further growth, they tell shareholders, can be achieved through sales in new markets with developing or recovering economies, growing middle classes, and population growth among young adults. China, in particular, is seen to have great sales potential because, as Anheuser Busch's 2005 report stated, 'current per capita consumption levels are only 20% of the levels of many developed countries.'

Yet the World Health Organization reports that in developing countries with overall low mortality, alcohol is already the leading risk factor for injury and disease (WHO 2002b). A WHO study has shown that alcohol problems increase with development. Developing countries often lack alcohol laws and policies or do not adequately enforce them. It is often assumed that an industrialized alcohol supply will have positive economic effects in low income countries, but the evidence for this is ambiguous, particularly on job creation. Any benefits are likely to be outweighed by the negative social and economic effects from increased alcohol consumption (Room and Jernigan 2000; Room *et al.* 2002). For example, a WHO study of the socio-economic impacts of alcohol in India estimated that the government earns 216 billion rupees a year from alcohol taxes but is spending around 244 billion rupees a year on managing the direct consequences of alcohol use (Gururaj *et al.* 2006).

With surplus operating profits growing 7–12% a year in the early 2000s, the global companies have had money to spend on entering new markets—through distribution partners, joint ventures where this is required, buying shares in existing companies, building new plants, or, quite typically, by simply buying the local competitor. Local acquisitions provide the global corporation with production facilities, distribution networks and cultural knowledge for marketing purposes. An even faster route to new markets is to buy a global competitor to obtain its profitable brands and share of established and new markets, as Pernod Ricard, Heineken and Carlsberg, and Inbev all did in 2008.

The goal is global growth, not national monopoly. Any anti-trust requirements are met by selling a few brands on to a co-operative competitor. Profitability comes from owning the most successful brands in a market, not all of them. The strategy, identified from annual reports, is to acquire the most successful local products in each country and market them alongside higher priced international brands (Hill 2008).

Recent industry analyses contrast 'global brands' with local 'commodity' products (International Center for Alcohol Policies 2006; Impact Databank 2007). But annual reports reveal that local brands, not just global ones, are important to the profitability of global companies. They are part of a two-pronged 'value and volume' strategy.

SABMiller's explanation of this in its 2005 report suggests that the strategy also applies to new drinkers:

> We now have a continuum of businesses from emerging to mature; enabling us to benefit from both value and volume growth. In many cases, there's also an upward trend towards higher value brands as consumers enter the market at the bottom end and others progress towards the premium end.

The entry of global alcohol companies into new markets is well illustrated by what investors call the BRIC countries—the fast growing economies of Brazil, Russia, India, and China (see Boxes 5.2 to 5.5). For example, in 2005 Diageo reported that spirits volume increased 21%, 51%, 26% and 78% in Brazil, Russia, India and China, respectively, compared with 3% globally. It planned to increase investment in these emerging markets, anticipating that in 10 years' time they would account for an even larger share of Diageo's profitability (Walsh 2005). Since 2002, population size has made China the largest and fastest-growing beer market. By 2004 Russia and Brazil were among the top five, with significant growth also in Thailand and the Philippines (Kirin Research Institute of Drinking and Lifestyle 2004). Once established in these BRIC countries, the global corporations report using their base to extend production, marketing, distribution and sales to neighbouring cities, states or countries in the region.

5.7 **The alcohol 'commodity chain'**

The wider perspective on globalization can contribute to our understanding of what a globalized alcohol industry means for effective alcohol policy. The concept of commodity chains—production networks of multiple firms operating across multiple countries—can be used to analyse the modern dynamics of power and profit-taking. Globalization takes advantage of cost variations between labour markets, supported by advances in communications and transport. These shape decisions about which links in the chain need to be owned directly by the corporation, rather than subcontracted. Jernigan applies this concept to the alcohol industry's networks of local producers, importers, advertisers and distributors. Exports, distribution agreements, brewing under licence, joint ventures, part-ownership or purchase of local plants or companies are all options in the international expansion of alcohol companies. Commodity chain analysis concludes that, to ensure that profits accrue to their shareholders, corporations should retain direct control over two links in the chain: design/recipe and advertising/marketing (Jernigan 2000a).

As designs/recipes for lager or particular types of spirits are broadly similar, what makes a product 'premium' is partly a marketing strategy targeting the high end of the market. The brand image is tailored to attract a particular demographic group or market niche. Image, price and marketing strategy are just as important at the volume end of the market.

Marketing is the dominant feature of the global alcohol production network (Jernigan 2009). Its importance is verified by the proportion of revenue devoted to 'investment in brands', as described in these companies' annual reports. In 2006 Heineken reported spending 12.6% of net sales (about US $1,985 million) on marketing;

Box 5.2 Brazil and the Latin American market

In Brazil, alcohol consumption now averages 6 litres per adult aged ≥15 years, up from 2 litres in the 1960s but below the average for mature alcohol markets. In Brazil 18–29-year-olds are 35% of the population compared with 16.5% in the USA (where they drink 45% of the alcohol sold). There is a high prevalence of binge drinking by teenagers, drink-driving and homicide while under the influence of alcohol. Alcohol dependence is estimated at 9.4–11.2% of the ≥18-year-old population, and the alcohol-related burden of disease in the region is far higher than the global average (Babor and Caetano 2005; Monteiro 2007).

In twelve Central and South American countries, global brewers now control more than half of the market and in eight of these account for more than 90% of beer sales (Caetano and Laranjeira 2005). In 2005 Inbev had 68% of the Brazilian beer market, with strong profitability in Brazil and southern South America driving its global growth. In 2006 Inbev moved from part to full ownership of Quinsa, a Luxembourg-based holding company for breweries in Argentina, Bolivia, Chile, Paraguay and Uruguay since 2002. In 2000 the Canadian brewer Molson bought Brazil's second largest brewery, Kaiser, and in 2004 bought the Bavaria brand and brewery, with Heineken taking a 20% stake. In 2005 SABMiller acquired a controlling share of Bavaria, and Molson passed most of its share on to Femsa when it merged with Coors, retaining 15%. Molson, Heineken, and Femsa also have co-operative arrangements in Central and North America. Pernod Ricard, including its Allied Dolmecq brands, had the largest share of the Brazilian spirits market, with sales up 12% in 2005. In 2006 and 2007 Diageo reported growth in whisky and ready-to-drink products in Brazil, Paraguay and Uruguay, driven by wider distribution and new advertising campaigns. Its Johnnie Walker brand grew by 40%, benefiting in Brazil from investment both 'above and below the line'—that is, from marketing such as sponsorship and direct promotions as well as advertisements.

Throughout the region, wine consumption is falling while consumption of spirits and beer is increasing, reflecting consolidation of ownership and intensive marketing of these beverages (Caetano and Laranjeira 2005; Jernigan 2005). In 2001, for example, $106 million was spent on advertising and marketing in Brazil. Production costs are low, alcohol is widely available and a can of beer costs half the price of Coca-cola. Of 25 countries in the Americas, Brazil's alcohol policies are rated most in need of improvement (Babor and Caetano 2005).

Diageo spent 15.5% (about US $2,246 million) in 2006, and Pernod Ricard spent 17% (about US $3,367 million) in 2006.

Policies that limit exposure to advertising and other marketing can affect sales, consumption levels and profits. This lies behind industry lobbying to retain self-regulation of alcohol advertising and voluntary codes of marketing practices, as discussed later in Chapter 15.

Box 5.3 Russia

Russia has a tradition of heavy spirits consumption and of state control and taxation. As described in Chapter 4, the anti-alcohol campaign from 1985 to 1987 reduced state-store alcohol sales by 63%. Because of an increase in home distilling, estimated total consumption decreased by 25%, from 14 litres to 10.5 litres per capita. Within 3 years male life expectancy increased from 62 to 65 years. In 1992 pro-market reforms were introduced and the state monopoly on alcohol was abolished. Consumption fluctuated but by 2001 was up to 15.0 litres per capita and male life expectancy was down to 59 years. Alcohol was identified as the major factor in deteriorating health statistics and increased violence (Nemtsov 1998, 2005; Pridemore 2002).

Liberalization of this large alcohol market attracted the global companies. Pernod Ricard is now Russia's largest spirits company, with its cognac sales growing by 19% per year and its local brands also reporting double-digit sales growth. In 2006 it negotiated a partnership to market Russian vodka brands worldwide. Diageo sells spirits and beers in Russia through 75% ownership of a joint venture company. This enabled it to fully purchase the local Smirnov vodka brand in 2006 and unite it with its own global Smirnoff brand. In 2005 and 2006, Diageo was 'throwing a lot at Russia' to establish this presence and expand distribution to 74 cities. In 2007 volumes and sales revenue increased by around 25%.

Russia's relatively low consumption of beer attracted the brewers. In 1992 Carlsberg and Scottish & Newcastle acquired an originally Swedish/Finnish joint venture, Baltic Beverage Holdings (BBH), to target the Russian Federation, the Ukraine, Kazakhstan, and the Baltic States. Russia is now the second largest and fastest-growing beer market in Europe and the fifth largest in the world. Consumption has risen from 37 litres per capita in 1999 to 51 litres in 2003. BBH has 38% of the beer market, and its volume and operating profits are increasing at around 18-20% a year. BBH's stated strategy is to 'promote local brands with a local identity for volume share, and national and international premium brands for increasing value share.' The sale of Scottish & Newcastle to Heineken and Carlsberg means that BBH is now fully owned by Carlsberg.

Inbev and Heineken also have been buying Russian breweries. Inbev is the second largest brewer in Russia, with eight breweries showing double-digit annual growth and another under construction in Siberia. Heineken is third, aiming for 20% of the market with its ten breweries, some bought with cash after downsizing holdings in Germany and Belgium. Since 2006 Heineken has also brewed Budweiser under licence for the Russian market.

When Russia increased taxes and extended its ban on spirits advertising to beer, allowing beer advertisements only on television after 10 p.m., BBH's response was to organize twenty 'massive' beer festivals in sixteen cities from Moscow to Vladivostok, featuring different areas tailored to each of its fifteen brands and their target audience.

Box 5.4 India

Low per-capita consumption and perceptions of India as an abstaining, religious culture mask traditions of drinking, high current use by male drinkers and a falling average age of initiation (Prasad 2009). Around 95% of alcohol consumed is spirits, legal or illicit, and the remainder mainly beer. Under colonial rule, *arrack* (sugar-cane spirits, 'country liquor') began to be replaced by licensed and taxed production of stronger, more expensive products. Alcohol policy in India is devolved to state level. Although the Constitution calls on states to prohibit intoxicating drugs, only two jurisdictions currently prohibit alcohol. In other states, alcohol taxes, usually on selling price, provide 15–20% of states' revenue, their largest source after sales tax. In several states, renewal of retail licences is contingent on meeting stiff sales quotas (Benegal 2005). A recent study of Bangalore showed, however, that direct and indirect costs of alcohol misuse are costing the state more than three times what it earns from alcohol taxes (Prasad 2009).

Globalization, economic liberalization and World Trade Organization (WTO) membership have contributed to greater normalization of alcohol use. Village production has stagnated but sales of non-traditional beer, white spirits and wine grew by 7–8% in the early 2000s, with drinking rates increasing among urban middle and upper socio-economic groups. Beer in smaller packs, new flavoured products and new advertising depicting good times and desirable lifestyles targets women and young people (Benegal 2005; Euromonitor 2005).

India has its own alcohol giant, the UB Group, with breweries and distilleries as well as other interests. UB sells the top spirits and top beer brands. Its acquisition of European distilleries ('bringing the spirits of the world to India') and mergers among global corporations mean that it is now the world's third largest spirits producer. SABMiller is the second largest brewer in India, entering the market in 2000 by buying the Narang brewery. In 2003–2005, UB's McDowell Spirits bought Indian company Shaw Wallace for its spirits production, with its breweries going to SABMiller's subsidiary Mysore Breweries. UB and SABMiller then together accounted for more than 50% and 74% of sales volume in beer and spirits, respectively. This was part of a flurry of mergers and acquisitions after India joined the WTO in 2001. In 2006 SABMiller bought Foster's India operations and brand for US $127 million.

In 2002 Scottish & Newcastle entered a strategic alliance, then partnership with UB, taking a 37.5% share in it. When Scottish & Newcastle was bought in 2008, its India holdings went to Heineken. Heineken markets local and global brands in India through its half share of Asia Pacific Breweries, with plants in Maharashta and Goa. In 2006 Carlsberg formed a joint venture called South Asia Breweries, acquiring a brewery in Himachal Pradesh, near New Delhi, followed by construction of plants in Rajasthan, Maharashtra, and West Bengal. Ten percent of South Asia Breweries is held by the Danish Industrialization Fund for Developing Countries, despite a World Bank Note cautioning against alcohol as a development project (World Bank Group 2000). In 2007 Inbev formed a joint venture with RKJ in Mumbai and Anheuser-Busch with Crown Beers in South India.

Box 5.4 India *(continued)*

Pernod Ricard describes itself as the largest foreign wine and spirits operator in India. While high tariffs continue, it markets local brands as well as imports and in 2006 was India's fourth largest local spirits producer, reporting 18% growth in volumes. Diageo sells its global brands through distributors, but in 2006 formed a joint venture with Radico Khaitan, India's second largest drinks company, to produce local brands of Indian-made foreign liquor. It noted the market opportunity for 'aspirational products', and that one in 20 Indians now drank alcohol, compared to one in 300 two decades ago.

With 'high decibel activity' by multinationals and the rapid growth of UB (United Breweries 2006–7), alcohol sales are currently growing by about 20% per year. Beer consumption increased by 51% from 2002 to 2006 while consumption of Indian-made foreign spirits grew by 53% (Lal Pai 2008).

Box 5.5 China

China has a long history of alcohol production and drinking, particularly spirits. Consumption varies considerably by region, with drinking more common in Northern China, in urban areas, and among some ethnic minority groups. More than 25% of men and 60% of women do not drink, but in a large WHO-sponsored survey in five areas of China heavy drinkers were 6.7% of the sample but accounted for 55.3% of alcohol consumed (WHO 2001b). Alcohol consumption more than doubled in the 1980s and 1990s, with alcohol advertising growing over the same period, particularly on television, prompting government intervention. Industry consolidation, including global companies, contributes to increased marketing of branded drinks. In 2003, US $357 million was spent on television advertising for alcohol (Zhang 2004; Euromonitor 2006).

In 1994 SABMiller negotiated joint control of China's second largest brewery with the government agency China Resources Enterprises. More acquisitions included a 30% share in Harbin, leading brewer in Northwest China (later sold) and joint ventures begun by Australasian brewer Lion Nathan (now controlled by the Japanese brewer Kirin). In 2004 SABMiller was the largest foreign brewer in China, with thirty-three breweries. In 2006 China Resources Snow became China's largest brewer by sales volume and brewing capacity, with Snow the country's leading beer brand.

Anheuser-Busch entered the market in 1993 with a 5% stake in China's largest brewer and brand Tsingtao. It then built its own Budweiser brewery at Wuhan. In the 2000s it expanded rapidly. Budweiser and Bud Ice sales in China increased 21.5% in 2002 and by 2003 had nearly half the premium-priced beer market. In 2003 Anheuser-Busch formed a strategic alliance with Tsingtao (50 breweries) and increased its shareholding to 27%. In 2004 it bought Harbin (thirteen breweries) and is using its Budweiser wholesale network and increased marketing capacity to

Box 5.5 China *(continued)*

expand Harbin's sales territory. In 2007 it began selling Corona in China for its Mexican partner, Grupo Modelo. Anheuser-Busch's 2007 report noted that China had accounted for 45% of the growth in global beer volumes over the past 5 years and the company was well positioned to take part in substantial future long-term growth.

After providing technical support to Chinese breweries in the 1980s, Inbev bought two breweries in 1997 and acquired part-ownership of other Chinese companies, later increasing its share. By 2004 it had thirty-nine sites producing nearly 35 million hectolitres and the largest market share in each of the provinces in which it operated. China was a major contributor to 8–11% returns on investment in Inbev's Asia Pacific region during 2002–2004. Two more acquisitions in 2006 consolidated its position in Central and East China. Its strategy is to focus on the most profitable segments of the China market, strengthening local brands while building multi-regional brands. The Japanese alcohol companies Asahi and Kirin also have a well-established and growing presence in China.

Lower tariffs and great sales potential also attracted global spirits producers, selling mainly through the on-premises and city supermarkets (Euromonitor 2006). Since 2003, Pernod Ricard has reported exceptional volume growth by marketing brandies to business elites through sponsorship and lifestyle campaigns. China is also a growth driver for Diageo, who reported a 57% increase in sales in 2007. A significant proportion of this is Johnnie Walker whisky, which is marketed with a high-profile 'Walk On' campaign throughout Asia.

5.8 **Current marketing practices**

Whereas small producers market principally on quality and price, the global alcohol industry is 'marketing-driven' (Room *et al.* 2002). In mature markets, alcohol is now heavily promoted relative to many other products. In the USA, for example, growth in measured alcohol advertising since 1975 has outstripped inflation by 20% (Jernigan and O'Hara 2004). Global and local brands are promoted through integrated brand campaigns using advertising, sponsorships and direct marketing.

Traditional media such as television, radio and print are important in the promotion of alcohol, and there are many commonalities in the content of alcohol advertisements around the world. Advertisements emphasize sexual and social stereotypes and lack diversity. Common elements are humour, sociability, physical attractiveness, success, romance, adventure, fun activities, celebrity endorsers, animation, and music. More recently, irony and subversive messages have become part of the repertoire. Alcohol is almost never associated with food and negative outcomes are not shown (Austin and Hurst 2005; McCreanor *et al.* 2005; Zwarun 2006).

While traditional media remain important, an estimate for the USA is that only one-third to one-half of total expenditure on alcohol promotion is in the measured media (Jernigan 2005). Alcohol sponsorship of sports, music and cultural events is a marketing strategy that inserts alcohol brands and products directly into people's enjoyment of leisure activities (Buchanan and Lev 1989; Klein 2000). It is associated with heavier drinking by individual players, teams and clubs (O'Brien and Kypri 2008), but its main purpose is to link alcohol brands to the buying public's favourite sports. Anheuser-Busch, Heineken, and Carlsberg regularly spend around US $20 million to sponsor a major international sports event that attracts a global fan base. For example, Budweiser was the official international beer of the Beijing Olympics in 2008, and began Olympics-related marketing in China in mid 2007. Marketing via international sports events involves integrated campaigns that stress brand personality and include branded merchandise and ticket competitions at retail outlets around the world, utilizing all media, unpaid sports coverage and direct promotion opportunities at the event itself.

There has been an increase in unmeasured marketing activities involving the Internet, including brand websites (Montgomery 1997), sponsored television sites (Hurst 2006) and social networking sites. For example, two Diageo advertisements placed on YouTube.com were viewed more than three million times each (Jernigan 2009). Electronic marketing includes direct and **viral marketing** via cell phones as well as the Internet (Casswell 2004). Alcohol is promoted indirectly via televised coverage of alcohol-sponsored sports (Madden and Grube 1994; Zwarun 2006) and through depictions of drinking and branded product placement in films (Dal Cin *et al.* 2008). Direct marketing includes point-of-sale promotions such as discount pricing (Center for Disease Control and Prevention 2003; Jones and Lynch 2007; Kuo *et al.* 2003b), branded merchandise, and promotional items (Hurtz *et al.* 2007; Henriksen *et al.* 2008), including alcohol-themed toys (Austin and Knaus 2000).

Young people are a key growth sector for the alcohol industry and of strategic importance in building brand loyalty (Jackson *et al.* 2000). In the USA, research on alcohol advertising shows disproportionate exposure of younger people (Jernigan 2005), and of lower average consumption groups such as African-Americans (Alaniz 1998; Dal Cin *et al.* 2008) and young women (Jernigan *et al.* 2004). Alcohol marketing is likely to be particularly important for younger people because of the role that brands play in their lives (Klein 2000; Casswell 2004) and because of methods that will be attractive to them, such as new technology or brand sponsorship of rock concerts and hip-hop artists (Herd 2005: Mosher 2005; Van den Bulck and Beullens 2005). These marketing strategies reach their young target audience but may be largely invisible to older groups and policymakers, with implications for the appropriateness of current policies intended to protect vulnerable populations (Casswell 2004).

Young people are also being targeted by alcohol marketers through the design of new beverages and packaging (Mosher and Johnsson 2005). In the UK, analysis of the distribution and promotional strategies for particular alcohol products has shown how these strategies target particular segments of the market such as starter drinkers (11–15-year-olds) and young established drinkers (16–24-year-olds) (Jackson *et al.* 2000). In Australia, sweet ready-to-drink alcohol products appeal to young people, particularly underage drinkers, who do not always detect the alcohol content (Copeland *et al.* 2007; Choice 2008). Following heavy marketing in the USA, by 2005 these sweet alcoholic drinks were the preferred beverage for binge-drinking 17- and 18-year-old girls (Jernigan 2009).

Expenditure on alcohol marketing may be particularly effective in emerging markets, which are not yet saturated by advertising. Diageo's 2006 annual report noted that, following a 28% increase in its marketing expenditure, the volumes it sold outside its European and US markets were up 14% compared with 6% worldwide.

5.9 **Conclusion**

The globalization of the alcohol industry over the past decade has transformed not only the structure of alcohol production and distribution, but also the nature of alcohol marketing. The size and profitability of these companies supports integrated marketing on a global scale. Size also allows considerable resources to be devoted, directly or indirectly, to promoting the policy interests of the industry, as will become apparent in Chapter 15.

The supply-side developments described above have implications for how we understand national alcohol markets and the need for effective alcohol policies. Most global alcohol corporations originate in industrialized countries with long traditions of drinking and of regulating the retail sale of alcohol. The challenge these countries face are highly sophisticated, integrated marketing strategies and well-funded efforts to influence policy outcomes.

Global companies now seek most of their growth and profitability in the emerging markets for alcohol in developing economies, where drinking has not been a daily norm and where few effective preventative or harm reduction policies are in place. This challenges researchers, the public health sector and governments alike to respond with both national and global public health strategies to minimize the health consequences and social harms resulting from expanded use of alcoholic beverages.

Chapter 6

International context of alcohol policy

6.1 Introduction

The basic premise of this book, as laid out in Chapter 2, is that alcohol is no ordinary commodity. Many countries have a history in which alcoholic beverages have been or are still treated as special commodities. Some countries have had (and some still have) a total prohibition on alcoholic beverages. Many countries have limited (and are still limiting) the availability of alcoholic beverages, and most countries currently levy special taxes on alcoholic beverages (Hurst *et al.* 1997; Österberg and Karlsson 2002; WHO 2004b; Anderson and Baumberg 2006a; Karlsson and Österberg 2007). There was even a moment in history, a century ago, when a series of agreements at the international level attempted to control the market in 'trade spirits' by forbidding exports to Africa (Bruun *et al.* 1975a).

In recent decades the operating assumption in international agreements has been to treat alcoholic beverages as ordinary commodities like bread and milk or coffee and tea. In a world of increasing international trade and, as we have seen in Chapter 5, globalization of the alcohol industry, this has meant that national and local alcohol control policies have increasingly come under pressure because of decisions at the international level. This chapter describes how these pressures have arisen and how they affect national and local alcohol policies and the prospects for alcohol control at the international level. It is argued that the current situation in international trade and market regimes can be changed by purposive action in the interests of public health and social welfare. Much of the material on which this chapter is based comes from the European Union (EU), but the lessons learned from the European countries are relevant to other parts of the world as well. To deal with the burden of illness resulting from alcohol, and to counter the view that alcohol is an ordinary commodity, public health organizations have begun to formulate strategies and interventions that can be used by governments to protect the health of their populations. Thus the final part of this chapter discusses the role of the World Health Organization in providing a broader perspective on the international context of alcohol policies.

6.2 International trade agreements and economic treaties

Many international trade agreements and economic treaties have been drafted and signed at a regional level since World War II to promote free trade in commodities. At the beginning of 2000, there were altogether 127 regional and other trade agreements registered at the World Trade Organization (WTO) (Andriamananjara 2001). At the global level, multilateral trade agreements are now the business of the WTO, which in 1995 succeeded the General Agreement on Tariffs and Trade (GATT). The GATT was signed in 1947 and in 1994 it was subscribed to by 125 governments, which together accounted for nearly 90% of world trade (WTO 2008). In July 2008 the WTO had 153 members (WTO 2009). Since 1995, new countries joining the WTO come under both GATT and its extension, the General Agreement on Trade in Services (GATS). Any bilateral or regional trade agreement to which a WTO member country is party must be based on similar WTO rules and principles (Kelsey 2008).

The WTO's principal objective is to liberalize and stabilize international trade in the interest of stimulating economic growth and development. The WTO institutionalizes a code of rules for trade agreements and provides enforcement mechanisms for resolving trade disputes. WTO's ministerial and officials' meetings are forums in which countries can discuss trade problems and negotiate on trade liberalization. The purpose of WTO trade agreements is to reduce controls on market access and various national restrictions on international trade. This is achieved through a requirement for progressive liberalization in successive rounds of negotiations (Kelsey 2008).

In many respects the EU, formally started in 1951, is the most important multinational economic agreement at a regional level. In 1993 it founded a single European market. Later the EU developed beyond this, so that stimulating trade in the region has become a part of a more comprehensive international structure and co-operation (Österberg and Karlsson 2002). As the number of the EU member states has grown from six to 27 and additional countries are negotiating or considering membership in the EU, the EU treaties and decisions affect alcohol policies in almost all European countries (Anderson and Baumberg 2006).

The most economically important regional trade agreement outside Europe is the North American Free Trade Agreement (NAFTA) among Canada, Mexico and the USA, which came into effect in 1994. Besides trade with goods, the NAFTA deals with trade in services as well as with investments. There are numerous other regional and bilateral trade agreements at various stages of development, along with the membership of the WTO, which apply to trade in alcoholic beverages and may also influence national and local alcohol control policies.

6.3 Effects of equal treatment principle on alcohol policies

Trade agreements require governments to reduce and eventually abolish all tariff and non-tariff barriers to international trade. One of the core principles of the WTO is that the participating countries have to extend the most favoured treatment that is afforded to domestic buyers and sellers to buyers and sellers from foreign signatories (Grieshaber-Otto et al. 2006). This ensures that internal tax and regulatory measures are applied equally to domestic and imported products without protection for domestic production. This national treatment principle has been extended beyond goods in the GATS (Grieshaber-Otto and Schacter 2002). Its objective is to reduce barriers for trade in services, and its implications for alcohol policy are reviewed in Box 6.1. Negotiations on GATS stalled in 2006 for reasons largely due to trade in agriculture,

Box 6.1 General Agreement on Trade in Services (GATS)

Purpose	To promote free movement of services worldwide.
Services included	All aspects of international services that are provided, traded, and shared between countries. Companies can compete for provision of services in partner countries, including specifically government procurement, and for public services at any level of government if there is already any contracting out.
Domestic regulation	Specific requirements with regard to domestic regulations not more burdensome or restrictive than necessary to ensure the service.
Examples of alcohol-related services	Alcohol production, distribution, and marketing; grain production; transportation of grain to breweries and distilleries; marketing and serving alcohol products; investments in alcohol production facilities.
Implications for alcohol policies	The GATS does not distinguish between alcohol-related services, which may have important public health consequences, and any other service.
	Although the treaty contains exceptions and exclusions, they may be interpreted narrowly and may not provide significant and lasting protection for preventive alcohol control measures. And like other international treaties, the GATS effectively restricts future possibilities for certain alcohol policy measures. For example, rules on alcohol monopolies must conform to the most-favoured nation rule.

but a number of bilateral and regional agreements have now extended the national treatment principle beyond goods.

The treatment of domestic and foreign goods on equal terms brings up the question of what should be construed as substitutes or like commodities. The European Court of Justice (ECJ) has dealt with this question several times with regard to alcoholic beverages (Österberg and Karlsson 2002). Two examples are given in Boxes 6.2 and 6.3.

The issue of whether certain alcoholic beverages are substitutes for each other, and thus need to be treated on equal terms, has also arisen under the GATT and the WTO, usually in terms of the equitability of the tax treatment of different local and imported alcoholic beverages. In 1996, the traditional Japanese liquor *shochu* was deemed to be a like product to vodka, and subsequently also to other imported distilled spirits like gin, rum, brandy, and whiskey. As a result, equal tax treatment was given to all of these beverages. In 1999 the EU successfully used the WTO rules to overturn South Korea's tax system for distilled spirits. In a case against Chile, the WTO panel ruled that imported spirits with higher alcohol content than the Chilean liquor *pisco* could not be taxed at higher rates because this had the effect of protecting domestic liquor

Box 6.2 Aquavit and pickled herring sandwiches

Case 171/78, 'European Commission versus Denmark', dealt with the Danish rules according to which the excise duty for Danish aquavit was 35% lower than the excise duty for other distilled spirits like gin and whiskey. The Danish government argued that Danish drinking habits provided adequate cause for distinguishing aquavit from other distilled alcoholic beverages, as aquavit was consumed mainly at meals as an accompaniment to certain typical Danish dishes like pickled herring sandwiches. Therefore, aquavit could not, according to the Danish government, be placed on the same footing as other distilled spirits, as the real consumer choice was between aquavit and beer or aquavit and wine, and not between aquavit and other distilled spirits. In other words, aquavit and distilled spirits were not substitutes or like products. The European Court of Justice (ECJ), however, did not accept this interpretation. In the ECJ's view, aquavit could well serve as a substitute for other distilled beverages in some cases and could therefore be classified as a product competing with other distilled spirits (Germer 1990, p. 482).

production (Grieshaber-Otto *et al.* 2000; Zeigler 2006). Given the political dynamics following such decisions, the result is usually a lowering of the net tax rate on the affected group of beverages.

6.4 Single market, open borders and tax harmonization in the EU

In 2009 there still was a great variation in alcohol excise duty levels across EU member states, with a zero excise duty rate for wine in 15 EU member states in South

Box 6.3 Can wine be taxed more than beer?

Case 170/78, 'European Commission versus the UK',examined whether the UK could tax wine more than beer. In this case the UK government denied the existence of a competitive relationship between wine and beer, and thus the possibility of substitution, whereas the Commission argued that wine and beer were at least potential substitutes for each other. Both could be used for thirst-quenching and to accompany meals, and both also belonged to the same category of alcoholic beverages, i.e. products of natural fermentation (cf. Germer 1990, p. 485). The ECJ decided that the argument of the Commission was well founded. It stated, furthermore, that 'the tax policy of a member state must not crystallize existing consumer habits so as to be biased in favour of the relevant national industries' (Germer 1990: 485). On the other hand, the ECJ did not accept the Commission's proposal for accepting a single criterion for comparison in setting beer and wine excise duties. It stated that no matter which guideline for comparison was used, the UK's tax system protected domestic beer production for imported wines, and had to be altered.

and Central Europe, and relatively high alcohol taxes in Denmark, Finland, Ireland, Sweden, and the UK. This was the situation, despite the fact that the EU Commission has made repeated attempts in the last three decades to harmonize alcohol excise duty rates in its member states on the grounds that different excise duty rates interfere with the efficient operation of the single European market (Österberg and Karlsson 2002).

A common structure for excise duties was adopted in the EU at the beginning of 1993, which has made it much easier to compare alcohol excise duty rates in different EU member states. It also means that since that year EU member states have not been able to put a special tax on a certain brand that would deviate from the general excise duty rates in that beverage category. For instance, in Finland before its EU membership in 1995 it was possible to raise the price of a certain brand of alcoholic beverage if that brand were favoured by young people or heavy consumers and caused special harms. EU rules have also restricted Sweden from continuing to tax beer up to 3.5% alcohol by volume at a rate clearly lower than stronger beers because the highest alcohol content for untaxed or reduced-tax beer in the EU is 2.8% alcohol by volume, and all beer stronger than this must be taxed on the basis of its alcohol content with a similar rate for each centilitre of ethyl alcohol (Holder *et al.* 1998).

Since 1993, in all EU member states, all brands within each of the four alcoholic beverage categories (i.e. beer, wine, intermediate products, and spirits) must be treated the same with regard to excise duties. However, there are some exceptions for alcoholic beverages from small breweries or distilleries, low-alcohol-volume products inside the four beverage categories, and certain beverages in certain countries like *ouzo* in Greece. The exceptions to the general rule are usually in the direction of reduced excise duty rates. However, **alcopops** or Ready-to-Drink (RTD) products, which tend to attract youthful drinkers, have a special extra tax in some EU member states (see Excise Duty Tables: European Commission 2009).

When the EU Commission did not succeed in harmonizing alcohol excise duty rates through administrative decisions, the Commission started to resort to market forces. The Commission was hoping that increasing travellers' rights to take alcoholic beverages across the borders without paying any additional taxes in the home country would put pressure on neighbouring countries to equalize their alcohol excise duty rates by forcing down higher taxes (Tigerstedt 1990). In creating the single European market in 1993, quantitative quotas for travellers' tax-free alcohol imports were removed (Österberg and Karlsson 2002). This policy has led to decreases in alcohol excise duty rates especially in the Nordic countries.

The EU's insistence on essentially free import of alcoholic beverages for private use between EU countries has had its intended effect on forcing down alcohol taxes. To counter the effects of the low alcohol excise duty rates in Germany, Denmark decreased its excise duty rates for beer and wine by half in 1991 and 1992, and the rate for distilled spirits by half in October 2003 (Karlsson and Österberg 2009). After it became clear that Estonia, with low alcohol excise duty rates would join the EU in May 2004, Finland lowered its excise duty rates for alcoholic beverages by an average of 33% in March 2004 in order to combat the expected increase in travellers' alcohol imports (Mäkelä and Österberg 2009).

During recent years the ECJ has also had its say concerning sales, taxation, and imports of alcoholic beverages from one EU country to another. In the Joustra case the ECJ ruled in November 2006 that consumers who buy alcohol from another EU country are exempt from excise duties in their home country only if they transport the beverages over the border by themselves (Baumberg and Anderson 2008). Furthermore, in the Rosengren case the ECJ ruled in June 2007 that the Swedish ban on private imports of alcoholic beverages via the Internet is an unjustified barrier to the movement of goods, and therefore contradictory to EU law. Consequently, buying alcoholic beverages from other EU countries via the Internet is perfectly legal as long as excise duties are paid in the home country.

When opening of the borders has led to tax changes in the neighbouring countries, the usual case has been that the country with higher alcohol excise duty rates has lowered its duty levels. A related situation was created by the Uruguay Round Agreement which came into force in July 1995 and changed radically the EU's trading system for wine by making it possible to import low-price wine from non-EU countries into the EU (Österberg and Karlsson 2002). This is one more reason why it is very difficult to put a positive excise duty rate on wine in the EU, and as long as the excise duty rate for wine is low or zero in the majority of EU member states it is difficult to raise excise duty rates for beer, intermediate products and distilled spirits.

6.5 Effects on the control of alcohol supply and marketing

A number of international trade agreements and economic treaties have affected the activities of state enterprises and monopolies. While most such agreements recognize the right of partner countries to run monopolies, their activity is restricted. This is because monopolies, by definition, reduce opportunities for private international traders. Finland, Iceland, Norway, and Sweden were thus compelled to privatize their import, export, wholesale, and production monopolies for alcoholic beverages when they entered the European Economic Area (EEA) agreement, although they have managed to retain their off-premises retail monopolies for alcoholic beverages (Holder et al. 1998). Also trade complaints by the EU and the USA under the GATT about the operation of Canadian provincial alcohol monopolies resulted in a weakening of the Ontario monopoly and a decrease in the minimum price for beer (Giesbrecht et al. 2006).

Whereas complaints in the WTO must be brought by national governments, complaints in the EU context can also be brought by commercial enterprises or private persons. Two cases that were instrumental in settling the status of the Nordic alcohol monopolies are described in Boxes 6.4 and 6.5. As these examples indicate, the principles of free market competition and the free flow of goods, services, labour, and capital affect major elements of national alcohol policies, such as using state alcohol monopoly systems as an instrument for public health and social welfare.

EU oversight of retail licensing procedures has also weakened national control of privately owned retail sales outlets for alcoholic beverages. For instance, Finland has been forced to give up needs assessment in licensing on-premises retail outlets for alcoholic beverages (see The Supreme Administrative Court 1526/7/96). In most EU

Box 6.4 The Restamark case

This case played an important role in the partial de-monopolization of the alcohol market in Finland (Holder *et al.* 1998; Ugland 2002). In January 1994, a Finnish enterprise, Restamark, which was owned by the Finnish Restaurant and Cafeteria Association, tried to import a shipment of alcoholic beverages into Finland. This was not allowed, as it was against the current Finnish Alcohol Act. But the importer claimed that it was justified according to the EEA Agreement, which had been in force since the beginning of 1994. The case was bought to the Court of the European Free Trade Area. The Court concluded in December 1994 that the Finnish import monopoly on alcoholic beverages was not compatible with the EEA Agreement, and had to be abolished (Alavaikko and Österberg 2000). This ruling also doomed the Icelandic, Norwegian, and Swedish alcohol import monopolies. Finland and Sweden abolished their monopolies on production, imports, exports, and wholesale in 1995, and Iceland and Norway followed suit in 1996.

countries, licensing policy has become a formal procedure whereby every applicant fulfilling some basic requirements, for instance, no criminal record and no unpaid taxes, automatically receives a retail licence for alcoholic beverages.

At the EU level the content of television broadcasting is regulated by a Council directive (89/552/EEC) called 'Television without Frontiers'. The main objective of this directive, originally approved in 1989, is to create the necessary conditions for free movement of television broadcasts within the single market, to guarantee cultural diversity and to protect consumers, especially minors. Consequently, the directive

Box 6.5 The Franzén case

On January 1, 1994, a Swedish shopkeeper, Harry Franzén, tried to sell wine in his store. In a chaotic situation, he ended up donating the bottles to his customers without being able to collect payment for them. As Franzén's aim was to be prosecuted, he tried to break the law again on April 7, 1994, and on January 1, 1995. On these two occasions Franzén sold wine in his grocery store, was stopped by the police, and was prosecuted in the district court of Landskrona. In court Franzén claimed that he could not be convicted because the prevailing Swedish Alcohol Act was contrary to the EU Treaty. Consequently, the Landskrona court asked the ECJ for a preliminary ruling. In this case the ECJ found that the operation of the Swedish off-premises retail alcohol monopoly, Systembolaget, was organized in a non-discriminatory manner and was not against the EU treaties (Holder *et al.* 1998). The Franzén case's effect on the Nordic alcohol control system was very important because it ended the legal struggle to try to prove that the off-premises retail alcohol monopolies were in conflict with the EU treaties.

includes some restrictions on the content of alcohol advertising in broadcast media (Österberg and Karlsson 2002).

Alcohol advertising has also been dealt with in the ECJ. In a case dealing with alcohol advertising in Catalonia in the early 1990s the ECJ found legislation banning advertising of alcoholic beverages of more than 23% by volume in certain places proportional to its objective and thus not against the EU Treaty (Österberg and Karlsson 2002). In 1998 Sweden asked the ECJ for precedent related to a case concerning *Gourmet*, a magazine meant for professionals and as such lawfully including alcohol advertisements. However, the magazine including alcohol advertisements was also sent to some Swedish consumers, contrary to the Swedish law on alcohol advertising. The ECJ ruled that under the EU treaty, freedom to provide services did not preclude a prohibition on alcohol advertising to protect public health unless this could be achieved with less effect on EU trade. The ECJ then referred the case back to the Swedish court on this question of proportionality (ECJ C-405/98). The Swedish court did not find the prohibition of alcohol advertising proportional to its goals, and in 2003 the Swedish government amended the Alcohol Act to apply the ban of advertising in all media only to alcoholic beverages of more than 15% alcohol by volume. Beverages with less than 15% alcohol may be advertised in periodicals and other journals (Baumberg and Anderson 2008).

In 1991, with the Loi Évin, France introduced the most restrictive measures on alcohol advertising in the European Community (EC) by banning almost all direct and indirect alcohol advertising. The alcohol industry has regarded this as an infringement of the single market rules. In 2002 the EU Commission and Bacardi each filed cases against France arising from the Loi Évin's restriction of alcohol sponsorship of sports and related advertising, including advertisements and signage on international sports coverage. The ECJ ruled that the Loi Évin is compatible with freedom to provide services within the EU and was both justified and proportionate to its purpose of protecting public health (ECJ C-262/02, C-429/02).

Despite these examples in which restrictions on advertising have been upheld, it is possible that trade agreement memberships have had chilling effects outside of the formal policy process (Baumberg and Anderson 2008). In Thailand, for example, a newspaper reported that a group of foreign operators threatened that the Thai government would be taken to the WTO if a proposed ban on alcohol advertising came into force (Casswell and Thamarangsi 2009).

Economic integration has also affected other measures that are interpreted as barriers to trade. In the Cassis de Dijon case in the late 1970s, the ECJ ruling led to the general interpretation that a beverage lawfully marketed in one EU member state can be lawfully marketed in other EU member states. One practical result of this ruling is that the Swedish alcohol off-premises retail monopoly had to include alcopops or RTD drinks in its range (Romanus 2000).

6.6 International financial organizations and national alcohol policies

Until recently, relatively little attention has been paid to the intersection between alcohol issues and the operations of international development and financial agencies like the International Monetary Fund (IMF) and the World Bank, which have often had major effects on alcohol policies at national and local levels.

International agencies concerned with economic development have had a strong ideological bias against government ownership of production or distribution functions. They have often encouraged dismantling or sale of government monopolies as a condition of development grants, particularly in structural adjustment programmes for countries with financial difficulties without any differentiation of alcoholic beverages from other commodities.

To a limited extent, international financial bodies have also intervened in the alcohol market by financing new or modernized alcohol production plants as part of a general strategy to promote economic development. For instance, the World Bank Group once financed breweries and wineries, though not distilleries. Alcohol production may also result from government-to-government aid projects. For example, in the early 2000s New Zealand assisted Bhutan in adding value to its grain crop by making alcohol. Part way through, the New Zealand team became aware of local problems with alcohol and sought advice on adding a health promotion strand to their aid project.

In an important precedent in 2000 the Word Bank Group adopted a policy recognizing that investment in alcoholic beverage production was highly sensitive. World Bank staff was mandated to be very selective in supporting only those projects 'with strong developmental impacts which are consistent with public health issues and social policy concerns' (World Bank Group 2000).

6.7 **Alcohol control at the international level: the public health perspective**

Thus far we have considered the international context of alcohol control from the perspective of the international trade organizations, which often operate in ways that favour the interests of the alcohol industry. This section considers the role of international agencies charged with the promotion of health and well-being.

Since World War II there have been almost no international-level agreements that seek to limit alcohol-related harms. An exception to this is the Convention Concerning the Protection of Wages of the International Labour Organization (ILO), which forbids 'the payment of wages in the form of liquor of high alcoholic content' (Article 4, Section 1; ILO 1949) and the 'payment of wages in taverns' except for the tavern's own employees (Article 13, Section 2; ILO 1949). It is clear that economic policies at the international level have considerably limited the ability of nations and local governments to control alcohol consumption and related problems, and virtually nothing has been done at the international level that would enhance the ability of governments to control alcohol problems.

The situation for alcohol is quite different from other drugs that have implications for public health. A series of international agreements, dating back to the European colonial era at the beginning of the twentieth century, has established a common system for the control of opiates, cocaine, and marijuana. Since 1971, the market in common psychoactive pharmaceuticals such as benzodiazepines and amphetamines has also been controlled by an international convention, with nations pledging to support control efforts at national and local levels. Since 1988, the control regime has been progressively extended also to cover chemical precursors to control psychoactive drugs (Room and Paglia 1999).

The path forward for alcohol at the international level is unlikely to include an International Alcohol Control Board modelled on the International Narcotics Control Board. However, the contrast between alcohol and controlled drugs is stark, particularly when the WHO Global Burden of Disease study estimate for alcohol is almost six times greater than the drugs under international control, taken together (Murray and Lopez 1996a).

A more likely model for future international agreements on alcohol is the Framework Convention on Tobacco Control (FCTC), the first treaty negotiated under the auspices of the WHO (Room 2006a). The WHO FCTC reaffirms the right of all people to the highest standard of health, and represents a paradigm shift in developing a regulatory strategy to address addictive substances (WHO 2009a). In contrast to the previous drug control strategies, the WHO FCTC asserts the importance of demand reduction strategies as well as supply issues as described in Box 6.6. The Convention entered into force on February 2005 and had then 168 signatories. By mid-June 2009 it had been ratified or approved by 164 of these parties (WHO 2009b).

There are several similarities between the situations of alcohol and tobacco. Both are widely available and commonly used psychoactive substances, with substantial dependence potential and devastating effects on health. For both, the present customary levels of consumption will be difficult to change. And many of the issues that are on the agenda in the WHO FCTC also apply to problems in regulating the alcohol market. These issues include:

- international harmonization of taxes in a direction that will promote public health;
- provisions to reduce smuggling, including expectations of comity between nations in enforcing anti-smuggling laws;
- agreement on abolishing duty-free travellers' allowances and tax-free sales;
- restrictions on advertising and sponsorship by brands and companies;
- international standards for testing the product for purity, and for warning labels and controls on packaging; and
- a shift away from agricultural subsidies for raw materials (Joossens 2000).

At the international level of alcohol policy issues, the prime mover until now has been the WHO, a division of the United Nations (UN). While the WHO's role in alcohol issues has been limited in the past (Room 1984a), the WHO Regional Office for Europe (WHO EURO) was particularly active in the 1990s in its promotion of the European Alcohol Action Plan (Gual and Colom 2001), which provides an example of a co-ordinated effort to develop national alcohol policies through international collaboration between the WHO and its member states. Box 6.7 gives a list of WHO activities in the alcohol field during the last 15 years.

Box 6.6 Measures to control the tobacco market according to the WHO Framework Convention of Tobacco Control

A. Domestic measures

Licensing of production, distribution, retailing	Optional (§15.7)
Testing, measuring, regulating contents	Required (§9)
Labeling contents	Required for constituents and emissions (§11.2); and for where to be sold (§15.2.a)
Warnings on or in packaging	Required, detailed (§11)
Taxation	Urged as 'effective and important' (§6)
Distribution free or in small quantities	Prohibited (§16.2 & 3)
Sales in vending machines	Optional commitment to prohibit (§16.5)
Self-service sales	Optional ban (§16.1.b)
Sales to minors	Prohibited (§16)
Liability of producers or sellers	Encouraged 'for the purpose of tobacco control' (§19)
Legislation against illicit trade	Required (§15.4.b)
Advertising	Banned if constitutionally allowed; otherwise restricted (§13)
Other promotion, sponsorship	Banned if constitutionally allowed; otherwise restricted (§13)
Limits on times, occasions of use	Protection required from tobacco smoke in indoor public & workplace (§8)
Providing and promoting treatment	Encouraged (§14.2)
Promoting public awareness	Required (§12)

B. Co-operation on international control

Enacting and strengthening legislation against illicit trade	Required (§15.4.b)
Co-operation with other countries and with international organizations	Encouraged 'as appropriate' on policies (§5), and 'as mutually agreed' on expertise and assistance (§22)
Requiring and exchanging import and export authorizations	To consider 'developing a practical tracking and tracing regime' (§15.2.b)

Box 6.6 Measures to control the tobacco market according to the WHO Framework Convention of Tobacco Control *(continued)*

Sales and imports of tax- and duty-free products	May prohibit or restrict 'as appropriate' (§6.2.b)
Marking products with destination and origin	Required (§15.2)
Monitoring and controlling of goods in transit or bonded	Required for products held or moving 'under suspension of taxes or duties' (§15.4.d)
Seizure and confiscation of manufacturing equipment and goods in illicit trade	Destruction of seized equipment and goods required (§15.4.c)
Confiscation of proceeds derived from illicit trade	To be adopted 'as appropriate'
Elimination of cross-border advertising, promotion, sponsorship	May ban and penalize such cross-border promotion on basis equal to penalties on domestic promotion (§13.7)
Assistance to other countries on civil or criminal liability	Encouraged (§19.3)
Reporting requirements to international bodies	Periodic reports, on a schedule to be agreed on, on laws, surveillance, taxation, trade, etc. (§21)

In 2001, the Director-General of the WHO named an Alcohol Policy Strategy Advisory Committee to aid in the development of the WHO's work in this area. In 2005 the 58th World Health Assembly adopted a resolution on Public Health Problems Caused by Harmful Use of Alcohol, and three years later the 61st World Health Assembly adopted a resolution on Strategies to Reduce the Harmful Use of Alcohol. This resolution has led to the drafting, in consultation with governments, of a strategy on Global Alcohol Policy which will be presented to the 63rd World Health Assembly in May 2010.

In 2006, regional meetings of health ministers of member states in WHO's Western Pacific Region and South-East Asia region adopted resolutions recommending policy options to governments for reducing alcohol-related harm. The Western Pacific Regional Strategy to Reduce Alcohol Related Harm recommended effective policies and processes and was based on a full consultation procedure.

In the European context, the EU's attention to the public health aspects of alcohol has increased. In 2001 the EU adopted a ministerial resolution concerning the promotion of alcohol to youth, and in 2006 the EU published a formal Communication on an EU strategy to support member states in reducing alcohol-related harm (COM/2006/625 final). Related to this Communication the EU also initiated an Alcohol and Health Forum, including both public health NGOs and alcohol industry agencies. This kind of attention to alcohol reflects the fact that, under the Amsterdam

Box 6.7 World Health Organization actions in the alcohol field

WHO—EURO

◆ Since 1992, the European Alcohol Action Plan (EAAP) has provided a basis for alcohol policy development and implementation in WHO Member States throughout the European Region.

◆ European Charter on Alcohol was accepted at the European Ministerial Conference on Health, Society and Alcohol in Paris, France, 12–14 December 1995.

◆ Second European Alcohol Action Plan covered the years 2000–2005.

◆ Declaration on Young People and Alcohol was accepted during the Ministerial Conference on Young People and Alcohol in Stockholm, February 2001.

◆ Framework for alcohol policy in the WHO European Region was endorsed by the 55th session of the WHO Regional Committee for Europe in September 2005, Bucharest, Romania.

WHO—Western Pacific

◆ Regional Strategy to Reduce Alcohol Related Harm, adopted 21 September 2006 (WPR/R57.R5).

WHO—South-east Asia

◆ Alcohol Consumption Control—Policy Options in South-East Asia Region, adopted 25 August 2006 (SEA/RC59/15).

WHO—Geneva

◆ World Health Assembly resolution (A58/26), May 2005. Public-health problems caused by harmful use of alcohol.

◆ WHO Expert Committee on Problems Related to Alcohol Consumption. 2007. *Second Report.* Geneva: World Health Organization, Technical Report Series No. 944. Available at: http://www.who.int/substance_abuse/expert_committee_alcohol_trs944.pdf.

◆ World Health Assembly resolution (A61/13), May 2008. Strategies to reduce the harmful use of alcohol.

Treaty enlarging the responsibilities of the EU, public health has now become an official EU concern (Österberg and Karlsson 2002). However, the approach taken in the Alcohol and Health Forum, of attempting to find consensus between conflicting interests held by industry and public health, has resulted in a lack of effective initiatives (Anderson 2008).

6.8 **Conclusions: alcohol, trade agreements and public health**

Most international trade agreements and economic treaties since World War II have been built on the idea of free trade and a global free-market economy. They aim to support economic growth through the reduction of obstacles to free trade and production such as tariff barriers, taxation favouring domestic products, quantitative trade restrictions, state or private monopoly arrangements, and state subsidies to domestic industries.

In these international trade agreements and economic treaties, alcoholic beverages are almost always treated like ordinary consumer goods. Even when an alcoholic beverage (e.g. wine) is treated as a special commodity, this is usually because this type of beverage falls within the category of subsidized agricultural products, not because it is considered harmful to public health. Equal treatment obligations constrain government measures developed to control alcoholic beverages as special commodities. From a public health and social policy perspective, it may be eminently sensible to freeze preferences for traditional commodities and to discourage consumers from developing a taste for new types of beverages. But increasingly, the WTO or the EU and NAFTA consider such measures illegal protectionism. The increasing application of the equal treatment standard to services and investments, combined with the doctrine of effective equality opportunities for foreign investments or service producers, could prove especially problematic for alcohol control policies in the future.

Since World War II there have been almost no international-level agreements that seek to limit alcohol-related harms. At the international level of alcohol policy issues, the prime mover has been the WHO, and there are signs that its activities with regard to alcohol are increasing. Many alcohol-related problems do not, however, commonly fall under the rubric of health, but are concerns of other governmental agencies such as law enforcement and social welfare agencies. There is thus a need to expand the scope of international collaborative action on alcohol problems beyond the World Health Organization.

As Chapters 2–4 have shown, alcohol is a commodity that causes social, health, and economic problems to the drinker and to society as a whole. Because of these problems, many countries and smaller communities have implemented a wide variety of policies to decrease problems caused by drinking alcoholic beverages, as will be discussed in Chapters 7–14. The most effective strategies include raising the prices of alcoholic beverages with special alcohol taxes, as well as restricting the physical availability of alcohol by controlling the market, either by maintaining state monopolies or by licensing the production and trade of alcoholic beverages. Restrictions on marketing activities are also likely to have an impact. The more effective strategies are also those most likely to be threatened or weakened by international trade agreement disputes. To the extent that alcohol is considered to be an ordinary commodity, these agreements and treaties often become severe obstacles for conducting purposeful and efficient alcohol control policies. For example, this chapter has shown that with the growing emphasis on free trade and free markets, international organizations like the WTO have pushed to dismantle effective alcohol control measures, such as state alcohol monopolies and other restrictions on the supply of alcoholic beverages.

On the other hand, at least thus far, many alcohol control measures, such as minimum legal age limits for purchasing alcoholic beverages and blood alcohol limits for driving, have not been affected by international trade or common market agreements, and some have withstood challenges. It should be remembered that the WTO, the EU and NAFTA cannot overstep the areas of their competence, and cannot act, for instance, on alcohol control measures motivated purely by public health or social policy goals. Governments can also specify some industries or products as temporary exceptions to international trade agreements, although these may be hard to maintain over time. However, the impact of international trade agreements and economic treaties cannot be blamed entirely for the lack of effective alcohol control policies at the national level. Even if international trade agreements and economic treaties restrain the ability of governments to implement alcohol control measures, nation states and international health organizations have ample possibilities to reduce alcohol-related harms, which may not currently be used to full advantage.

Chapter 7

Strategies and interventions to reduce alcohol-related harm

7.1 Introduction

As indicated in Chapter 1, alcohol policy is broadly defined as any purposeful effort or authoritative decision on the part of governments or non-government groups to minimize or prevent alcohol-related consequences. Policies may involve the implementation of a specific strategy with regard to alcohol problems (e.g. increase alcohol taxes), or the allocation of resources that reflect priorities with regard to prevention or treatment efforts. This chapter sets the stage for the chapters to follow by describing how research is conducted to evaluate the effects of specific alcohol policies, and to assess the impact of prevention strategies (e.g. alcohol education in schools) and other interventions (e.g. screening and brief counselling for high-risk drinkers) that precede formal alcohol policies.

In some cases policies persist despite evidence that the strategy is flawed, and the outcome with regard to reducing alcohol-related problems is thus inconsequential. To understand why policies succeed or fail to accomplish their aims, the field of alcohol policy analysis has begun to consider the mechanisms that relate policies to outcomes, as demonstrated by the research discussed in this chapter.

7.2 Rules of evidence

A variety of methodological approaches have been used to assess the impact of alcohol policies as well as policy-relevant prevention and treatment strategies. These include experimental studies, survey research, analysis of archival and official statistics, **time-series analyses**, qualitative research, and **natural experiments**. In many studies **quasi-experimental** research designs have been used. This type of research typically involves before and after measurement of a group, community, or other jurisdiction that is exposed to an intervention (experimental condition), with similar measurement conducted in comparable groups or communities where no intervention took place (control condition). It is called quasi-experimental because it lacks the random assignment to conditions that is part of a true experiment. Natural experiments, a type of quasi-experimental design, have played a particularly important role in the evaluation of some interventions. For example, when sobriety checks (see Chapter 11) are implemented in one jurisdiction and not in an adjacent one, the relative impact of the policy can be examined over time through comparative analysis of archival data such as accident rates or drink-driving arrests.

The appropriateness of any given research methodology for alcohol policy evaluation depends on the phenomena under study, the current state of knowledge, the availability of valid measurement procedures, and the ways in which the information will be put to use (McKinlay 1992). Generally, the most conclusive evidence in the behavioural and medical sciences derives from **randomized clinical trials** or randomized control experiments where an untreated control group is compared to an intervention group. An example of this design in the policy/prevention field is the evaluation of a school-based preventive intervention that randomly assigns some students to a non-intervention control group and other students to a programme that teaches alcohol resistance skills. Yet even such a well-accepted design has pitfalls when applied to alcohol prevention research because the individual is often not the proper unit of analysis. For instance, the teaching of resistance skills in a school-based intervention will usually be done by a teacher in a classroom full of students, and the social interaction taking place at the level of the class should be taken into account as part of the design and the analysis. Though they are still rare, there are now some evaluation studies that take the community as the unit to be randomized (e.g. Wagenaar *et al.* 2000b). Some studies even tested the effects of an alcohol control measure by random assignment of different regions of a country to the intervention and the control condition (e.g. Skog 2000; Norström and Skog 2005).

Randomized controlled studies are rare in the alcohol policy field because of political, ethical, and cost considerations. For example, it is usually not possible to randomize a group of communities to pay higher taxes on alcohol while a comparison group of communities pays lower taxes. Therefore, most of the evidence on alcohol policy comes from quasi-experimental studies where the possibility of bias and **confounding** always exists. For example, when a policy change occurs naturally rather than as part of a planned experiment, it is sometimes difficult to assess how much of the change in outcomes is due to the policy change rather than to other factors such as attitude change, enhanced enforcement, and so on, that may have precipitated or accompanied the policy change. For this reason, it is particularly important to undertake several studies, each with a different design, to strengthen the conclusions that can be drawn.

The most direct evidence on the effects of alcohol policies comes from studying what happens when the intervention is applied or removed, in comparison with another time or place when there is no change in the intervention. When a study of such an intervention is planned in advance, consideration can be given to the kinds of data that will be most appropriate to collect. Useful data would likely include population surveys before and after the change (if possible with least a part of the survey including the same respondents followed up after the intervention), the compilation of event data on cases coming to the attention of health, police, and other social response agencies, and observational and qualitative interview material concerning social processes in the period of change. However, a useful evaluation can often be done even in the absence of such planning, when the political process creates what, from the researcher's perspective, is a natural experiment. In this case, the researcher is dependent on matching post-intervention data with data that were collected for other purposes prior to the change. Evaluation research is often dependent on the availability of such data, and these data are most available in developed economies with mature alcohol markets. In the absence of data collection capabilities and research resources in many emerging markets for alcohol (e.g. parts of Asia, Africa, and Latin America), policymakers may have to rely on evidence from country situations that may or may not match their own.

Studies of what happens when there is a change—an implemented or discontinued intervention—provide the most valuable evidence on the effects of alcohol policy. Yet one can also learn from cross-sectional studies comparing sites where different policies are in effect. Given the potential sources of confounding, however, data from such studies provide only weak evidence of effectiveness.

The various modes of data collection have different advantages and drawbacks. Social surveys, for example, generally measure attitudes and behaviours through the direct questioning of individual drinkers. Studies based on survey data tend to be descriptive, correlational, and subject to the limitations of self-report methods. Data collected by social and health agencies (e.g. police statistics, hospital discharge data, mortality records) have different strengths and weaknesses. By definition, they give a good picture of the agency response in an area, but the available data are influenced by cultural perceptions, agency priorities, and recording practices.

Quantitative research methods, such as social surveys, can be complemented by qualitative studies, such as ethnographic interviewing, participant observation, case studies, and focus group activities. As long as standard scientific principles of confirmation, refutation, causal inference and generalizability are applied, research that uses a number of methods and strategies can produce a firm evidence base on which effective alcohol policy can be developed.

The value of combining different types of evidence is that each method has its own advantages. In general, as one moves from individual-level to population-level interventions, the utility of experimental methods becomes problematic. One reason is that controlled experiments may not be the best way of evaluating behaviours and outcomes in complex real-life settings. It is often not feasible to experimentally manipulate people or policies at the level of the general population or even the community. For this reason different research approaches, measurement procedures, and data collection techniques can all contribute to an understanding of alcohol policy.

Evaluation research is necessary in order to measure whether the policy has any impact, and to provide a 'reality check' to high expectations often attached to promising new initiatives in this area. Evaluation also needs to be ongoing. Evidence from one time period may not necessarily be applicable to situations emerging in another era. And evidence from developed countries may not always be applicable to developing countries. Furthermore, communities often want locally based evidence, or at least evidence that is close to home, to justify their policies rather than relying on dated findings from far afield. While there may be general agreement about supply and demand, and the role of access to alcohol in curtailing problems, there may be doubt among policymakers that these findings will apply to their jurisdiction.

Evaluation research provides a useful but often under-utilized resource to decision-makers. Should resources be devoted to those policies that have at best a modest effect, or should they be directed to policies that have a chance for a broader and more substantial impact? Decisions about which strategies to implement, phase out, or modify should be informed by findings from systematic evaluation.

With these methodological considerations in mind, the policies, strategies, and interventions discussed in Chapters 8–14 of this book were systematically evaluated on the basis of the following rules of evidence. First, the authors reviewed and critically appraised the world literature on each area, with other experts serving as external reviewers. Special attention was given to research developments during the last decade, in part because of the dramatic increase in research since the first edition of this book was published. The emphasis was always on studies with better research designs (e.g. experimental or quasi-experimental designs with control groups or comparison conditions). The variety of approaches, wide scope of the literature searches, and expert involvement have led to detailed evaluations and careful weighting of the existing evidence. Still, potential biases may be present due to missed studies and selectivity of inclusion. And for some policies and interventions, the research basis is relatively small.

One limitation of an undertaking of this kind is that, given the origins of the scientific literature in the alcohol field, most of the research reviewed in the intervention chapters of this book originated in English-speaking countries. To compensate for the relative lack of research in other parts of the world, the authors were asked to give careful consideration to the cross-national generalizability of findings from particular studies. Finally, a series of meetings was held to review and critique the contents, findings, and conclusions of each chapter.

7.3 Overview of intervention chapters

The policies, strategies, and interventions discussed in the next seven chapters cover the most currently favoured policy options where there is a related research base capable of review. Chapter 8 focuses on policies aimed at changing the affordability of alcohol through price controls and taxation. Chapter 9 examines policies aimed at changing the physical availability of alcohol. Chapters 10 and 11 address a broad range of strategies aimed at preventing or minimizing important alcohol-related harms and consequences. Chapter 12, which examines the evidence on impact of marketing and current approaches to regulating alcohol promotion, and Chapter 13, on education and persuasion approaches to primary prevention, both cover strategies that generally try to influence individual perceptions about alcohol. Finally, Chapter 14 discusses from a public health perspective the effectiveness of treatment programmes and early interventions designed to prevent the progression of alcohol problems.

Box 7.1 summarizes the theoretical assumptions that underlie the broad areas of alcohol policy covered in these chapters. The assumptions suggest that alcohol consumption and alcohol-related problems can be reduced by a variety of mechanisms, including demand reduction, supply control, environmental constraints, deterrence, punishment, social pressure, health information, reducing exposure to social modelling, treatment, and early intervention. The extent to which these theoretical assumptions are valid, generalizable, and applicable to the prevention and treatment of alcohol-related problems in different parts of the world is considered in Chapters 8–14.

Box 7.1 Theoretical assumptions underlying seven broad areas of alcohol policy

Policy approach	Theoretical assumption
Alcohol taxes and other price controls	Increasing the economic cost of alcohol relative to alternative commodities will reduce demand.
Regulate physical availability through restrictions on time, place, and density of alcohol outlets	Reducing supply by restricting physical availability will increase effort to obtain alcohol, and thereby reduce total volume consumed as well as alcohol-related problems.
Alter the drinking context	Creating environmental and social constraints will limit alcohol consumption and reduce alcohol-related violence.
Drink-driving countermeasures	Deterrence, punishment, and social pressure will reduce drink-driving.
Education and persuasion: provide information to adults and young people especially through mass media and school-based alcohol education programmes	Health information that increases knowledge and changes attitudes will prevent drinking problems.
Regulate alcohol advertising and other marketing	Reducing exposure to marketing, which normalizes drinking and links it with social aspirations, will slow recruitment of drinkers and reduce heavier drinking by young persons.
Conduct screening and brief intervention in health care settings; increase availability of treatment programmes	Alcohol dependence will be prevented by motivating heavy drinkers to drink moderately; various therapeutic interventions will increase abstinence among persons who have developed a dependence on alcohol.

How these interventions and the assumptions on which they are based can be used to guide the development of effective alcohol policies is considered in the final chapter of the book.

Although alcohol is no ordinary commodity with respect to harmful consequences, it is very much an ordinary commodity when it comes to effects of control measures. For example, alcohol consumption responds to changes in price and availability. What we will show in the following intervention chapters parallels the findings from other areas of public health research, such as tobacco control. As one of the emerging success stories in addressing a global disease epidemic, tobacco control demonstrates that when sound epidemiological research is complemented by policy-relevant studies on prevention and treatment, significant reductions can be made in the disease burden.

Chapter 8

Controlling affordability: pricing and taxation

8.1 Introduction

Among the various measures by which states and nations affect alcohol-related problems, the most common one is the regulation of alcohol taxes and prices. This is in part because governments need financial resources and mostly acquire them by taxation, including taxes on alcohol. There are long national traditions of customs tariffs on alcohol imports and excise duties on domestic production. As alcohol production became more commercial and centralized, collecting the taxes became easier. For more than a century, taxation of alcoholic beverages has also been used by governments to reduce rates of harm from drinking. Economic studies conducted in many developed and some developing regions of the world have demonstrated that increased alcohol taxes and prices are related to reductions in alcohol use and related problems.

This chapter considers the aims, mechanisms, and effects of alcohol taxation and pricing, two important economic strategies that have strong implications for the prevention of alcohol-related problems. Economic research and other studies are reviewed to evaluate how alcohol prices affect alcohol consumption and what aspects moderate the effects of price changes. Some economists use the term 'full price' of alcohol, incorporating both the monetary cost and the time and effort required to obtain it (Chaloupka *et al.* 2002). However, this chapter focuses solely on monetary costs, with non-monetary restrictions being the focus of the following chapter.

8.2 Aims of formal controls over beverage prices

In the absence of any formal controls over production, distribution, and sales, prices of alcoholic beverages would be set by market conditions purely on the basis of supply and demand. However, most countries increase alcoholic beverage retail prices over their production and distribution costs and control profit through special alcohol taxes or other price controls. Quite often there is no explicitly stated public health rationale for taxes on alcoholic beverages, such as special excise duties, value-added taxes, or sales taxes higher than the normal rate. But in many countries, alcohol and other dependence-producing substances have been treated differently from other consumer products because of public health and social policy considerations.

During certain time periods, taxation of alcoholic beverages has been a very important source of state revenue. Between 1911 and 1917, for example, more than one-third of the total revenues from taxes levied by the US government came from alcoholic beverages (Landis 1952). Similar figures can be found for Ireland, The Netherlands, the UK, and the Nordic countries (Denmark, Finland, Iceland, Norway, and Sweden). The relative importance of alcohol taxation as a source of state revenues declined in most established market economies during the twentieth century, particularly after the advent of modern income taxation and general value-added taxes. In many market economies, the share of alcohol taxes in state budgets has also declined because of decreases in alcohol tax rates. For instance, Ireland experienced a clear decrease in alcohol tax revenues relative to total state revenues between 1970, when its share was 16.5% (Davies and Walsh 1983), and 1996, when it was estimated at 5.0% (Hurst *et al.* 1997). Despite these trends, alcohol tax revenues are still of considerable fiscal significance in many developed countries (Hurst *et al.* 1997).

In some developing countries, alcohol taxation remains an important source of government revenue. In India, alcohol taxes are one of the main sources of revenue at the state level, accounting for as much as 23% of the total tax revenue collected in some states (Room *et al.* 2002). In Cameroon, 43% of government revenue in 1990 came from taxes on beer and soft drinks. In many other developing countries, the proportion of government revenue is in the same range as in the developed economies: 2% in Nigeria, 2.3% in South Africa, 4% in Sri Lanka, and 10% in Kenya (Room *et al.* 2002). The equivalent figure for the 12 countries of the European Community (EC) in 1991 was 2.4%. A crucial issue in many developing countries is the existence of a substantial parallel ('informal') market of alcoholic beverages in which alcohol tax is not collected, and which constrains the effect of tax increases.

8.3 Mechanisms: supply and demand

Basic economic theory posits that alcohol prices represent an equilibrium between the demand for alcoholic beverages and their supply or their availability through retailers (Pindyck *et al.* 1989). Reduced supply with a constant demand, or increased demand with a constant supply, will result in higher prices. In a similar manner, increased supply with a constant demand, or decreased demand with a constant supply, will result in lower prices. It is also the case that deliberate changes in prices will affect supply-and-demand relationships. Alcoholic beverage prices that are increased through means external to market forces, such as heavier alcohol excise duties, will reduce alcohol consumption, as consumers can only afford a smaller amount of drinking with higher prices.

In order to generate more revenue, a state may impose or increase alcohol excise duties, or increase the price of alcoholic beverages in some other way, to obtain more financial gain from each unit sold. Increased excise duty rates usually lead to increases in alcoholic beverage prices, and the increase in beverage prices usually leads to a reduction in alcohol consumption. If alcohol consumption remains unchanged despite increased tax rates and alcohol prices, the state receives all the new consumer expenditures on alcoholic beverages in the form of new tax revenues. In this example, the demand for alcoholic beverages is not at all responsive to any price change from the increased taxes. In reality, however, this is almost never the case. How responsive the demand for alcoholic beverages is to increases or decreases in price will determine how the change in price will affect alcohol consumption.

Economists use the term **price elasticity of demand** when measuring the sensitivity of consumption to changes in price. The price elasticity of demand is defined as the percentage change in consumption resulting from a 1% change in price. For example, price elasticity for alcohol of −0.5 implies that a 1% increase in its price would reduce alcohol consumption by 0.5%. If the price elasticity of demand has a value between zero and −1.0, the demand for a commodity is said to be inelastic with respect to its own price, as a change in its price results in a relatively smaller change in its consumption. With values below −1.0, the demand is said to be **price elastic**, as the change in its price leads to a proportionally greater change in its consumption. Obviously, commodities with very inelastic demand are the best alternatives for the purposes of revenue generation. As will be discussed later in this chapter, the demand for alcoholic beverages is often inelastic. However, a rise in price will produce some reduction in consumption even if the commodity is **price inelastic**, so long as the value is not zero or higher.

The responsiveness of alcohol consumption to its price affects not only the efficiency with which special alcohol taxes generate revenue, but also the potential health benefits to be reaped from higher alcohol prices. Highly elastic demand for alcohol would indicate more than proportionate decreases in alcohol use relative to increases in its price, suggesting that substantial health benefits may accrue with higher alcohol prices, assuming a monotonic positive relationship between overall alcohol consumption and related problems. As the elasticity value nears zero, these benefits decrease, and if it reaches zero, additional health benefits from increased alcohol prices are eliminated. Thus, though revenue generation and reduced alcohol problems are different goals with somewhat different relations to increases in alcohol prices, they can be optimized with respect to one another by how alcohol taxes are set and changed.

8.4 **Taxing alcoholic beverages**

Alcoholic beverages are viewed as especially suitable commodities for taxation because of their detrimental social and public health consequences. In many countries, alcohol taxation systems incorporate varying tax rates for different beverage categories. Usually, this entails higher tax rates per litre of alcohol for distilled spirits than for wine or beer, reflecting particular concerns relating to spirits consumption but also the fact that production and distribution costs per centilitre of alcohol are lower for distilled spirits than for wine and beer. Therefore, similar alcohol excise duty rates for distilled spirits, beer, and wine would mean that one litre of alcohol would be sold cheaper in the form of distilled spirits than in the form of wine or beer.

In some countries, very-low-alcohol content beverages have been taxed at very low rates (or not taxed as alcohol at all), to encourage their consumption ahead of higher-alcohol alternatives. Similarly, a number of countries have imposed special taxes on '**alcopops**' (premixed sweetened beverages) following concerns about their popularity with young drinkers. Except to the extent that the state requires otherwise, producers, wholesalers and retailers remain free to set prices to compete with each other, including considerable price differentiation between quality classes. In some places, price fixing and minimum pricing requirements are also allowed or imposed, which restrict pricing choices in the alcohol market. In Canada, for instance, minimum price levels set by the provinces of Quebec and Ontario for beer have been justified as contributing to public health and order (Giesbrecht *et al.* 2006).

In many countries real prices for alcoholic beverages have declined substantially since 1950 (e.g. Leppänen *et al.* 2001; Österberg and Karlsson 2003; Cook 2007). This trend has continued in recent years, with a review of alcohol prices relative to disposable income in Europe demonstrating increases in the affordability of alcohol between 1996 and 2004 in nineteen of the twenty countries examined (Rabinovich *et al.* 2009). A major cause of this decline is that excise duties are commonly set as a fixed amount of the local currency, so that inflation automatically reduces their value, unless there is new legislation to set a new tax level. A solution to the tendency of inflation to reduce the tax rate in real terms is to provide that the tax rate is tied to a cost-of-living index, rising and falling with it, rather than being set at a fixed value. This is the case in Australia, where alcohol excise duty rates are adjusted every six months in line with the Consumer Price Index (Australian Tax Office 2006).

8.5 Investigating and interpreting elasticity values

The effect of price changes on alcohol consumption has been more extensively investigated than any other potential alcohol control measure. Econometric methods have been the most common tool used to study these effects. Three recent reviews of published studies have attempted to summarize systematically the results of the econometric studies that have examined this issue (Fogarty 2006; Gallet 2007; Wagenaar *et al.* 2009b). Across these three reviews, studies have been identified from the following countries: Austria, Australia, Belgium, Canada, China, Cyprus, Denmark, Finland, France, Germany, Greece, India, Ireland, Italy, Japan, Kenya, The Netherlands, New Zealand, Norway, Poland, Portugal, Spain, Sweden, the UK, and the USA. Among this list, the majority of the studies come from Canada, the USA, the UK and the Nordic countries, indicating that information about the effects of changing alcohol prices on alcohol consumption chiefly derives from the developed countries.

All three reviews find similar results: alcohol demand is price responsive, inelastic and varies between beverage categories. Overall, total alcohol has an average short-run price elasticity of approximately –0.5, beer has an average elasticity of around –0.4 and both wine and spirits have an average elasticity of around –0.7 (see Table 8.1). A further large-scale study too recent to be included in these systematic reviews focused on the relationship between the affordability of alcohol (incorporating changes in both price and disposable income) in twenty European countries between 1996 and 2003, finding that alcohol had an affordability elasticity of 0.32 in the long term (Rabinovich *et al.* 2009). These results suggest that a 10% increase in the affordability of alcohol would result in a 3.2% increase in alcohol consumption.

The overall similarities in the results presented in the reviews conceal substantial variation between the results of the underlying studies, with considerable deviation in own-price elasticities both between countries and over time. Fogarty (2006) focused

Table 8.1 Elasticities reported in three meta-analyses of alcohol price and consumption

Report	Median price elasticity			
	Alcohol	Wine	Beer	Spirits
Fogarty (2006)	NA	−0.77	−0.38	−0.70
Gallet (2007)	−0.52	−0.70	−0.36	−0.68
Wagenaar et al. (2009b)	−0.51	−0.69	−0.46	−0.80

NA, not applicable.

on variation across countries, finding no specific country effects—instead demonstrating that elasticity is related to market share. In other words, in a society in which beer is the dominant alcoholic beverage, beer will be relatively inelastic, while wine and spirits will be less inelastic. This finding, combined with the fact that the majority of studies of alcohol price elasticity have come from beer-drinking countries, may explain the consistently lower price elasticity of beer found in the reviews discussed above. This suggests that the dominant beverage in each culture is treated more as a basic dietary requirement like bread and is thus less responsive to changes in price than the other beverages, which are treated more as luxuries or beverages not belonging to everyday diet (Österberg 1995; Leppänen et al. 2001). This is illustrated in Table 8.2, which shows the results of three Swedish studies of price elasticity. Spirits were the least price-elastic beverage in Sweden in the first half of the twentieth century when they were the most commonly drunk beverage. In the period from 1960 to 1986, both beer and spirits were much less price elastic than wine, reflecting the increasingly regular use of beer by Swedes. Finally, in the more recent study, beverage-specific price elasticities have evened out, reflecting the recent increases in the popularity of wine.

The variation in the effect of price on alcohol consumption between countries is demonstrated by the results of a European study undertaken by Leppänen et al. (2001), which are reproduced in Table 8.3. These results show clear variation between countries, with price having substantially less effect on consumption in the wine-producing countries (e.g. France, Italy, Spain, Portugal) in which wine is used more as a regular commodity consumed with meals.

Both Fogarty (2006) and Gallet (2007) explore the variation in elasticity estimates over time, suggesting that alcohol has become less price elastic in recent years. Further evidence that alcohol price elasticities have decreased over time comes from Finland

Table 8.2 Variation in alcohol price elasticity over time in Sweden

Period	Beer elasticity	Spirits elasticity	Wine elasticity	Source
1920–1951	−1.2	−0.5	−1.6	Bryding and Rosén (1969)
1968–1986	−0.4	−0.2	−0.9	Selvanathan (1991)
1984–2004	−0.9	−0.8	−0.6	Norström (2005)

Table 8.3 Variation in 1980 alcohol price elasticity between countries

Country	Alcohol price elasticity
Austria	−0.17
Belgium	−0.43
Denmark	−0.50
Finland	−0.86
France	−0.12
Greece	−0.17
Ireland	−0.62
Italy	−0.14
Netherlands	−0.52
Norway	−1.15
Portugal	−0.16
Spain	−0.13
Sweden	−0.97
UK	−0.63

Source: Leppänen *et al.* (2001).

(Ahtola *et al.* 1986) and the UK (Mazzocchi 2006). This trend could reflect increasing affluence, although it has also been suggested that elasticity may be lower when *per capita* consumption is higher (Holder and Edwards 1995). In addition, studies have suggested that the effects of price on consumption vary depending on the other alcohol control measures in place. Huitfeldt and Jorner (1972) found that the lifting of the Bratt rationing system in Sweden in 1955 made alcohol more price elastic. Similarly, in the USA, Trolldal and Ponicki (2005) found that alcohol was generally less price elastic in states with restrictive alcohol controls, and Laixuthai and Chaloupka *et al.* (1993) found that the effect of price on youth alcohol consumption decreased following the increase in the minimum legal drinking age to 21 years.

The few studies outside of the developed world suggest broadly similar relationships, with two studies from India estimating that the price elasticity of alcohol was between −0.4 (John 2005) and −1.0 (Musgrave and Stern 1988) and a study of beer demand in Turkey estimating beer price elasticity at −0.37 (Özgüven 2004). Studies in Africa have produced a variety of results. In Kenya, Partanen (1991) estimated western-style beer elasticity at −0.33 in the short run and −1.00 in the long run, while more recent analyses of Kenyan data (Okello 2001) examined traditional or other local brews and market beer (non-traditional beer), and found higher long-run elasticities of −1.11 and −5.49 respectively. In Tanzania, Osoro *et al.* (2001) found little difference between traditional and non-traditional beers, with elasticities of −0.44 and −0.31 respectively. Selvanathan and Selvanathan (2005a) used national accounts data to estimate alcohol price elasticity for 43 countries, resulting in a range of estimates from −0.014 (Belgium) to −1.422 (Puerto Rico). When the results are divided into developed and developing countries (24 and 19 respectively), the mean alcohol price elasticity estimates are −0.442 and −0.568, suggesting on the average similar price effects in the developing and developed world (Selvanathan and Selvanathan 2005a).

The econometric literature summarized above focuses on the effects of gradual price changes over long time periods or cross-sectional differences between regions. Only a few studies have examined the effects of abrupt changes in alcohol prices. The most dramatic natural experiment comes from Denmark in 1917, where spirits prices were increased by a factor of twelve and beer prices almost doubled due to tax changes in a situation of shortages during World War I. These price increases had immediate effects, with alcohol consumption falling by three-quarters within two years (Bruun *et al.* 1975a). Examining these changes, Skog and Melberg (2006) estimated spirits price elasticity at −0.5. Similarly, Kendell *et al.* (1983) found that an increase of around 11% in the price of alcohol (relative to other goods) in Scotland reduced total alcohol consumption among a sample of regular drinkers by around 15%, although the analysis failed to control for regression to the mean and thus may have overstated the effect. More recently, decreased import duties on spirits in Switzerland resulted in a reduction in the price of imported spirits of between 30% and 50%, although domestically produced spirits did not change much in price (Heeb *et al.* 2003). Two studies examining the results of these changes found significant increases in spirits consumption. Heeb *et al.* (2003) found that spirits consumption had increased by around 30% three months after the price changes, and a later follow-up by Kuo *et al.* (2003a) found a 40% increase. On the other hand, Mäkelä *et al.* (2008) and Mäkelä and Österberg (2009) present a summary of the impacts of alcohol tax decreases (along with increased traveller's allowances) in Denmark and Finland. The tax changes were limited to spirits in Denmark, but affected all beverage categories in Finland. Analysis of individual-level data from a panel study found no detectable increase in consumption in either Finland or Denmark following the tax changes. According to aggregate level estimates, spirits consumption increased in Denmark, but overall consumption fell. In Finland total alcohol consumption increased by 10% (Mäkelä and Österberg 2009).

The considerable variation in elasticity values, including some instances where changes in taxes apparently had little or no effect, provides a caution that predictions of effects based on past studies are always conditioned on *ceteris paribus*: other things being equal. Some conditions which can change elasticity values are discussed above (e.g. whether the supply is rationed) and below (e.g. the extent of affluence in the society). Structural and cultural changes in a society are among the other factors which could influence the effect of a change in taxes on consumption (Room *et al.* 2009). Variation in the elasticity between countries is highly influenced by the cultural role of alcohol within societies, with cultures in which alcohol is more of a luxury likely to see larger price effects on consumption than cultures where alcohol is a more everyday product. By themselves, elasticity values thus give general guidance on what is to be expected, rather than an exact prediction.

8.6 Differential prices by beverage

As already mentioned, governments have often used differential taxation as a means to favour one beverage type over another. The most common differentiation has been a higher tax rate per unit of alcohol for strong spirits drinks. Such a differentiation contributed to all of the Nordic countries eventually changing from spirits-drinking to beer-drinking countries in the course of the twentieth century—a change which is viewed in present-day Russia, for instance, as desirable from a public health perspective (Treisman 2008). Mäkelä *et al.* (2007) reviewed the association between consumption of particular types of alcohol and alcohol-related harm. They found that, while spirits are more likely to be associated with alcohol poisonings than other beverages, in general the level of harm for a given amount of alcohol did not vary much between beverage types. On the other hand, they found evidence that the consumption of spirits was associated with higher overall alcohol consumption, and thus worthwhile discouraging through higher pricing. While the amount and pattern of alcohol consumption are more important than the form of alcohol for most alcohol problems, there are some problems particularly associated with strong beverages, notably alcohol overdose deaths.

In a similar vein, some governments have attempted to encourage substitution of low-alcohol beverages for higher-alcohol alternatives via tax concessions. In Sweden, for instance, no alcohol tax is charged on beer of 2.8% alcohol by volume or lower (Olsson *et al.* 2002), and in Australia, the first 1.15% of alcohol in beer is not taxed, thereby favouring weaker beer (Econtech 2004). A study in Norway (Skog 1988) examined how the introduction of cheaper low-alcohol beer influenced overall consumption, finding some evidence that it was consumed in place of stronger beer. In Australia, state-level taxes were considerably lower for low- and mid-strength beer until 1997, when state alcohol taxes were ruled illegal. This, combined with the lower federal excise rates for light beer, led to significant price advantages for low-alcohol beer and resulted in substantial substitution from higher-alcohol products to light beer, and thus a reduction in the amount of alcohol consumed as beer (Stockwell and Crosbie 2001), although a small experimental study of on-premises drinking found that providing cheap low-alcohol beverages had little impact on the overall level of consumption (Mugford 1984). There is thus some evidence that increased prices for high-alcohol beverages and decreased prices for low-alcohol beverages can result in reductions in the total amount of alcohol consumed and thus reductions in alcohol-related problems.

In recent years, there has been growing concern about the role of alcopops, also known as premixed spirits, ready-to-drink spirits, or designer drinks, in youth alcohol consumption and related harms (Sutton and Nylander 1999). There is some evidence that the sweet taste of these drinks is attractive to young people (Copeland *et al.* 2007) and that the marketing of them has targeted youth (Jackson *et al.* 2000), although in a review of the literature Metzner and Kraus (2008) found little evidence that alcopops were any more problematic than other alcoholic beverages. In recent years a number of countries have increased taxes on alcopops in attempts to reduce risky drinking, particularly among young people (Metzner and Kraus 2008). Studies in Germany (Deutsche Bundesregierung 2005) and Switzerland (Niederer *et al.* 2008) found substantial reductions in consumption of these beverages, although similar reductions in Austria without an accompanying tax increase raise some doubts about causality (Uhl 2007). Early evidence in Australia suggests that a recent increase in the excise duty on alcopops has resulted in substantial reductions in sales of these beverages and an overall reduction in total alcohol consumption (Chikritzhs *et al.* 2009). Thus, the evidence suggests that increases in the price of alcopops result in reductions in consumption of these beverages. However, there is no evidence available regarding the effect of these changes on measures of alcohol-related harm.

Focusing price-related interventions on particular beverages makes cross-beverage substitution an important issue. If taxes are raised on a particular type of beverage, do drinkers simply transfer their drinking to a different beverage, or is an actual reduction in consumption achieved? There have been no systematic reviews of cross-price elasticities between alcohol beverage categories, and most studies have focused on gradual price changes over time or price changes in different regions. Selvanathan and Selvanathan (2005b) examined cross-price elasticities in ten developed countries over more than 30 years, finding significant but low cross-price elasticities, suggesting that consumers do shift their consumption between beverages when prices change, but that substitution is not total. This finding has been supported in a number of other econometric studies (Okello 2001; Osoro *et al.* 2001; Özgüven 2004; Ramful and Zhao 2008), although not consistently, with some studies finding no evidence of a substitution effect (Godfrey 1988; Huang 2003; Mangeloja and Pehkonen 2009). No study has found complete substitution between beverage types following price changes.

As with estimates of own-price elasticities, studies of beverage substitution have generally used econometric methods and have focused on gradual price changes, with few studies examining the impacts of large changes in beverage-specific taxes. In the Danish example from 1917 discussed previously, beer consumption increased slightly in response to the huge increase in spirits prices, but overall consumption of alcohol still dropped substantially (Skog and Melberg 2006). In Switzerland, increases in the tax rate on spirits and the corresponding reduction in spirits consumption was not offset by any significant substitution to other beverages (Heeb *et al.* 2003). The issue of beverage substitution has been a key concern in debates over specific alcopop taxes, with suggestions that consumers will simply switch to mixing their own spirits-based drinks. Unfortunately, there have been only limited analyses of the impacts of alcopop taxes, so the degree of substitution remains unclear. Data from Switzerland suggest that the substantial reduction in spirit-based alcopop consumption was largely offset by increases in beer and wine-based alcopop consumption and in consumption of bottled spirits (Niederer *et al.* 2008). Results from Germany are less clear. Initial analyses found very little evidence of beverage substitution (Deutsche Bundesregierung 2005), while a more recent follow-up study suggested that the reduction in alcopop consumption had been offset by increases in beer and spirits consumption. In Australia, the early evidence suggests that the increased alcopop tax has resulted in small increases in consumption of spirits and beer, but an overall decrease in total alcohol consumed (Chikritzhs *et al.* 2009).

Inconsistencies in effects of alcopop taxes may be explained in part by the complexity of the alcohol market. Cross-price elasticities are generally calculated using average prices across broad beverage categories, neglecting the possibility of substitution within a beverage category based on quality or price differences. But studies have demonstrated that consumers have a wide range of prices available to them within beverage categories. In California, Treno *et al.* (1993) showed that even among just the ten most popular products in each beverage category, prices varied by a factor of 60. Furthermore, prices paid for alcoholic beverages bought for on-premises consumption (e.g. at a restaurant or bar) are significantly higher than those paid for alcohol purchased for consumption elsewhere (Donnar and Jakee 2004; Gruenewald *et al.* 2006), so that switching the place of consumption can substantially affect what is paid. Among young adults in many countries, this price disparity has resulted in large amounts of drinking taking place before attending night-time entertainment venues like bars or clubs, and thus often arriving at these venues already intoxicated (e.g. Brunet 2007; Hughes *et al.* 2008; Wells *et al.* 2009). Clearly consumers can offset changes to the price of alcohol in a variety of ways. There has been little research into how price changes affect the amount of alcohol consumed on- and off-premises, although it has been shown in the UK, where more beer is drunk on- than off-premises (Huang 2003), that on-premises beer consumption is substantially less price-responsive than off-premises consumption and that there is significant substitution between the two. In terms of quality substitution, Gruenewald *et al.* (2006) demonstrate that consumers respond to price changes both by substituting between beverage categories and by substituting different quality products within beverage categories. In particular, their results demonstrate that price changes at the cheapest end of the price spectrum are the most likely to result in reduced levels of consumption, suggesting a government-set minimum price may be the most effective way of ensuring price increases result in decreased consumption.

It is also worth noting that there are substantial differences between prices of recorded and unrecorded alcohol consumption in many parts of the world, with unrecorded consumption an important part of the market particularly in the developing regions (cf. Table 3.1). To the extent that existing capabilities for home production and smuggling can respond rapidly to price changes, elasticity values of commercial alcohol beverages may be affected. For example, Andrienko and Nemtsov (2005) estimate that total vodka consumption in present-day Russia is unaffected by price changes, with substitution to moonshine replacing retail vodka purchases when prices increase. Similarly, studies in Africa report high levels of cross-price elasticity between market beer and locally brewed (and often untaxed) beer, suggesting that increases in market beer prices produced substantial increases in consumption of local beer. In Zimbabwe, an increase in alcohol taxes was quickly rescinded following a net drop in taxation revenue due to cheap and readily available illegal alcohol supplies (Jernigan 1999). Similarly, tax changes in one country can influence cross-border purchases of alcohol. For example, Asplund *et al.* (2007) show that tax reductions on spirits in Denmark by 45% in 2003 reduced spirits sales in Sweden by around 2%.

Consistent with the strong evidence that changes in alcohol prices overall result in changes in alcohol consumption and related harms, there is also reasonable evidence that interventions focused on the prices of specific beverage categories can be effective. In particular, policies which result in very-low-alcohol products (e.g. low-alcohol beer) being sold at relatively low prices and high-alcohol products at particularly high prices are likely to reduce the total amount of pure alcohol consumed and thus reduce alcohol-related harm. In addition, there is good evidence that increases in alcohol prices result in substitution towards cheaper forms of alcohol, suggesting that increases in price at the lower end of the price spectrum (e.g. increases in the minimum price of alcohol) are likely to be among the most effective ways of reducing consumption.

8.7 Discounting and minimum pricing

The discounting of alcoholic beverages has raised concerns in a number of ways. In on-premises settings, alcohol discounting usually takes the form of 'happy hours', periods of time in which alcohol is sold at low prices. There is some evidence that these kinds of promotions increase alcohol consumption. Experimental studies by Babor *et al.* (1978, 1980) found that consumption of alcohol doubled during happy hours, while an ecological study by Kuo *et al.* (2003b) found associations between binge-drinking rates of college students and the number of discount alcohol promotions near their residence. Two studies by Thombs and colleagues demonstrate significant associations between patron intoxication and drink specials, particularly 'all-you-can-drink' specials (Thombs *et al.* 2008, 2009). Similarly, Van Hoof *et al.* (2008) found some self-reported associations between happy-hour specials and higher levels of alcohol consumption among teenagers in The Netherlands. While a number of jurisdictions have restricted or banned happy-hour style promotions, there has been little research into the effects of these restrictions. Smart and Adlaf (1986) and Smart (1996b) have examined the impact of happy-hour bans in Canada and the USA, finding little impact in terms of consumption levels or alcohol-related motor vehicle accidents, although neither study had a strong design.

In off-premises settings, particularly when sold in chain grocery stores, alcohol is often heavily discounted to encourage people into a store, acting as a loss leader. In the UK, the use of alcohol products as loss leaders has been widespread, with grocery stores regularly selling alcohol at below-cost prices (SHAAP 2007). In response to these practices, the Scottish government has announced the intention to introduce minimum pricing of alcohol (Scottish Government 2009). As discussed above, Gruenewald *et al.* (2006) have shown that changes in the price of the cheapest alcohol products have the most impact on consumption, suggesting that setting a minimum alcohol price could be an effective method for reducing alcohol-related harm. Although minimum pricing (or floor pricing) has been implemented in some jurisdictions (e.g. see Giesbrecht *et al.* 2006 for a discussion of floor pricing in Quebec and Ontario), there has been almost no research into its impact on consumption or harm. Some remote Australian communities have banned the sale of large wine casks, the cheapest form of alcohol, a policy that amounts to a *de facto* increase in the minimum price of alcohol. Evaluations in these communities have generally found reductions in overall harm, but at the same time significant substitution of fortified wines, the next cheapest beverage, has also been observed (Hogan *et al.* 2006). Despite the lack of research in this area, a complex modelling process using data from England and Wales suggests that minimum prices for a standard unit of alcohol would be one of the most effective ways to reduce alcohol-related problems (Meier *et al.* 2008b).

8.8 Income, economic conditions and alcohol consumption

While the focus of this chapter is on alcohol taxation and pricing, economic theory suggests that broader economic conditions will also have an impact on alcohol consumption. It is well established that alcohol consumption increases with income (see Gallet 2007 for a review of income elasticities), and that alcohol consumption at the aggregate level is generally pro-cyclical. In other words, drinking rises when the economy booms and declines during economic recessions (Ruhm 1995; Freeman 2001; Ruhm and Black 2002; Krüger and Svensson 2008), although some studies have found that problematic drinking is counter-cyclical (Dee 2001; Johansson *et al.* 2006). By contrast, there has been little examination of how the impacts of price changes vary depending on levels of prosperity.

Selvanathan and Selvanathan's study (2005a), already referred to above, found that the income elasticity of alcohol was substantially higher in developing than in developed countries, providing some evidence that prices are most effective at reducing consumption when aggregate income is low, as proposed earlier in this chapter. Even at the individual level there has been little examination of the differences in alcohol price elasticity by socio-economic status. It has often been suggested that alcohol taxes are regressive, that is, they have greater fiscal impact on the poor than on the rich. There remains some debate around the extent of this disparity, with studies from New Zealand (Ashton *et al.* 1989), five African countries (Younger 1993; Younger and Sahn 1999) and Russia (Decoster 2005) finding little evidence of regressive effects of alcohol taxes, in part because abstention from alcohol is more common among the poor. However, there is good evidence from the USA (Lyon and Schwab 1995) and Australia (Webb 2006) that alcohol taxation is proportionally more demanding for poorer households. Even if alcohol taxes are fiscally regressive, increased taxes may reduce overall inequalities through more substantial health impacts on economically disadvantaged people, as Kotakorpi (2008) demonstrates theoretically (using a tax on unhealthy food as an example). This reduction in health inequalities depends on the poor altering their consumption more than the rich when prices change. In a study of the effect of an increase in the price of alcohol on regular drinkers (Kendell *et al.* 1983), those with lower incomes reduced their consumption more markedly than those earning more money. Similarly, another study (Sutton and Godfrey 1995) found that alcohol consumption was more price-responsive among people with lower income levels. More recently, studies from Finland found no systematic difference across income groups in the effect of a spirits tax reduction on alcohol consumption (Mäkelä *et al.* 2008), but substantially greater increases in alcohol-related mortality among less privileged people (Herttua *et al.* 2008).

8.9 Price elasticities for particular groups of drinkers

In econometric studies based on time-series data, the price-elasticity values reflect the average reactions of consumers to changes in prices. This treatment of consumers as one group has raised political concerns about the relevance of price elasticity estimates in alcohol policymaking. One example of these concerns is the disagreement in the literature on whether heavy drinkers are responsive to changes in alcohol prices.

In response to these issues, a growing literature examines the effects of alcohol taxes and price on individual measures of alcohol consumption (typically by means of surveys) in an attempt to ascertain how price changes affect consumption among particular subgroups of drinkers. In their review, Wagenaar *et al.* (2009b) found that studies based on individual-level data generally produce smaller elasticity estimates than aggregate studies, largely because of the greater variability in data at the individual level.

There is a substantial body of literature, predominantly from the USA, examining the impact of alcohol price on young drinkers, with youth-specific studies consistently finding that changes in alcohol price were related to changes in youth drinking (see Grossman *et al.* 1994 and Chaloupka *et al.* 2002 for reviews). Gallet (2007) included 13 studies of young adult drinking in his meta-regression, with a median price-elasticity of −0.39, slightly less elastic than adult consumption. Two studies based on longitudinal survey data found that alcohol taxes reduced youth alcohol consumption particularly among more frequent young drinkers (Coate and Grossman 1988; Laixuthai and Chaloupka 1993). Some studies have shown that price increases reduce heavy episodic or binge drinking among youth (Williams *et al.* 2005), although Chaloupka and Wechsler (1996) found that this effect was not significant for males in their college student sample. Outside of the USA, the decreases in spirits taxation in Switzerland discussed previously were shown to particularly increase consumption by young male drinkers (Heeb *et al.* 2003). Whereas these general findings seem robust, several studies have not supported the role of alcohol taxes in reducing youth consumption. Dee (1999) found no effect for beer taxes on drinking among high-school seniors, while Saffer and Dave (2006) found significant price effects on consumption among the same sample but not on the drinking of a sample of 12–16-year-olds. Nelson (2008b) examined the impact of beer taxes on consumption among youth, young adults, and adults, finding that the amount of state beer tax was not significantly related either to drinking prevalence or to binge drinking, once state-level fixed effects and other alcohol control policies were controlled for. At least some of these disparities may be due to the ways in which price is measured in these studies, with proxies such as beer taxes shown to be quite poor measures of actual price (Young and Bielinska-Kwapisz 2002).

The extent to which adult heavy and problematic drinkers are responsive to changes in alcohol prices has been the subject of a relatively small number of studies. Manning *et al.* (1995) argued that they are not, at least for the very heaviest consumers, but with an analysis using cross-sectional data, which is weak in terms of causal inference. In a later study using longitudinal data, Farrell *et al.* (2003) examined the relationship between alcohol prices and three dimensions of alcohol misuse—heavy consumption, physical and other consequences of drinking, and increased salience of drinking—finding that both heavy drinking and consequences of drinking were significantly related to alcohol price, with elasticities of −1.325 and −1.895 respectively. Heeb *et al.* (2003) studied the impacts of the spirits tax reduction in Switzerland three months after its introduction, finding that the subsequent increases in consumption were predominantly confined to low- and medium-volume drinkers. Over four waves of panel data, Gmel *et al.* (2008) found that heavier drinkers increased their consumption more sharply in the short term, but declined to pre-tax change levels in the longer term. Recent reductions in alcohol taxes in the Nordic countries have also been examined using panel data, with little evidence that heavy drinkers reacted differently than lighter drinkers (Mäkelä *et al.* 2008; Ripatti and Mäkelä 2008). However, studies of the effects of tax changes on problem indicators, reviewed in the next section, provide much stronger evidence that changes in taxes do influence rates of problem drinking.

8.10 **Alcohol prices and problems related to alcohol use**

Whereas alcohol sales data are not routinely available for subgroups of the population, measures of alcohol-related problems are often more specific. These include statistics on morbidity and mortality focusing on alcohol-related liver disease, traffic accidents, violence, and suicide. Thus, one way to study the effects of price policy on heavy drinkers is to examine harmful outcomes related to heavy use, such as cirrhosis mortality (Cook and Tauchen 1982). One benefit of this approach is that it takes into account the possible substitution of recorded alcohol consumption by unrecorded alcohol consumption like homemade or privately imported alcoholic beverages (see Nordlund and Österberg 2000).

Studies of cirrhosis mortality have found that tax increases reduce mortality and thus impact on the consumption of the heaviest drinkers in society (Cook 1981; Cook and Tauchen 1982; Seeley 1988; Cook 2007). Similarly, Skog and Melberg's (2006) analysis of the effects of the huge increases in alcohol taxes in Denmark in 1917 found that rates of mortality for delirium tremens were reduced substantially. In the USA Markowitz *et al.* (2003) examined suicide rates between 1976 and 1999, finding that male suicide rates, particularly among young adults, were reduced by increases in the beer tax. In Finland, the recent reduction in alcohol taxation had a substantial effect on alcohol-related sudden deaths, with an estimated increase of 17% in mortality following the tax change (Koski *et al.* 2007), while a study of all alcohol-related mortality found a 16% increase among males and a 32% increase among females, with a particular concentration among those in lower socio-economic groups (Herttua *et al.* 2008). In addition, criminality and hospitalizations increased in Finland following the tax decrease (Mäkelä and Österberg 2009). A recent study in Alaska (Wagenaar *et al.* 2009a) found that alcohol excise tax increases in 1983 and 2002 were each associated with substantial reductions in alcohol-related disease mortality. These effects immediately followed the excise increases and were sustained over the entire study period, resulting in reductions in alcohol-related mortality of between 11% and 29% (see Figure 8.1).

The 'Living With Alcohol' programme in the Northern Territory (Australia) involved a small levy on alcoholic drinks >3% alcohol by volume. The money collected by means of this *de facto* tax was then used to fund a variety of alcohol harm reduction programmes. A rigorous evaluation of the programme found that the combination of the price increase and the programme implementation significantly reduced acute alcohol-related mortality, whereas the effect did not persist when the levy was removed. A reduction in chronic mortality was also found, but this effect did

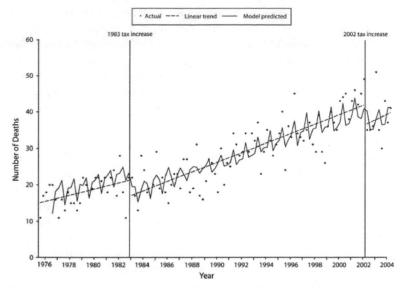

Fig. 8.1 Rate of quarterly alcohol-related disease mortality per 100 000 population aged ≥15 years: Alaska, 1976–2004. Reproduced from Wagenaar (2009a), with permission.

not appear until six years after the programme commenced, making it difficult to assign causality (Chikritzhs *et al.* 2005). Ohsfeldt and Morrisey (1997) focused on workplace accidents in the USA between 1975 and 1985, finding that an increase of 10% in beer taxes would have resulted in 1.7% fewer workdays lost through injuries.

A substantial body of literature has examined the links between alcohol taxes, alcoholic beverage prices, and road traffic accidents, predominantly in the USA. One study (Cook 1981) found that states that had increased their alcohol taxes between 1960 and 1975 experienced less than average increases in road traffic fatalities. Advances in econometrics and data availability allowed subsequent researchers to combine cross-sectional and longitudinal data into single studies, controlling for the impacts of other alcohol and traffic policies. These cross-sectional time-series analyses have found significant relationships between taxes and fatality rates for both youth (Saffer and Grossman 1987a) and the general population (Saffer and Grossman 1987a; Evans *et al.* 1991; Ruhm 1996), although some studies have found inconsistent or non-significant relationships (Dee 1999; Mast *et al.* 1999; Young and Likens 2000). Young and Bielinska-Kwapisz (2006) suggest that these inconsistencies may be due to differences in measures used to represent the price of alcohol, which vary from using just the beer tax to the use of estimates of the average price of alcohol. Using advanced statistical models to study the links between taxation rates, prices and traffic fatalities, their work shows a significant negative relationship between the price of alcohol and traffic deaths. Other recent studies have produced reasonably consistent findings. McCarthy (2003) used 18 years of data from California, finding that crashes were more related to alcohol prices when younger drivers were involved, although the effect of price was still significant for drivers aged ≥60 years. Similarly, Eisenberg (2003) found that beer taxes were most strongly related to crashes involving young people (aged ≤21 years) and to crashes that occur on weekends at night. Ponicki *et al.* (2007) examined data from 48 US states between 1975 and 2001, finding that alcohol prices were significantly related to youth traffic fatalities, although this effect had diminished somewhat since the introduction of the minimum legal drinking age of 21 years. There has been very little research in this area outside the USA, with Adrian *et al.* (2001) in Canada and Arranz and Gil (2008) in Spain finding significantly negative relationships between alcohol prices and traffic accidents.

Several studies have examined the impact of the price of alcoholic beverages on homicides and other crimes, including rape, robbery, assaults, motor vehicle thefts, domestic violence, and child abuse (Cook and Moore 1993; Markowitz and Grossman 1998; Grossman and Markowitz 1999; Markowitz 2000; Markowitz and Grossman 2000; Chaloupka *et al.* 2002; Sen 2006; Sivarajasingam *et al.* 2006). These studies suggest that raising the price of alcohol is likely to result in a reduction in violence. Finally, there is a growing literature linking alcohol regulation and sexually transmitted diseases, with a number of studies in the USA finding significant relationships between alcohol taxation rates and rates of gonorrhoea (Chesson *et al.* 2000; Grossman *et al.* 2004; Markowitz *et al.* 2005).

A review of studies focusing on the direct link between alcohol taxation and alcohol-related harms identified twenty-two studies in this area (Meier *et al.* 2008a). The review concluded that there is clear evidence that alcohol taxation is related to alcohol-related harms across the range of outcomes discussed above.

8.11 **Summary**

This chapter has evaluated the role of alcohol prices and taxes as a means to curb total alcohol consumption and alcohol-related problems. Dozens of studies conducted in both the developed and developing countries have demonstrated that alcohol prices do have an effect on the level of alcohol consumption and related problems, including mortality rates, crime and traffic accidents. Consumers of alcoholic beverages respond to changes in alcohol prices, and the evidence suggests that this applies to all groups of drinkers, including young people and heavy or problem drinkers.

Apart from tax rates, some governments have used other means to influence price, such as establishing minimum sale prices or restricting discounted sales in order to reduce rates of alcohol problems. Although somewhat limited, the evidence suggests that raising the minimum price of the cheapest beverages is especially effective in influencing heavy drinkers, and in reducing rates of harm. There is little evidence that limiting or banning periods of discounted sales in on-premises drinking establishments (happy hours) has any impact on consumption or harm at the aggregate level.

There are only preliminary evaluations of recent attempts to reduce alcohol-related harm among young people by increasing the price of premixed drinks (alcopops). There is reasonable evidence that increasing the price of premixed drinks can reduce the consumption of these beverages, but there remains uncertainty about the extent of substitution to other beverages. There have been no studies assessing whether increasing the prices of premixed drinks has had an impact on levels of alcohol-related harm among young people.

Despite the apparent effectiveness of measures to influence price, the real price of alcoholic beverages has decreased in many countries during the last decades, at a time when other alcohol control measures have been liberalized or abandoned completely. A major reason for this price decline has been the failure of governments to increase tax levels in accordance with inflation and rising standards of living. On the contrary, in some cases alcohol taxes have been reduced to compete with cross-border smuggling and imports, or as required by trade dispute decisions (see Chapter 6).

Alcohol taxes are thus an attractive instrument of alcohol policy, as they can be used both to generate direct revenue for the state and to reduce alcohol-related harms. Even setting aside their contribution to government revenue, they are among the most cost-effective ways for a government to reduce alcohol-related harm in both developed and developing countries (Chisholm *et al.* 2004; Collins and Lapsley 2008; Anderson *et al.* 2009a). The most important downside to raising alcohol taxes is the possibility of potential alternatives or substitutions to taxed alcoholic beverages, particularly in terms of illegal smuggling or illegal in-country alcohol production. The net effects of taxation and price increases, however, are to reduce alcohol use and related problems.

Chapter 9

Regulating the physical availability of alcohol

9.1 **Introduction**

This chapter reviews the scientific evidence on limiting the physical availability of beverage alcohol as an approach to reducing alcohol consumption and problems. We consider alcohol in terms of its availability both as a retail product and as beverage obtained through social sources. In general, availability refers to the ease or convenience of obtaining alcohol. Availability policies are based on the assumption that easier access to alcohol increases overall consumption in a population, which, in turn, increases alcohol problems. Restricting alcohol availability through law is a key policy in many parts of the world (Kortteinen 1989; WHO 2004b) and has a long history as a means of controlling alcohol problems. For example, the Code of Hammurabi, dating from 3800 years ago, included three articles governing the behaviour of tavern-keepers and their customers in Mesopotamia (Hammurabi 2000).

The retail markets that make alcoholic beverages available to people can be described as either formal or informal. Formal alcohol markets are regulated by government, whether at the community level or at the regional or national levels. The special regulation of alcoholic beverage sales often reflects social concerns about health, safety, and public order; it includes general limits on opening hours, days for retail sales, the placement and location of retail markets, who may purchase alcohol, and how alcohol can be advertised and promoted (which is discussed in Chapter 12).

Informal markets provide alcohol largely through unregulated social and commercial networks (e.g. through home production and distribution and sale of alcohol). Informal alcohol markets are a relatively small part of total consumption in most of the developed world, though their importance has grown in Europe (Moskalewicz 2000; Leifman 2001). In developing countries, informal retail markets are important, accounting in some places for as much as 90% of total consumption (Room *et al.* 2002).

Social availability of alcohol refers to access through non-commercial social networks, including acquaintances, friends, relatives, and strangers. Social sources for alcohol may be particularly important for underage youth. Thus, a study of more than 10 000 schoolchildren under the legal drinking age in England (Bellis *et al.* 2007) concluded that youth tend to obtain alcohol from adults (both family members and strangers), older siblings, and peers as well as from commercial outlets. Although social sources of alcohol often do not entail a direct cost to the drinker, this is not always the case. Adults, for example, may charge minors to purchase alcohol for them or a social host may charge an entrance fee to a party where alcohol is available.

Overall, young and underage drinkers most often obtain alcohol from social sources and are adept at using a wide variety of such sources (Dent *et al.* 2005; Rossow *et al.* 2005; Hearst *et al.* 2007; Paschall *et al.* 2007). As commercial access to alcohol becomes more difficult, social sources may become relatively more important (Paschall *et al.* 2007; Treno *et al.* 2008). Successful strategies to reduce access to alcohol thus need to address both commercial and social availability of alcohol, especially to youth.

9.1.1 Why availability matters

Availability-limitation approaches to prevention attempt to reduce drinking and drinking problems by increasing the economic and opportunity costs associated with obtaining alcohol (Chaloupka *et al.* 2002). Such approaches thus focus on price (see Chapter 8) and on regulating the places, times, and contexts where consumers can obtain alcohol (Gruenewald 2007). The object of such policies is to reduce overall drinking in the population and thus drinking-related problems. In general, research strongly indicates that when alcohol is readily available through commercial or social sources, consumption and associated problems increase. Conversely, when restrictions are placed on availability, alcohol use and associated problems decrease (e.g. Anderson and Baumberg 2006a; Cook 2007; Grube in press). Alcohol availability received considerable attention worldwide during the early part of the twentieth century with the passage of prohibition laws in many countries. In more recent years there has been considerable public discussion in many countries about the advisability of increasing or relaxing restrictions on the retail availability of alcohol, such as that occurring in the EU in the context of harmonizing alcohol trade policies (see Chapter 6). There is, of course, great variability worldwide in policies regulating access to alcohol. A number of countries have monopolies for at least some form of retail sale. For example, in North America, many Canadian provinces and some US states operate monopolies for distilled spirits and sometimes wine. Sweden, among other countries, has a retail monopoly that is intended to regulate availability by such policies as limiting the number of outlets and restricting opening hours. Total prohibition is practiced in many Muslim countries. By contrast, in many developing countries there is concern that availability of alcohol and the alcohol market are largely unregulated (Pinsky and Laranjeira 2007).

9.2 Changes in retail availability

Alcohol availability is often regulated by enacting partial or total bans, restricting hours and days of sale, and controlling the location, type, and **number of retail outlets**. This approach is based upon the assumption that reductions in supply increase the full costs of alcohol and thereby reduce alcohol consumption (Chaloupka *et al.* 2002). That is, as alcohol availability decreases, convenience costs to the consumer increase, and vice versa. Thus physical availability has the potential to influence the consumer's demand for alcoholic beverages as well as the supply.

9.2.1 Total or partial bans

Total prohibition of alcohol sales on a countrywide basis is uncommon in the modern world. All modern countries with total prohibition, such as Saudi Arabia and Iran, are Islamic. Other countries with strong Muslim majorities, such as Pakistan, allow non-Muslims to purchase alcohol. Still others, such as Indonesia, do not have alcohol prohibition even for Muslims. Modern-day prohibition is much more common in subnational jurisdictions. For example, one Indian state, Gujarat, has had prohibition since 1947, and has been joined by other states for shorter periods (Rahman 2002). In Canada and the USA, many First Nations and Native American tribes living on designated lands have implemented total prohibition of alcohol within the boundaries of the reservation. Aboriginal groups in Australia have also applied partial or total bans on alcohol (d'Abbs and Togni 2000; Chikritzhs et al. 2007).

Although prohibition is never completely effective at eliminating alcohol availability, it is clear from historical evaluations of the prohibition periods in North America and the Nordic countries (e.g. Paulson 1973) that total bans on alcohol production and sales can reduce alcohol-related problems. In India, where prohibition has been in force in a number of states, research indicates that overall alcohol consumption decreases substantially when total prohibition is introduced, and that prohibition of *arrack*, the local spirit, reduces its consumption by as much as 76% (Rahman 2002). Thus there is evidence that complete prohibition reduces consumption and alcohol-related problems; however, where there is a substantial demand for alcohol, it may be filled partly by illegal operators. There may be considerable violence associated with the illegal market, as well as other undesired consequences, such as organized crime (Johansen 1994; Österberg and Haavisto 1997). One study (Jensen 2000) found that whereas prohibition in the USA was associated with reduced alcohol consumption, there were also elevated rates of homicide.

Prohibition is easier to enforce in isolated areas, where alcohol imports into the 'dry' (i.e. no-alcohol) area can be effectively controlled. Restrictions have often occurred on islands or in isolated towns or communities that have particularly severe alcohol problems (Brady 2000). For example, when the possession or importation of alcohol was banned in the small Alaskan town of Barrow, the number of outpatient visits for alcohol-related causes fell significantly. When the ban was subsequently lifted, rates of outpatient visits returned to their former levels, falling again with the reintroduction of the prohibition (Chiu et al. 1997). Complete bans on alcohol have also been implemented in some remote Australian communities, usually producing reductions in alcohol-related problems (Chikritzhs et al. 2007). Partial alcohol bans have often been used as an alternative to complete prohibition in remote communities in Australia. These bans typically restrict the sales of cheap cask wine, acting as a *de facto* minimum pricing policy. While there is evidence of significant substitution of the next cheapest beverage type (fortified wines), the prohibitions may have produced some reductions in alcohol-related harm (Chikritzhs et al. 2007; d'Abbs and Togni 2000). An example of a more extensive ban is shown in Box 9.1. Restrictions in remote communities have often been implemented as part of an extensive programme, following widespread community concern relating to alcohol. They seem to be most successful when implemented with full community support (Brady 2000; d'Abbs and Togni 2000). The fact that these total and partial bans often have been implemented as part of more comprehensive community programmes, however, makes it very difficult to attribute the observed reductions in consumption and problems to the restrictions themselves.

Box 9.1 Partial ban on alcohol as a harm reduction measure

In September 2007, the take-away sale of any alcoholic beverage with an alcohol content higher than 2.7% was banned in the small Western Australian town of Fitzroy Crossing. Prior to the restrictions Fitzroy Crossing had particularly high rates of alcohol-related problems and members of the Indigenous community had campaigned strongly for the restrictions. An evaluation of the restrictions found that in the months following the ban, off-premises alcohol sales fell by 88%. In conjunction with this fall in sales, domestic violence incidents dropped by 28% and emergency department presentations fell by 48%. Qualitative and quantitative analyses found little evidence of displacement, with alcohol problems in surrounding towns not increasing notably (Henderson-Yates *et al.* 2008).

For most of the developed world, total prohibition is not a politically acceptable option even if the potential for reducing alcohol problems does exist. However, as described later, bans on alcohol sales for specific persons in the population (e.g. children and adolescents), or in specific circumstances (e.g. at sporting events), have been applied with demonstrated success.

9.2.2 Regulating retail outlets for alcohol

Alcoholic beverages are sold in two ways: either for consumption on the premises, such as at a bar, café or restaurant, or to take away for consumption elsewhere, as in the case of a liquor store or a supermarket. In mature markets for alcohol, both 'on-premises' and 'off-premises' sales are typically regulated through laws on sale of alcohol and **licensing systems**. These laws and policies specify who may sell alcohol, to whom alcohol may be sold (e.g. restricting sales to minors or intoxicated customers), conditions of sale (e.g. purchase quotas or sales over the counter), and days or hours of trading. Regulation of 'on-premises' sales offers additional opportunities to influence what happens during and after the purchase (see Chapter 10). This may include specifying drink sizes, disallowing discount drink promotions, or requiring staff to receive server training in **responsible beverage service**. Regulations or licence conditions may also cover food service, availability of entertainment, and other non-alcohol-related matters and may even regulate the design and furnishing of the bar or restaurant. 'Off-premises' sales offer fewer opportunities to influence drinking behaviour, but may influence consumption by controlling the type, strength, packaging and price of take-away alcohol sales. Restricting the location of outlets can also affect alcohol problems. For example, a Brazilian study of banning alcohol sales in outlets having access to major highways found some effect on rates of traffic injuries (Room *et al.* 2002). The number and location of different types of outlet may also be controlled through sale of liquor licenses or through local planning systems.

9.2.3 Densities of retail outlets

Restricting the number of places where alcohol can be sold has been widely used to reduce alcohol-related problems by limiting consumption. In general, this has been accomplished using the state licensing apparatus, with limitations either formally legislated or emerging through individual licensing decisions. In much of the world, these kinds of restrictions have been seen increasingly as anti-competitive, and in many cases licensing laws have been liberalized, resulting in substantial increases in outlet numbers (e.g. Marsden Jacob Associates 2005).

There is strong evidence that substantial changes in the number of alcohol outlets result in significant changes to alcohol consumption and related harm. The strongest evidence generally comes via **natural experiments**, when significant changes in legislation result in major changes to the number of places at which alcohol can be purchased. Such changes (e.g. the introduction of alcoholic beverages for sale in grocery stores) have mostly occurred when retail sales of one or several types of alcoholic beverage have been moved from a very limited number of state monopoly outlets to a large number of private outlets (e.g. grocery stores) or vice versa.

In recent years, a growing number of studies have examined the effect of more gradual changes in outlet density on alcohol consumption and related harms, such as those brought about through ongoing relaxation of liquor licensing regulations. There is a substantial body of evidence linking gradual changes in outlet density to alcohol-related problems, particularly violence. In Norway, changes in on-premises outlet density over a 35-year period were related to changes in assault rates, even when *per capita* consumption was controlled (Norström 2000). More recent studies have used shorter time-periods and smaller geographic units to undertake cross-sectional **time-series analyses**, finding significant relationships between outlet density and violence rates over time (Gruenewald and Remer 2006; Livingston 2008). A study of the sharp reduction in off-premises outlets in parts of Los Angeles following the civil unrest in 1992 (Yu *et al.* 2008) indicated that for every 10% reduction in outlets in a census tract, assaults were reduced by 2.6%. A related study of the same reduction in outlets (Cohen *et al.* 2006) found significant reductions in rates of gonorrhoea in areas where liquor stores had been closed. A longitudinal study from California (Freisthler and Weiss 2008) found that greater alcohol outlet density was related to higher child maltreatment rates, with annual changes in outlet numbers varying significantly with county-level referrals to child protection. Other studies have found significantly positive correlations between outlet densities, drink-driving (Gruenewald *et al.* 2002; Treno *et al.* 2003), car crashes (Scribner *et al.* 1994), and pedestrian injuries (LaScala *et al.* 2001). The effects of outlet density on drink-driving, however, appear to be modest. A recent longitudinal analysis found that a 10% increase in off-premises outlet density was associated with a 0.9% increase in alcohol-related fatalities (Treno *et al.* 2007b). Overall, the evidence of an association between outlet density and alcohol-related harms is quite consistent. A growing number of studies has found higher rates of alcohol-related problems in areas with higher outlet densities (see Stockwell and Gruenewald 2004; Gruenewald 2007; and Livingston *et al.* 2007 for reviews).

Studies have been less consistent in terms of the association of outlet density with alcohol consumption. For example, Scribner *et al.* (2000) and Truong and Sturm (2007, 2009) found positive relationships between outlet density and consumption at the census tract level, whereas Pollack *et al.* (2005) and Abbey *et al.* (1993) found no significant relationship. Godfrey (1988) examined licensing and demand for alcohol in the UK over a period of 25 years, finding that licence numbers and demand for beer (but not for wine or spirits) were related, with increases in outlets leading to greater beer consumption. In Canada, Trolldal (2005c) conducted time-series analyses for four provinces, finding a significant increase in spirits sales with increased number of spirits outlets, whereas little evidence was found for the effect of outlet density on consumption of wine and beer. Gruenewald *et al.* (1993, 2000) have used cross-sectional time-series models to examine gradual changes in outlet densities. In the initial study (Gruenewald *et al.* 1993), data from 38 states were used to examine the relationship between outlet density and consumption over a ten-year period. The study found significant effects for outlet density and for the geographic spread of outlets, suggesting that the number of outlets was related to alcohol sales. A follow-up study using self-reported consumption data at the neighbourhood level over five years (Gruenewald *et al.* 2000) found no relationship between outlet density and drinking behaviour. Alcohol outlet density was found to be related to both perceived ease of access to alcohol and to alcohol consumption among youth in California (Treno *et al.* 2008). There is substantial evidence that outlet density is related to rates of heavy episodic drinking by youths and young adults (e.g. Chaloupka and Wechsler 1996; Weitzman *et al.* 2003; Huckle *et al.* 2008a; Livingston *et al.* 2008; Kypri *et al.* 2008; Scribner *et al.* 2008).

As noted above, gradual changes in alcohol outlet density are related to levels of alcohol consumption, particularly among younger drinkers. There is more compelling evidence that alcohol outlet density is related to violence rates, although the precise mechanisms behind this relationship are unclear. A simple explanation is that outlets affect levels of consumption, which in turn affect violence rates. However, the mixed results from analyses of consumption suggest that outlet densities may influence violence rates without necessarily increasing consumption. Several explanations have been proposed to account for these findings. Gruenewald (2007, 2008) proposes that higher densities allow the emergence of niche establishments, some of which attract violence-prone patrons and thus increase the likelihood of violent encounters. Routine activities theory (e.g. Roncek and Maier 1991; Smith *et al.* 2000; Parker 2004) suggests that one role of outlet density in violence is to bring together more people (particularly young, intoxicated males) who can fulfil the roles of both victim and aggressor.

These interpretations of the outlet density–violence association have important implications for policies aimed at controlling outlet density. Specifically, they suggest that dense clustering of alcohol outlets in entertainment districts is likely to be particularly problematic because it increases niche environments or the number of interactions among drinkers, thus increasing the likelihood of violent incidents. These entertainment districts often involve large numbers of drinkers moving from premises to premises throughout the night, increasing the likelihood of alcohol-related aggression.

Clustering of premises into high-density entertainment districts is increasingly common. Hadfield (2006) documents the commercial value of bunching, with pub properties located in close proximity to other licensed premises worth twice as much as those further removed from drinking circuits. While governments in the UK and Australia have attempted to reduce the impact of clustered premises by restricting additional licenses in particular areas (Herring *et al.* 2008; Victorian Government 2008), these policy changes have not been evaluated.

In summary, there is reasonably strong evidence that alcohol outlet density is related to alcohol-related problems, especially violence. The evidence supporting an association between density and consumption is mixed.

9.2.4 Hours and days of trade

Restricting the days and times of alcohol sale reduces opportunities (and availability) for purchasing alcohol. Although such restrictions have been a common strategy for reducing alcohol-related problems, in recent years there has been a trend to liberalize days and hours of sale in many countries (e.g. Drummond 2000; Stockwell and Chikritzhs 2009). This trend has developed at the same time as increasing evidence emerges that availability restrictions prevent or reduce alcohol-related problems.

A recent review of the effects of changes in hours of sale included 48 studies from eight countries across four decades with a wide variety of research designs (Stockwell and Chikritzhs 2009). However, only 14 of the studies were published in peer-reviewed journals and included baseline and control observations. A clear majority (79%) of these studies found that changes in hours of sale affected at least one outcome measure. Acute harms (closely associated in time with drinking events) were most likely to change and chronic problems such as liver cirrhosis were unlikely to be impacted in the short term. The authors concluded that, based upon controlled studies, the evidence supports the expectation that changes in hours of sale will be associated with changes in alcohol-related harms.

Recent studies using more advanced statistical tools and proper controls have typically investigated the effects of increased late-night trading hours. For example, Chikritzhs and Stockwell (2002, 2006, 2007) studied the extension of hotel closing times from midnight to 1 a.m. in Western Australia. They found significant increases in assaults and in impaired driver road crashes to be associated with the extended hours. The study also found increased blood alcohol concentrations (BACs) among male drivers aged 18–25 years who were apprehended during the later trading hours (though female drivers who were stopped had lower BACs). Recent studies from Canada and Iceland have found that adding late night trading hours is associated with alcohol-related problems. Vingilis *et al.* (2005, 2007) examined the extension of trading hours from 1 a.m. to 2 a.m. in Ontario using a variety of data sources, finding no impact on motor vehicle injuries across the province, but significant increases in other injuries (such as assault and fall-related injuries). Ragnarsdóttir *et al.* (2002) used a simple pre/post evaluation to study the impact of a change to unrestricted opening hours in Reykjavik compared with the prior policy of relatively early closing times (11:30 p.m. on weeknights, 2:00 a.m. on weekends). The extended hours were related to significant increases in injuries, police work, and drink-driving. These events were distributed over a longer period of time, however, and thus reduced the peak demand for police and emergency personnel at 2 a.m. on weekends.

Other studies have evaluated changes in UK trading hours. Earlier studies of the liberalization of trading hour restrictions in Scotland in 1976 showed mixed results. Two studies (Duffy and Plant 1986; Duffy and Pinot de Moira 1996) found no increases in chronic problems such as liver cirrhosis, alcohol dependence, total alcohol-related deaths, alcohol pancreatic disease, and hospital admissions which would not be unexpected with only one hour increases in trading hours. Duffy and Pinot de Moira (1996) did find significant increases in alcohol poisonings, i.e. acute harms, which corroborates findings by Northbridge et al. (1986). The most recent change in UK licensing laws occurred in late 2005, which allowed 24-hour trading. Evaluation of this change is difficult because of incremental extensions in trading that had taken place prior to the new legislation (Hadfield 2006) and the relatively limited uptake of extended hours by licensed premises (Hough and Hunter 2008). One study based upon a single emergency department in London found increased numbers of alcohol-related emergency cases associated with the change (Newton et al. 2007). A report produced for the UK Home Office (Babb 2007) compared 12-month periods before and after the changes. The study found a 1% rise in the overall number of violence, criminal damage and harassment incidents occurring between 6 p.m. and 6 a.m. (typical night-time drinking hours) and a 25% rise in those which occurred between 3 a.m. and 6 a.m. (typical heavy drinking late hours). These two increases occurred during a time when there was an overall 1% fall in recorded incidents and a fall of 5% in serious violent crimes. An evaluation by Hough and Hunter (2008) found similar increases in night-time incidents yet concluded that expanded opening hours had little effect on crime. This conclusion is surprising since there appears to be an overall downward trend in such events over the two years (possibly for other reasons) yet night-time events increased, which runs counter to this overall downward trend. It should also be noted that these evaluations are largely based on only one year of post-intervention data and therefore should be interpreted with some caution. The recent UK change provides a less clear-cut picture than that seen in most other jurisdictions, but evaluations do find increased rates of alcohol-related acute problems following increases in trading hours.

Whereas most studies have evaluated the effect of increasing hours of sale, a Brazilian study examined how restrictions on hours of sale affected the rates of alcohol-related harm (Duailibi et al. 2007b). A new law in Diadema (an industrial city near São Paolo in Brazil) mandated all on-premises alcohol outlets to close at 11 p.m. Prior to the law most bars traded 24 hours per day. The study found a reduction of around nine murders per month after the restrictions were imposed. Box 9.2 provides another example of how sales restrictions influenced alcohol-related problem rates.

In addition to changes in daily trading hours, other policy changes have added or removed entire days of sale. Norström and Skog (2005) found a 3.7% increase in total alcohol consumption following the 2001 removal of a Saturday sales ban in Sweden, but did not find significant impacts on indicators of assaults or drink-driving. A US study of the removal of a state-wide ban on Sunday sales by off-premises alcohol

Box 9.2 'Feed the children first!': the impact of Thirsty Thursday in Tennant Creek

In Tennant Creek, an outback community in Australia, an Aboriginal community group mounted a long and eventually successful campaign to close the local pubs and off-premises outlets on the day pay checks arrived. On Thursdays, off-premises alcohol sales were banned, and on other days take-away sales were limited to the hours of noon to 9 p.m. In addition, bars were closed until noon on Thursdays and Fridays. 'Feed the children first!' was the slogan of the campaign. Two evaluations of the effects of this much-contested change found a 19.4% decrease in drinking over a two-year period, with a concomitant reduction in arrests, hospital admissions, and women's refuge admissions (Gray *et al.* 1998; Brady 2000). D'Abbs and Togni (2000) also found a 34% reduction in alcohol-related hospital admissions and a 46% decline in women's refuge admissions in the first and more stringent phase of the restrictions. Although the effects of the closing hour restrictions may have been confounded with price increases and other interventions, this example suggests that concentrated efforts to control alcohol availability can produce substantial reductions in alcohol-related problems.

outlets in the state of New Mexico (McMillan and Lapham 2006) documented a 29% increase in the daily rate of alcohol-related crashes and a 42% increase in alcohol-related crash fatalities on Sundays. The policy also provided for local elections by individual counties to reinstate the bans if desired. A natural experiment was thus possible with some counties continuing Sunday sales and some reinstating the ban. McMillan *et al.* (2007) found that counties which reinstated the ban experienced a subsequent reduction in alcohol-involved crashes, with the benefits greatest in counties with older populations. The study concluded that passing the local option law allowing jurisdictions authority to change these regulations reduced the rate of alcohol-related crashes at the county level and may also have benefits for surrounding counties.

One of the few studies focusing on youth (Baker *et al.* 2000) found that temporary bans on the sale of alcohol from midnight Friday through 10 a.m. Monday (because of federal elections in Mexico) reduced cross-border drinking by young Americans. In particular, the early closing on Friday night was associated with a 34% net reduction in the number of persons with BACs of ≥0.08% (our calculations based on Table 2 data in Baker *et al.* 2000). In a similar study Voas *et al.* (2002) found that after bar closing hours in Juarez, Mexico were changed from 5 a.m. to 2 a.m., the number of young American pedestrians returning with BACs of ≥0.08% from Juarez at 3 a.m. or later was reduced by 89%.

Importantly, restrictions on hours of sale appear to affect heavier as well as lighter drinkers. Several studies from the Nordic countries have shown that Saturday closing seems to have a stronger impact on heavy drinkers and marginalized groups compared to the general population (Mäkelä *et al.* 2002). A decrease in violence resulting from Norway's 1984 Saturday closing suggests that the people most affected by this temporary unavailability were those who were more likely to be involved in domestic violence and disruptive intoxication (Nordlund 1985). Similarly, Smith (1986a) demonstrated that patrons of extended-hours taverns are an especially heavy drinking segment of the population.

In sum, there is strong and reasonably consistent evidence from a number of countries that changes to hours or days of trade have significant impacts on the volume of alcohol consumed and on the rates of alcohol-related problems. When hours and days of sale are increased, consumption and harm increase and vice versa. This evidence comes from studies in Australia, Brazil, Canada, the Nordic countries, and the USA. A small number of studies suggest that trading hour restrictions affect heavy drinkers in particular. The weight of evidence suggests that restrictions on opening hours and days of sale are important policy levers for managing alcohol-related harm. Increasing the hours and days of sale is typically related to increased consumption and alcohol harms (usually acute harm) and studies of reduced hours of sale or bans on days of sale are associated with reduced problems.

9.2.5 State retail monopolies

One form of alcohol sales regulation used in many countries is for the government to monopolize ownership of one or more types of retail outlet. The idea of government ownership of alcohol sales outlets in the interest of public order or public health first arose in the nineteenth century. The original form, known as the 'Gothenburg system', involved municipally owned taverns, and this later became the basis for the Swedish off-premises monopoly stores. Monopoly systems existed at one time or another in parts of Britain and Australia, and they still operate in parts of the USA and much of Canada, as well as in fifteen other countries around the world (WHO 2004b). In Iceland, Norway, Sweden, and Finland, state monopoly systems were implemented in the early twentieth century with substantial powers over the production, sale, and distribution of alcohol. The entry of Sweden and Finland into the EU in 1995, and Iceland and Norway's special treaty relationship with the EU, caused a substantial weakening of these integrated monopoly systems (Holder *et al.* 1998), although the off-premises retail monopolies have been retained in all four countries (Cisneros Örnberg and Ólafsdóttir 2008). Government monopolies also operate in Eastern Europe (e.g. Russia), southern Africa, and Costa Rica as well as a number of Indian states (Room 2000a).

Retail alcohol monopolies can influence alcohol consumption in a variety of ways: by limiting the number of outlets, limiting their hours of sale, and removing the private profit motive for increasing sales. The evidence is quite strong that off-premises monopoly systems limit alcohol consumption and alcohol-related problems, and that elimination of government off-premises monopolies can increase total alcohol consumption (Her *et al.* 1999). A number of studies have addressed the impact of taking an alcoholic beverage out of, as well as into, a monopoly system. In Finland, the most notable change was observed in 1969 when beer up to 4.7% alcohol was allowed to be sold by grocery stores and it became easier to get a restaurant license to sell beer and wine. At the same time the legal drinking age was lowered from 21 to 18 years for wine and beer and to 20 years for all alcoholic beverages. There was also a significant expansion of state alcohol monopoly stores in rural areas. The number of off-premises outlets increased from 130 to about 17 600, and the number of on-premises outlets grew from 940 to more than 4000 (Österberg 1979). The overall consumption of alcohol increased by 46% from 1968 to 1969. In the following five years, mortality from liver cirrhosis increased by 50%, hospital admissions for alcoholic psychosis increased by 110% for men and 130% for women, and arrests for drunkenness increased by 80% for men and 160% for women (Poikolainen 1980). A more recent study using sales data from 1960 to 2004 (Mangeloja and Pehkonen 2009) showed that increases in consumption appeared to be particularly marked for beer and somewhat less so for spirits. Changes in the number of monopoly stores and in the numbers of groceries and restaurants selling beer each contributed independently to the increase in consumption.

In Sweden, research has been conducted on the effects of allowing the sale of 'medium strength' beer (around 4.5% alcohol) in grocery stores in 1965, and reversing this policy in 1977. The change in 1965 greatly increased the number of outlets for medium strength beer. An analysis by Noval and Nilsson (1984) concluded that introducing 4.5% beer to the grocery stores in Sweden raised total consumption by about 15%, and that moving it back to monopoly outlets reduced total consumption by about the same amount. Ramstedt (2002b) examined just the retraction of the right to sell 4.5% beer in grocery stores, finding a 15% reduction in traffic injuries. There is some evidence that the effect of removing medium strength beer from grocery stores was greatest among young people (Hibell 1984).

Wagenaar and Holder (1995) found that privatization of wine sales in five US states produced an increase in wine sales from 42% to 150% in four of these states and a more modest (13%) increase in one state. No significant substitution effects were observed and hence a net increase in total consumption followed the privatization of wine sales. However, analyses of data from one of these states, conducted by another group of researchers (e.g. Mulford et al. 1992), suggested no impact of privatization; the different conclusions may be explained by different data utilization and technical approaches (Her et al. 1999). Other studies of the dismantling of retail alcohol monopolies in Canada and the USA found modest increases in consumption (Wagenaar and Holder 1995; Adrian et al. 1996; Trolldal 2005a,b). Trolldal's study (2005b) also examined traffic crashes in Alberta, Canada after a tripling in outlet numbers following privatization, but found no significant increase. It is unclear, however, whether the observed effects are due to increased outlet density or to other changes related to privatization. It has been noted (Her et al. 1999) that privatization of retail alcohol sales has been implemented with different kinds of deregulation. In some cases (e.g. in Alberta, Quebec, Washington, and Virginia) privatization led to increased prices, which may have countered the effect of increased physical availability.

Elimination of a private profit interest may also facilitate the enforcement of rules against selling to minors or intoxicated patrons, yet evidence in this respect is only found regarding sales to minors. Rossow et al. (2008) found that monopoly stores in Finland and Norway were one-third as likely as private stores to sell alcohol to underage-appearing 18-year-olds without checking identification. Using cross-sectional data, Miller *et al.* (2006) found that underage drinking, binge drinking and motor vehicle fatality rates were substantially lower in states with retail monopolies than in those with privatized retail systems.

Over-the-counter sales (where an alcohol purchase has to be requested from a sales clerk) has been a further restriction on alcohol availability within the state retail monopolies in several countries. The transition from over-the-counter sales to self-service sales in Swedish monopoly outlets was evaluated by Skog (2000) applying an experimental design. Skog (2000) found that introduction of self-service led to a net increase of about 10% in wine sales and 6% in spirits sales. Applying the same research design, Horverak (2008) evaluated the transition from over-the-counter sales to self-service in Norwegian monopoly outlets and found fairly similar effects, i.e. a net increase in alcohol sales by 10%.

Taking into account the potential impact of a retail monopoly (via restrictions on number of outlets, days and hours of sale, etc.), Holder *et al.* (2008) estimated what would be the potential effects of privatizing a state monopoly of retail alcohol sales in Sweden. Projecting two different scenarios of privatization, retail sales in specialized private stores and retail sales in grocery stores, they estimated that privatization could lead to a 25–60% increase in deaths from explicitly alcohol-related illnesses and a 10–20% increase in assaults.

Whereas, in principle, state-run retail monopolies have the potential to curtail sales of alcohol and thereby alcohol-related harm, in recent years some of the government-run retail systems, especially in North America, have increasingly focused on increasing sales volume, and have devoted substantial resources to advertising and other promotion techniques to increase sales. These developments are likely to undercut the potential for reducing harm and high-risk drinking.

9.3 Restrictions on eligibility to purchase and sell alcohol

At various times throughout history restrictions have been placed on those who buy and sell alcohol. These restrictions are generally intended to exclude one group or another from purchasing alcoholic beverages and to regulate the clerks and sellers of alcohol. For instance, sales of alcoholic beverages to Aboriginal populations were forbidden in many European settler societies (Brady 2000). The most common restriction on sales in effect throughout the world at the beginning of the twenty-first century are the prohibition of alcohol sales to children and youths and the denial of sale to persons who are intoxicated.

9.3.1 Limiting alcohol sales on an individual basis

Fifty years ago, broad restrictions on who could purchase alcohol were fairly common. The most elaborate example of such controls was the **Bratt system** in Sweden, in effect until 1955, where a **rationing** scheme assigned a limit to each male adult on how much spirits could be purchased (Norström 1987). There was also a list of those barred altogether from purchasing. Such lists were also maintained in Finland and Norway (Tigerstedt 2000), and this procedure was included in laws in some

English-speaking jurisdictions. These individual banning orders were abolished in the Nordic countries in the 1970s, and until recently had also fallen out of favour in English-speaking jurisdictions as impermissible intrusions on civil liberties.

Now there are signs of a revival of such approaches. In Britain, exclusion orders can be made against 'habitual drunkards' or violent offenders, preventing them from entering particular premises for up to two years (Home Office 2008). In Australia, the Victorian Government has recently introduced laws allowing police to issue banning orders to 'troublemakers', preventing them from entering designated entertainment precincts for up to 24 hours, and allowing the courts to issue exclusion orders for up to 12 months for particularly problematic offenders (Victorian Government 2008). In addition to these formal measures, informal banning orders exist in many countries, for example, through agreements between licensees (e.g. Pubwatch in the UK: Pratten and Greig 2007) or through conditions imposed on parole by a court. There has been little evaluation of these measures.

There is clear evidence that general alcohol-rationing schemes, such as Sweden's Bratt system (Norström 1987) and a similar system in effect in Greenland from 1979 to 1982 (Schechter 1986), were responsible for reducing liver cirrhosis mortality, violence, and other consequences of heavy drinking. During a political crisis situation in Poland in 1981 to 1982, alcohol rationing that limited each adult to half a litre of spirits per month was introduced. Heavy drinkers were affected most. Periods of binge drinking became much shorter. Along with a 60% drop in mental hospital admissions for alcoholic psychosis, deaths from liver diseases dropped by one-quarter, and deaths from injuries by 15% (Moskalewicz and Swiatkiewicz 2000).

Many countries ban alcohol sales to persons who are already intoxicated. All 50 US states have criminal or civil laws against such sales (Holder *et al.* 1993). There has been no evaluation of these particular legislative bans, but there are studies on increased enforcement of such bans (see Chapter 10).

9.3.2 Minimum alcohol purchasing age laws

Almost all countries have legal restrictions on the age at which young people may purchase or possess alcohol. These restrictions vary widely, ranging typically from 16 to 21 years of age (WHO 2004b). Changes in minimum legal drinking age (MLDA) laws can have substantial effects on youth drinking. Klepp *et al.* (1996) found that implementation of the uniform minimum legal drinking age of 21 years in the USA reduced the overall prevalence of drink-driving. Other evaluations (Wagenaar 1981, 1986; Wagenaar and Maybee 1986; Saffer and Grossman 1987a,b) indicate that raising the minimum legal drinking age from 18 to 21 years decreased single vehicle nighttime crashes involving young drivers by 11–16% at all levels of crash severity. Voas and Tippetts (1999), using data from all 50 US states and the District of Columbia for the years 1982–1997, concluded that the enactment of the national uniform age 21 years minimum drinking age law was responsible for a 19% net decrease in fatal crashes involving young drinking drivers, after controlling for driving exposure, beer consumption, enactment of zero tolerance laws, and other relevant changes in state laws during that time period. Additional studies have shown that changes in the minimum drinking age are related to alcohol-related injury admissions to hospitals

(Smith 1986b), injury fatalities (Jones *et al.* 1992), and overall mortality (Carpenter and Dobkin 2007).

A comprehensive review (Wagenaar and Toomey 2002) based on all published studies on legal drinking age published between 1960 and 2000 (a total of 135 documents) concluded that increasing the legal age for purchase and consumption of alcohol to 21 years is the most effective strategy for reducing drinking and drinking problems among high-school students, college students, and other youth, compared to a wide range of other programmes and efforts. Based on national data from the Monitoring the Future (MTF) survey from 1976 to 1987, which sampled high-school seniors each year throughout the USA, it was concluded that having a minimum drinking age of 21 years in the USA is associated with a 5.5% lower prevalence of 30-day alcohol use and a 2.8% lower prevalence of heavy alcohol use among high-school seniors and recent high-school graduates (O'Malley and Wagenaar 1991). Similarly, increasing the drinking age from 18 resulted in a 13.8% decrease in the frequency of alcohol consumption. An analysis of state-level data in the USA found that raising the MLDA to 21 years reduced alcohol-related crashes among youth by as much as 19% (Voas *et al.* 2003). Similarly, the MLDA of 21 years has been associated with 47% decrease in fatal crashes involving young drivers with BAC ≥0.08% and a 40% decrease in such crashes involving young drivers with BAC ≥0.01% (Dang 2008). Conversely, a review of research indicated that the trend to decrease the MLDA in the USA from 21 to 18 years during the 1970s was associated with a 7% increase in traffic fatalities for the affected age groups (Cook 2007). Other studies have provided similar findings (Voas *et al.* 2003; Carpenter and Dobkin 2007; Carpenter *et al.* 2007; Fell *et al.* 2009). Miron and Tetelbaum (2007), however, suggest that the impact of the minimum drinking age increase to 21 years in the USA has been overstated, finding that the effect was largely concentrated in the states that voluntarily raised their drinking ages prior to federal intervention. An alternative interpretation is that later adopters of the age 21 years MLDA were less enthusiastic about the law and put fewer resources into enforcing it.

The literature on the effectiveness of drinking age restrictions is largely from North America. How well do these restrictions apply in other societies? One study from Denmark (Møller 2002) evaluated the effect of introducing a minimum 15-year age limit for off-premises purchases (after having had no minimum age limits for such purchases). The imposition of the law was associated with a 36% drop in the proportion of youth aged <15 years who had consumed alcohol in the previous month. In addition, there was also a 17% decline in the proportion of drinkers among students aged ≥15 years. The author hypothesized that the debate around the legislation may have sensitized parents of teenagers to pay more attention to their children's drinking. In Australia, several studies (Smith 1986b; Smith and Burvil 1986, 1987) found that the lowering of the drinking age from 21 to 18 years in three Australian states resulted in increases in traffic-related hospital admissions, other accident-related hospital admissions and rates of juvenile crime. More recently, the lowering of the drinking age in New Zealand from 20 to 18 years was associated with increased traffic injuries among 15–19-year-olds (Kypri *et al.* 2006) and in prosecutions for disorder offences among 14–15-year-olds (Huckle *et al.* 2006). A systematic review of 33 evaluations of

MLDA laws in Australia, Canada, and the USA found a median decline of 16% in crash-related outcomes for the targeted age groups following passage of laws to increase the MLDA (Shults *et al.* 2001).

However, even in the USA it is clear that the benefits of a higher drinking age are only realized if the law is enforced. Despite higher minimum drinking age laws, young people do succeed in purchasing alcohol (e.g. Grube 1997). Such sales result from low and inconsistent levels of enforcement, especially when there is little community support for underage alcohol sales enforcement (Wagenaar and Wolfson 1994, 1995). Even moderate increases in enforcement can reduce sales to minors by as much as 35–40%, especially when combined with media and other community activities (Grube 1997; Wagenaar *et al.* 2000a). This is illustrated in the project described in Box 9.3.

9.3.3 Controls on who can sell alcohol

Alcohol control agencies in countries with well-regulated markets typically spend a considerable part of their time checking the credentials of those seeking licenses to sell

---

Box 9.3 The CMCA project in the USA

The Communities Mobilizing for Change on Alcohol (CMCA) project was designed to reduce the accessibility of alcohol to youth below the legal drinking age of 21 years. Communities ranging in population from 8000 to 65 000 were matched and randomly assigned to the intervention or a control condition, resulting in seven intervention sites and eight comparison sites. The project employed a part-time local organizer within each community to implement interventions designed to reduce underage access to alcohol. Such interventions could include decoy operations with alcohol outlets (in which police typically have underage buyers purchase alcohol at selected outlets), citizen monitoring of outlets selling to youth, keg registration (which requires that purchasers of kegs of beer provide identifying information, thus establishing liability for resulting problems at parties where minors are drinking), developing alcohol-free events for youth, shortening hours of sale for alcohol, responsible beverage service training, and developing educational programmes for youth and adults. Evaluation data collected two-and-a-half years after the initiation of the intervention activities revealed that merchants increased checking for age identification and reported more care in controlling sales to youth (Wagenaar *et al.* 1996). Research using young-looking purchasers confirmed that alcohol merchants increased age-identification checks and reduced their propensity to sell to minors. A telephone survey indicated that 18–20-year-olds were less likely to consume alcohol themselves and less likely to provide it to other underage persons (Wagenaar *et al.* 2000a). Finally, the project found a statistically significant decline (intervention compared to control communities) in drink-driving arrests among 18–20-year-olds and disorderly conduct violations among 15–17-year-olds (Wagenaar *et al.* 2000a).

alcoholic beverages. Typically, there is a concern to keep those with criminal records or associations out of the trade. The minimum age of alcohol sellers that is set in some jurisdictions could affect whether underage sales might occur. Younger sellers, for example, may be more likely to sell to underage buyers. Treno *et al.* (2000) reported that among a community-based sample of alcohol establishments, off-premises sales were more likely from younger than older sales people. Similar findings have been reported by others, although some studies have found no association (see Rossow *et al.* 2008 for a review). Moreover, there have been no evaluations of minimum age-of-seller restrictions or other controls on who is permitted to sell alcohol.

9.4 Strength of alcoholic beverages

Lower-alcohol content beverages have been encouraged in many countries in recent years through policies that have made them more available or affordable, such as reduced rates of taxation. Lower taxation has been used in many Scandinavian countries, which have defined several classes of beer and at least two classes of wine according to their alcohol content. Putting 4.7% beer into the grocery stores in Finland in 1969, and allowing and then taking away such beer in grocery stores in Sweden, can be seen as experiments in changing the relative availability of different strengths of beverages. Part of the motivation for the Finnish change was to wean Finns from their traditional preference for strong spirits (Tigerstedt 2000). In the long run, both Finland and Sweden changed from spirits-drinking to beer-drinking nations (Leifman 2001). But the result of the Finnish change was the addition of a new beverage and new drinking occasions to existing ones, rather than the intended substitution.

A few studies have evaluated significant changes in the availability of specific beverage types. Holder and Blose (1987) found that allowing sales of distilled spirits (in addition to wine and beer) in restaurants in the US state of North Carolina (thus substantially increasing on-premises availability) led to a 6–7.4% increase in total sales of distilled spirits. Moreover, this increase in sales stimulated a 16–24% increase in night-time traffic crashes for male drivers (Blose and Holder 1987). In New Zealand, the introduction of wine into grocery stores in 1990 was associated with a 17% increase in wine sales, with little impact on the sales of other alcoholic beverages (Wagenaar and Langley 1995). The increase in wine sales was attributed to the increased physical availability of table wine as well as lower wine prices (due to increased competition).

Success has been reported in some places with the promotion of lighter beers. Skog (1988) analysed the effect of introducing light beer in Norway in March 1985, finding a substitution of lower- for higher-alcohol content beer, although the estimate was not statistically significant. He concluded that the data do not provide unequivocal evidence concerning whether the primary effect was substitution or addition. Another small-scale study conducted in Perth, Western Australia, indicates that changes in sales of high- vs low-strength beers are closely related to rates of alcohol-related crashes over time (Gruenewald *et al.* 1999).

Overall, the evidence is suggestive but not conclusive that making available and promoting beverages of lower alcohol content can be an effective strategy. With no tax on 2.8% beer in Sweden, it often costs half as much as the 3.5% beer, which is also available in the grocery stores. As a result, it has captured half the grocery sales market. Thus, such a strategy does have the potential to reduce the level of absolute alcohol consumed and associated intoxication and impairment.

9.6 Social availability and alcohol-free activities and events

Drinkers, especially young drinkers, use multiple sources to obtain alcohol. Social sources may be particularly important for underage drinkers (Dent *et al.* 2005; Rossow *et al.* 2005; Paschall *et al.* 2007). The 2007 survey of European school children (Hibell *et al.* 2009), for example, found that about 27% of students reported buying beer at an off-premises outlet for their own consumption and about 32% reported doing so at an on-premises establishment (pub, bar, restaurant, or disco). Large differences were found across countries, however, in the percentage of students buying at on- or off-premises outlets. Relatively few students (10–15%) in Finland, Sweden, or the UK reported buying beer in a store compared with students from Bulgaria, Romania, or Ukraine (46–55%). Given these data, it appears that a large percentage of young drinkers in many European countries must obtain alcohol from social rather than commercial sources.

Research in the USA suggests that parties, friends, and adult purchasers are the most common sources of alcohol among adolescents (Paschall *et al.* 2007). A major opportunity for underage drinkers to gain access to alcohol is parties. In one study, 32% of 6th graders, 56% of 9th graders, and 60% of 12th graders reported obtaining alcohol at parties (Harrison *et al.* 2000). Underage drinking parties frequently involve large groups and are commonly held in a home, an outdoor area, or other location such as a hotel room (Wagenaar *et al.* 1993; Jones-Webb *et al.* 1997). Such parties may be a particularly risky drinking context. Efforts to reduce alcohol availability thus cannot focus exclusively on commercial access but also must address social availability (Holder 1994b; Grube in press).

9.6.1 Dram shop liability

Dram shop liability laws allow individuals injured by a minor who had been drinking or by an intoxicated adult to recover damages from the alcohol retailer who served or sold alcohol to the person causing the injury (Mosher 2002). The term derives from the nineteenth century **temperance** era, but in the last 30 years the concept has been revived and remodelled by legislation or court decisions, particularly in the USA. Owners and licensees can be held liable for the actions of their employees under most or all dram shop liability laws. Many dram shop liability statutes include a 'responsible business practices defence'. This provision allows retailers to avoid liability if they can establish that they took reasonable steps to avoid serving minors and obviously intoxicated adults. Key to the defence is evidence that **responsible beverage service** training procedures and policies were fully implemented at the time of the illegal sale or service. Research suggests that implementation of dram shop liability may lead to significant increases in checking age identification and greater care in service practices (e.g. Sloan *et al.* 2000). Overall, dram shop liability has been estimated to reduce alcohol-related traffic fatalities among underage drivers by 3–4% (Chaloupka *et al.*

1993) in the USA. Sloan *et al.* (2000) analysed traffic fatalities across all states and found that imposing tort liability on commercial services resulted in reduced fatality rates for 15–20-year-old drivers. Utilization of data from all 50 states across time increases the strength of these findings.

9.6.2 Social host liability

Under social host liability, adults who provide alcohol to a minor or serve intoxicated adults in social settings can be held responsible for damages or injury caused by that minor or intoxicated adult (Grube and Nygaard 2005). One study of social host liability laws in the USA (Whetten-Goldstein *et al.* 2000) found such laws to be associated with decreases in alcohol-related traffic fatalities among adults, but not among underage persons. In a second study, social host liability laws were associated with decreases in reported heavy drinking and in decreases in drink-driving by lighter drinkers but had no effect on drink-driving by heavier drinkers (Stout *et al.* 2000). These mixed findings may reflect the lack of a comprehensive programme to ensure that social hosts are aware of their potential liability and that it is being enforced. Stout *et al.* suggest that the existence of social host liability must be effectively communicated before it can have a deterrent effect.

9.6.3 Bans on public drinking

Policies can also target specific events or locations where drinking occurs, such as drinking in parks or recreational locations, or in the workplace. Such restrictions have the potential for affecting youth drinking, in particular, since they often use public venues (e.g. public parks, beaches, lakes, etc.) for drinking (Hibell *et al.* 2004). Limiting drinking in such locations also holds the potential for reducing social access to alcohol (Giesbrecht and Douglas 1990; Conway 2002). More than half of local governments in New Zealand have implemented permanent ongoing liquor bans in public places. There are few studies of the effects of such bans.

A study by Bormann and Stone (2001) found sharp declines in arrests, assaults and ejections from the University of Colorado stadium in 1996 following a ban on alcohol sales. However, Spaite *et al.* (1990) found no significant changes in overall medical incidents following an alcohol ban at a football stadium. Despite the limited literature in this area, it has become common for alcohol to be restricted in sports stadiums, with patrons prevented from bringing alcohol into the stadium. A study by Gliksman *et al.* (1995) found that 86% of Canadian communities that adopted formal policies on the use of alcohol in public facilities experienced reductions in problems such as underage drinking, fighting, and vandalism. Other effects were seen in the reduced number of police interventions and public complaints involving alcohol. The authors concluded that policies needed to be in place for six months or longer before a community would experience significant problem reductions.

9.6.4. Other strategies to reduce social availability

A number of strategies to reduce social availability of alcohol are in use but have so far not been evaluated with respect to their effects on consumption or harms. 'Shoulder tap' operations use minors, working with police, to approach adult strangers outside of an alcohol outlet and ask them to purchase alcohol. If the older person actually makes the alcohol purchase and gives it to the youth, then he or she can be arrested or cited by the police. These interventions have been recommended in the USA as a strategy to directly reduce third-party alcohol transactions to minors (National Highway Traffic Safety Administration 1998; Stewart 1999).

'Party patrols' are a local enforcement strategy in which police arrive at a social event in which alcohol is being served and check age identifications of participants (Little and Bishop 1998; Stewart 1999). Police can use noise or nuisance ordinances as a basis for entering a social gathering to determine whether underage drinking is taking place. 'Keg registration' laws require the name of a purchaser of a barrel of beer to be linked to that keg. Keg registration is seen primarily as a tool for prosecuting adults who supply alcohol to young people at parties or for prosecuting retailers who sell kegs to minors. Keg registration laws have become increasingly popular in the USA.

Another strategy involves restricting the flow of alcohol at parties and other events to reduce the overall social availability of alcohol. Policies for preventing underage access to alcohol at parties can also be used to decrease the amount of drinking among young adults who may be of legal drinking age. Overlapping community policies include banning beer in kegs and prohibiting home deliveries of large quantities of alcohol. Overlapping policies for social events include limiting the quantity of alcohol per person and monitoring or serving alcohol rather than allowing self-service.

'Alcohol-free activities' are specific events or activities (e.g. 21st birthdays, New Year's Eve, etc.) that have traditionally been associated with particularly high levels of alcohol-related harm. To reduce these harms the events are organized either by promoting alcohol-free alternatives or by banning alcohol availability at them. Promoting alcohol-free events may be seen as a means of diminishing alcohol availability, although in many such cases no alcohol control legislation or authorities may be involved.

Approaches such as shoulder taps, party patrols, keg registration, and local bans on drinking locations need more extensive evaluation. Although such strategies may be useful as part of policy efforts to reduce physical availability of alcohol, little is known about their actual impact. A general foundation for local control of potential risks to public health and safety is provided by Ashe *et al.* (2003) who suggest that no strategy to affect the social supply side of alcohol will be consistently effective unless applied in practice and enforced.

9.7 Summarizing the impact of regulating alcohol availability

Studies of restrictions on alcohol availability support the conclusion that such strategies can contribute to the reduction of alcohol problems. The best available evidence comes from studies of changes in retail availability, including reductions in the hours and days of sale, limits on the number of alcohol outlets, and restrictions on retail access to alcohol. These studies consistently show that restrictions on availability are associated with reductions in both alcohol use and alcohol-related problems. Although total bans on alcohol sales have been found to markedly reduce alcohol consumption and problems, they can bring with them new problems, particularly through the development of an illegal market. Such measures also require comprehensive enforcement to ensure effectiveness.

For young people, laws that raise the minimum legal drinking age reduce alcohol sales and problems. This strategy has the strongest empirical support (Shults *et al.* 2001; Wagenaar and Toomey 2002), with dozens of studies finding substantial impacts on traffic and other casualties from changes to the drinking age. There is also good evidence concerning reductions in the number of outlets or outlet density. Research on large changes in the density of outlets has consistently found associations with consumption, and a series of longitudinal studies has found links between gradual changes in the density of alcohol outlets and alcohol-related problems. There is some evidence suggesting that the concentration of alcohol outlets into high-density clusters within entertainment precincts is particularly problematic, although this area requires further evaluation.

Reductions in hours or days of sale have generally been shown to reduce alcohol consumption and related problems. There is much less evidence on the effectiveness of measures such as bans on drinking in designated public areas and the implementation of lockouts at late-night licensed premises. Well-designed and conducted studies have not yet been undertaken to evaluate their effectiveness.

The research evidence from more economically developed countries supports the general conclusion that, as alcohol becomes more available in less developed countries, heavier drinking and alcohol problems are likely to increase. This suggests that as economies grow in low- and middle-income countries, likely changes in physical availability will follow the pattern observed in more developed countries.

The cost of restricting the physical availability of alcohol is low relative to the social and health costs related to drinking, especially heavy drinking. One obvious case is the minimum drinking age for alcohol. For example, the increased minimum drinking age in the USA was estimated to have saved thousands of lives over the past decade (Wagenaar *et al.* 1998). A WHO analysis of the relative cost of a 'restricted access' option estimated that a Saturday closing would have considerable societal benefit in most parts of the world, though less than what would result from a substantial rise in alcohol prices via higher excise taxation (Chisholm *et al.* 2006; Anderson *et al.* 2009a).

The strategies considered in this chapter are all measures that affect the drinker's environment. They provide evidence that regulations backed up with enforcement can be effective in reducing alcohol consumption and problems. The most direct and immediate enforcement mechanism in many jurisdictions is the requirement that the seller hold a specific license to sell alcoholic beverages. If there is effective power to suspend or revoke a license in the case of sales infractions, it can be an effective and flexible instrument for holding down rates of alcohol-related problems.

Chapter 10

Modifying the drinking context: licensed drinking environment and other contexts

10.1 Introduction

Alcohol is consumed in a variety of contexts including private residences, licensed premises and other settings such as parks, beaches, cars, and campsites. As described in previous chapters, licensing provides the opportunity to regulate retail alcohol sales for both on- and off-premises consumption. However, licensing of the environment where alcohol is actually consumed provides numerous opportunities to reduce harm over and above the licensing controls that apply to off-premises alcohol sales (Stockwell 1997). For example, licensed premises such as bars, pubs, and clubs may be subject to regulations of the training and licensing of staff, the forms of entertainment permitted and the maximum number of people who can be present at any time.

On-premises drinking establishments are referred to by many terms, including public houses or pubs, taverns, bars, hotels, nightclubs, and clubs. Because these terms differ among countries, in the following discussion we refer to all drinking contexts where people purchase and consume alcohol on the premises as commercial drinking establishments. Such establishments have long been the focus of preventive interventions not only because they are subject to regulation but also because they are often high-risk drinking settings for a number of alcohol-related problems, including heavy drinking (Snow and Landrum 1986; Martin *et al.* 1992; Single and Wortley 1993; Demers *et al.* 2002), driving after drinking (O'Donnell 1985; Single and McKenzie 1992; Fahrenkrug and Rehm 1995; Gruenewald *et al.* 1996), and violence and injury (Ireland and Thommeny 1993; Stockwell *et al.* 1993; Rossow 1996; Macdonald *et al.* 1999; Leonard *et al.* 2002). The high rate of problems in commercial drinking establishments make this drinking context a prime target for alcohol policies aimed at the prevention of alcohol-related problems.

10.1.1 Theoretical basis for modifying the drinking context

Reducing harm in the drinking context draws on routine activity and situational crime prevention theories (Graham and Homel 2008; Graham 2009) as well as responsive regulation theory (Ayres and Braithwaite 1992; Graham and Homel 2008). Routine activity theory, first developed to explain crime (Cohen and Felson 1979), posits that the occurrence of crime involves the confluence of a willing perpetrator, a suitable victim, and an absence of someone who can stop the crime, including 'guardians' who protect the victim, 'handlers' (people who know and can use the potential perpetrator's 'handles' to prevent the crime) (Felson 1995), and 'place managers' (those who control places where crimes might occur) (Eck and Weisburd 1995). Thus, at a most basic level, harms in the drinking context can be reduced by preventing the presence of those most likely to harm or be harmed (e.g. not admitting or serving minors or intoxicated persons) and ensuring that staff are capable of preventing harms from occurring (Graham *et al.* 2005a,b).

Situational crime prevention extends the basic situational determinants defined by routine activity theory by addressing specific environmental influences that deter or precipitate crime, or, for the present discussion, deter or precipitate behaviours that cause harm. Environmental deterrents include such factors as increasing the risk of getting caught and punished, making it less rewarding to engage in activities that lead to harms, removing excuses and increasing the amount of effort needed to cause the harm (Clarke 1997; Clarke and Homel 1997; Cornish and Clarke 2003). Examples of deterrents related to the drinking context are enhanced law enforcement that increases chances of licensees or bar staff being charged with serving minors or intoxicated persons, as discussed in Chapter 9. Perhaps the best example of situational deterrence is the successful reduction in driving after drinking in many countries (described in Chapter 11) where enhanced risk (and increased perceived risk) of getting caught, combined with increasing social disapproval, effectively decreased the reward (e.g. convenience) of driving after drinking.

Situational precipitants overlap with situational deterrents but are thought to function in a slightly different way, namely, by encouraging crimes or harms that may not have been planned or intended originally (Wortley 2001). These include environmental factors that provoke behaviours likely to lead to harm, social pressure to commit certain acts, social cues, and weak prohibitions. Within the drinking context, situational precipitants might include the pharmacological effects of alcohol itself, social pressure to consume large quantities (e.g. buying rounds of drinks) or to react to perceived insults with violence (Graham and Wells 2003), and weak proscriptions such as high tolerance for intoxication, violence, and other harmful behaviours. Addressing situational precipitants might involve reducing aspects of the environment that lead to provocation, setting higher standards for behaviour within the context through house policies and better management and staff practices, and cultural changes in the types of drinking behaviours that are considered acceptable.

The final theoretical framework that is relevant to preventing harm in the drinking context is responsive regulation (Ayres and Braithwaite 1992; Braithwaite 2002), an approach that takes into consideration the type of industry that is being regulated, including its history, culture, and key players. It adds education and persuasion to the regulation and the enforcement of liquor laws, with appropriate use of a hierarchy of sanctions for infringements by licensed premises. For commercial drinking establishments, this means that policies and regulations need to recognize the function of drinking as a 'time out' activity (Cavan 1966; Graham and Homel 2008) and the financial and other rewards relevant to operators and staff, as well as the key economic role of licensed premises, and the night-time economy generally (Hobbs *et al.* 2003), in some communities.

To the extent that commercial drinking establishments and other drinking contexts account for a disproportionate amount of heavy drinking and social harm, crime prevention theory provides a useful framework for organizing and evaluating interventions in these settings.

10.1.2 Measuring effectiveness of interventions focused on the drinking context

Approaches to reducing alcohol-related problems by modifying the context of commercial drinking establishments have focused on two distinct outcomes: (i) alcohol consumption by patrons and (ii) other behaviours such as drink-driving and violence. Strategies relating to the sale of alcohol typically focus on reducing service to individuals who are intoxicated or who are younger than the legal drinking age, and measure intoxication and underage drinking as outcomes. Strategies that focus on alcohol-related problems, on the other hand, may successfully reduce the problem without necessarily changing alcohol consumption. Thus, evaluations for these approaches use problem behaviours such as drink-driving and violence as outcomes. The present chapter includes interventions focused on reducing violence and other problem behaviour, whereas interventions specifically focused on drink-driving are discussed in Chapter 11.

Interventions focused on violence and injury go beyond changing serving practices. Although alcohol intoxication may play a causal role in aggressive behaviour (Bushman 1997) and be highly associated with violence in commercial drinking contexts (Homel and Clark 1994; Graham *et al.* 2006b), the characteristics of the drinker and the drinking context play key moderating roles in alcohol's effects (Graham *et al.* 2006a; see Graham *et al.* 1998). Certain aspects of the environment such as aggressive bar staff and their inability to manage problem behaviour (Homel *et al.* 1992; Wells *et al.* 1998; Lister *et al.* 2000; Winlow 2001; Winlow *et al.* 2001; Hobbs *et al.* 2002, 2003, 2007; Monaghan 2002; Graham *et al.* 2005a,b) may also contribute directly to aggression, independent of the effects of alcohol on patrons.

10.1.3 Types of interventions and programmes

Interventions or programmes to modify the commercial drinking environment can be conceptualized according to the breadth and nature of their focus. The first type is directed at individual drinking establishments or individual employees of drinking establishments. It includes training and licensing, as well as certification, and tools to help managers improve the drinking environment, such as risk assessment questionnaires and in-house policy guidelines. These interventions can be distinguished by whether they focus on (a) alcohol service or (b) other problem behaviours independent of alcohol service.

The second type of programme can be loosely referred to as 'enhanced enforcement'. Here the intervention addresses licensed premises generally through better or enhanced enforcement of existing laws and regulations, using enforcement as a strategy to identify and target high-risk establishments or using civil liability statutes to apply pressure to drinking establishments and their staff. These approaches sometimes focus on laws or regulations regarding alcohol service but tend to have generally broader prevention goals including violence and other problem behaviours.

The third category involves a comprehensive community approach directed toward a specific geographic entity (e.g. city, district) that includes interventions focused on individual establishments as well as enhanced enforcement. Community approaches involve more than just the first two types of interventions, however, in that they require a co-ordinated effort and commitment from community stakeholders and often look beyond the drinking establishments themselves to addressing street safety (e.g. lighting, transportation) and other community aspects of the drinking environment.

10.2 Interventions directed at establishments and bar employees

10.2.1 Responsible beverage service training and in-house policies

As described in Box 10.1, **responsible beverage service** (RBS) programmes (also referred to as 'server training' or 'server intervention' programmes) focus on attitudes, knowledge, skills, and practices of persons involved in serving alcoholic beverages in drinking establishments (see Carvolth 1995; Toomey *et al.* 1998). The primary goals of RBS are to prevent intoxication and underage drinking. Some programmes have also included separate or extended training for managers on policy development for the establishment.

Research on RBS programmes has occurred mostly in Australia, Canada, Sweden, and the USA. Nearly all evaluations have demonstrated improved knowledge and attitudes among participants (see reviews by Graham 2000; Lee and Chinnock 2006).

Box 10.1 Components of responsible beverage service (RBS) programmes

RBS programmes typically include the following four components:

◆ Attitude change: the benefits of preventing intoxication and not serving under-age patrons are stressed so that bar staff and management will take responsibility to prevent intoxication.

◆ Knowledge: the effects of alcohol, the relationship between alcohol consumption and blood alcohol concentration, the signs of intoxication, the laws and regulations related to serving alcohol, legal liability, strategies for dealing with intoxicated or underage patrons, and refusing service.

◆ Skills: the ability to recognize intoxication, refuse service, and avoid problems in dealing with an intoxicated person.

◆ Practice: checking age identification of young patrons, preventing intoxication, refusing service to someone who is becoming intoxicated, and arranging safe transport for intoxicated patrons.

These studies have also shown some effects on serving practices. In particular, servers are usually willing to intervene with customers who are visibly intoxicated (Gliksman *et al.* 1993), but generally will not intervene with individuals solely on the basis of the customer's estimated blood alcohol concentration (BAC) or number of drinks consumed (Howard-Pitney *et al.* 1991; Saltz and Stanghetta 1997). Also, training tends to decrease bad serving practices such as 'pushing' drinks and to increase 'soft' interventions such as suggesting food or slowing service, but training is less likely to increase actual refusal of service to intoxicated individuals (McKnight 1991; Gliksman *et al.* 1993; Krass and Flaherty 1994). The STAD (Stockholm Prevents Alcohol and Drug Problems) project, a multi-component programme that included RBS training, found a significantly greater increase in refusal of service to intoxicated patrons in establishments that received the programme compared with establishments in the control area (Wallin *et al.* 2005). However, because of the multiple components of the programme (training, enhanced enforcement, media coverage), the changes could also have resulted from other programme components.

With regard to reducing patron intoxication, several studies have found that server training generally results in lower BACs (Geller *et al.* 1987; Russ and Geller 1987; Dresser and Gliksman 1998) and fewer patrons with high BACs (Saltz 1987; Stockwell *et al.* 1993; Lang *et al.* 1998). Moreover, **time-series analyses** of mandatory server training (examining the effect of the state requiring server training by licensing regulations or law) suggest that training is associated with fewer visibly intoxicated patrons (Dresser and Gliksman 1998) and fewer single-vehicle night-time injury-producing crashes (Holder and Wagenaar 1994; see also review by Shults *et al.* 2001). However, other studies have found no effect of training on service to intoxicated patrons or on intoxication levels of patrons (Howard-Pitney *et al.* 1991; Krass and Flaherty 1994; Saltz and Stanghetta 1997) or mixed effects (Lang *et al.* 1998).

There has been increasing recognition of the need to focus on house rules and management support for RBS (see Stockwell 2001a). Many RBS programmes have included training for managers in the implementation of standard house policies or have used a 'risk assessment'approach to policy development (Saltz 1987; Mosher 1990). For example, the Australian 'FREO Respects You' Project, a voluntary programme involving local licensed premises (Lang *et al.* 1998), included a House Policy Checklist that covered the following topics: providing positive incentives for avoiding intoxication (e.g. food, cheaper prices for low- or non-alcohol drinks), avoiding incentives for intoxication (e.g. price specials), policies to minimize harm (e.g. increasing safe transportation options), and policies to minimize intoxication (e.g. providing and promoting food and non-alcoholic drinks, providing entertainment other than drinking, slowing and then refusing service to intoxicated patrons). A number of studies, however, have found limited effects of interventions focused on house policies (Howard-Pitney *et al.* 1991; Lang *et al.* 1998; Toomey *et al.* 2001, 2008).

In summary, although some studies have demonstrated an impact of server training and the development of house policies on the intoxication level of patrons, and one study found an association between state-mandated server training and lower rates of motor vehicle crashes, other studies have shown no measurable effect on alcohol consumption or other outcomes. Moreover, training programmes tend to be highly variable in quality and coverage (Toomey *et al.* 1998), and effects may diminish over time (Buka and Birdthistle 1999). On the other hand, a recent study of mandatory RBS training for licensed premises staff (Scott *et al.* 2007) in New South Wales, Australia found a significant increase in reported refusal of service to patrons who showed signs of intoxication.

Overall, the findings suggest that RBS training and house policies are likely to have at best a modest effect on alcohol consumption, and this effect will depend on the nature of the programme and the consistency of its implementation. The impact of RBS training on other outcomes is even less encouraging. A **Cochrane Review** (Lee and Chinnock 2006) concluded that there is no evidence that server training reduces injury, although few studies have actually examined injury or injury-related events.

10.2.2 Interventions to better manage aggression and other problem behaviour

Both training and licensing have been used to prevent aggression and injury by changing the way that bar staff deal with problem patrons. Although licensing of door staff is mandated in many countries, to date there is no evidence of its effectiveness (Lister *et al.* 2001; Graham and Homel 2008). Therefore, the following sections focus on the effectiveness of (a) freestanding training programmes for staff, and (b) programmes embedded in larger community action projects.

Training programmes specifically focused on dealing with aggressive patrons rather than serving practices have been developed for several reasons (Graham and Homel 2008). First, not all problems arise because patrons are intoxicated. For example, some bar settings attract patrons who may be looking for a fight. Second, individuals who arrive at the bar already intoxicated must be dealt with. Third, sometimes problems in bars are less related to intoxicated patrons and more related to aggressive or poorly trained bar or door staff. Fourth, when drinks are obtained from a busy serving bar, it is often not possible for even highly trained staff to monitor consumption levels. Fifth, factors within the drinking establishment such as over-crowding, 'macho' culture and competitive games can also play a role in stimulating violence.

Programmes have been developed in many countries to train security personnel and other bar staff in managing problem behaviour. However, most have never been subjected even to minimal evaluation. An exception is the *Safer Bars* programme developed in Canada for owners, managers and staff of licensed premises (described in Box 10.2). The three-hour training programme (Braun *et al.* 2000; Graham *et al.* 2008) is designed to increase early intervention by staff, improve teamwork and staff abilities in managing problem behaviour, and reduce the risk of injury to patrons. The *Safer Bars* training has been rated highly useful by bar staff and managers and has demonstrated a significant impact on knowledge and attitudes (Graham *et al.* 2005b). More importantly, a large-scale **randomized controlled study** (Graham *et al.* 2004) was able to demonstrate that the programme resulted in a significant reduction in physical aggression, as documented by trained observers.

Training programmes focused on preventing violence have also been implemented as a component of community projects. For example, the Queensland, Australia, community projects (Hauritz *et al.* 1998b; Homel *et al.* 1997) included a two-day

Box 10.2 The Safer Bars training programme

The *Safer Bars* training covers six broad areas related to preventing aggression and managing problem behaviour in commercial drinking establishments:

1. Understanding how aggression escalates and how to intervene early.
2. Assessing the situation and working as a team.
3. Keeping cool (that is, not losing one's temper).
4. Understanding and using effective body language (non-verbal techniques).
5. Responding to problem situations and dealing with intoxicated persons.
6. Legal issues related to preventing violence in licensed establishments.

training programme in crowd control and security for door staff as well as security management training for licensees and staff (Homel *et al.* 1997). In addition to the overall reduction in violence associated with the project, observational data in bars indicated friendlier but less permissive staff, more systematic checking of identification at the door, and an increase in staff controlling areas inside the bar as well as at the door (Homel *et al.* 1997; Hauritz *et al.* 1998b).

A similar effect was found for the multi-component STAD project (described in more detail in Box 10.3) which included a two-day training programme for bar staff and management personnel in conflict management and RBS, in addition to enhanced police enforcement relating to serving practices. The evaluation found a significant decrease in aggression in the intervention area compared with a slight increase in the control area (Wallin *et al.* 2003).

The other evaluated multi-component project that included staff training, Tackling Alcohol-related Street Crime (TASC), was conducted in Cardiff, Wales. This programme was unable to demonstrate a consistent reduction in violence (Maguire and Nettleton 2003; Warburton and Shepherd 2006) and found no effects that were specific to the training.

Overall, the evidence suggests that training programmes in managing problem behaviour and aggression may reduce aggression, but these results appear to depend on their quality and context. The effect of the *Safer Bars* programme on reducing aggression, although statistically significant, was modest (Graham *et al.* 2004). The training programmes within the Queensland studies and the STAD project were embedded in larger community action approaches that included a number of components, and these other components may have been at least partly responsible for the reductions in violence and even the changes in staff behaviour. Like training in RBS, the effects of training programmes in managing aggressive behaviour are likely to erode over time. For example, the evaluation of the *Safer Bars* programme found less of an impact among premises that had high turnover of managers and security staff. Similarly, the effects of the Surfers Paradise intervention quickly wore off in the two years after the intervention ended (Hauritz *et al.* 1998a). In this respect, the STAD project was notable because it included an intervention that was structured as a ten-year project, and the effects were not only sustained but appeared to increase over time.

10.3 Enhanced enforcement involving legal liability

Enforcement can be critical for the effectiveness of policies and training regarding RBS and other interventions. Several types of enforcement are potentially involved in the interventions discussed here, including administrative regulations, criminal law, and various kinds of civil law, including liability (tort) law. Besides the police, regulatory officials such as planning or liquor licensing inspectors are often involved as part of enhanced enforcement. These interventions usually try to persuade licensed sellers to organize their businesses differently, with regulatory sanctions (the threat of a licence loss or suspension) used as a strong incentive. Interventions involving enhanced enforcement have focused both on sales of alcohol and on preventing alcohol-related harm.

10.3.1 Increased enforcement of liquor laws and proactive policing

An evaluation of increased enforcement of laws prohibiting the sale of alcohol to intoxicated patrons in bars and restaurants (McKnight and Streff 1994) found a significantly higher rate of refusal of service to pseudo-patrons (i.e. actors who appeared to be intoxicated) in the county where enforcement was increased, compared with refusal rates in a comparison county that had no changes in enforcement. The US-based study also found a significant decrease in Driving While Impaired (DWI) charges in the experimental county, compared with no change in DWI charges in three counties for which comparison data were available. Moreover, the benefits of increased law enforcement greatly exceeded the costs (Levy and Miller 1995).

Proactive policing involving regular visits to licensees is a slightly different enforcement strategy that has been used to reduce offences relating to drunkenness and sales to minors. Although an early study in the UK found this to be an effective strategy (Jeffs and Saunders 1983), a later replication in Australia was unable to show a clear positive impact (Burns et al. 1995). Other research in the UK (Stewart 1993) and a study in New Zealand (Sim et al. 2005) found modest effects, although there appeared to be no carry-over beyond the period in which the enhanced policing occurred (see Graham and Homel 2008).

10.3.2 Targeted policing

Targeted policing has also been used to modify the drinking context. In the Alcohol-Linking project in Australia (Wiggers et al. 2004), police asked persons charged in police-attended incidents where they had consumed their last drink. These responses were used to target prevention efforts toward specific premises, although feedback was provided to all licensees in the area to inform them of the number of times their establishment had been identified relative to other establishments. As described in Box 10.4, this project was able to demonstrate a positive impact of the approach (although this effect was just short of statistical significance). It was also able

Box 10.3 Stockholm Prevents Alcohol and Drug Problems (STAD) project

This ten-year project was implemented in the northern part of central Stockholm (550 licensed premises) with the southern part serving as the control area (270 premises). The first part of the project included a survey of licensed premises and research documenting the extent of service to intoxicated persons. Led by an action group consisting of representatives from the county council, the licensing board, police, public health and bars and restaurants, the project included (1) a two-day training course in responsible beverage service and managing conflict for servers, security staff and owners and (2) enhanced enforcement by the licensing board and the police. A critical step in the project's evolution was the signing of a written agreement by high-ranking officials specifying how responsibilities for different parts of the intervention were to be distributed among participating organizations (Wallin *et al.* 2004).

The project appeared to gain momentum over time. Refusal of service to intoxicated persons increased from 5% in 1996 to 47% in 1999 and 70% in 2001 (Wallin *et al.* 2002, 2005). Although improvements in refusal of service also occurred in the control area (possibly reflecting some spill-over of the intervention), the refusal rate was higher for RBS-trained premises in the intervention area. The reduction in violent crimes was estimated at 29% for the intervention area compared with a slight increase in the control area (Wallin *et al.* 2003).

The success of the project seemed to be largely due to the strong support from the action group members, especially the head of the licensing board, positive media coverage, evidence provided by research data, and sustained and even increasing enforcement activity by police. The commitment to a ten-year time-frame which allowed the project to document and build on accomplishments and set up structures for continuing implementation appeared to have been a key factor in its success.

to implement the intervention in such a way that it became a permanent part of policing in the trial area, an important accomplishment given the transitory impact of short-term enhanced enforcement. New Zealand police have a similar Alco-Link Intelligence programme where data on place of last drink and observed intoxication level are collected on police charge sheets and analysed centrally, with results given to each police district. A continuing high profile in Alco-Link data, together with other evidence, may contribute to a premises losing its licence.

The TASC project in Wales also included a component whereby two venues with very high rates of assault were subjected to intensive police enforcement as well as shock tactics in the form of a presentation conducted by the local hospital emergency department showing graphic details of injuries (Warburton and Shepherd 2006). The intervention was associated with substantial reductions in emergency department admissions from these venues, but the weak study design involving pre–post measures in only two venues prevents conclusions about the broad effectiveness of this tactic.

10.3.3 Legal liability of servers, managers and owners of licensed premises

US laws that allow individuals injured by an underage or intoxicated individual to recover damages from the retailer who served or sold alcohol to the person causing the injury are referred to as **dram shop liability** laws (Mosher *et al.* 2002). Owners and licensees can also be held liable for the actions of their employees under these laws.

Research suggests that implementation of dram shop liability may lead to significant increases in checking age identification and greater care in service practices (e.g. Sloan *et al.* 2000). Several evaluations in the 1990s were able to show that states that held bar owners and staff legally liable for damage attributable to alcohol intoxication had lower rates of traffic fatalities (Chaloupka *et al.* 1993; Sloan *et al.* 1994b; Ruhm 1996) and homicide (Sloan *et al.* 1994a) compared with states that did not have this liability, with dram shop liability associated with reductions in alcohol-related traffic fatalities among underage drivers by 3–4% and among adult drivers by 4–7% (Chaloupka *et al.* 1993; Benson *et al.* 1999; Whetten-Goldstein *et al.* 2000). Importantly, dram shop liability appears to influence fatalities at both low and high BACs (Benson *et al.* 1999).

Several studies suggest that these changes are mediated by the attitudes and behaviour of bar owners and staff (Holder *et al.* 1993; Sloan *et al.* 2000). Consistent with this interpretation, Wagenaar and Holder (1991) found that when one state deliberately distributed publicity about the legal liability of servers, there was a 12% decrease in single-vehicle night-time injury-producing traffic crashes, a statistically significant change when compared with trends in other states. It should be noted that most of the research on holding the seller liable (under civil, tort law) for damage done by the drinker was conducted in the USA. Although there have been successful cases relating to server liability in Canada and Australia (Solomon and Payne 1996; Johnston 2001), legal systems in most countries have not accepted this extension of liability.

10.4 Community-level approaches

10.4.1 Community mobilization

Community mobilization programmes, also called community action projects, have been used to address problems associated with commercial drinking establishments, develop specific solutions to alcohol problems, and pressure owners of these establishments to take responsibility for issues such as noise level and patron behaviour (Homel *et al.* 1992; Putnam *et al.* 1993; Hauritz *et al.* 1998a,b). As with enforcement approaches, community action projects have typically included strategies and outcomes related both to alcohol consumption and to alcohol-related harms.

Box 10.3 describes the STAD project in Sweden, the most comprehensive community action project to date (Wallin and Andréasson 2005; Wallin *et al.* 2002, 2003, 2004, 2005). The success of this programme seemed to be due to its long timeframe, support from critical stakeholders and sustained police enforcement.

Another example of successful community mobilization is the Surfers Paradise project (Homel *et al.* 1997) and its replications (Hauritz *et al.* 1998b). The goal of the project was to reduce violence and disorder associated with the high concentration of licensed establishments in the resort town of Surfers Paradise in Queensland, Australia (Homel *et al.* 1997). The project involved three major strategies: (i) the creation of a Community Forum charged with the development of task groups and a safety audit; (ii) the implementation of risk assessments, 'Model House Policies', and a 'Code of Practice'; and (iii) enhanced monitoring of licensed premises by liquor licensing inspectors and law enforcement by police. This project and its replications in three North Queensland cities (Hauritz *et al.* 1998b) resulted in significant improvements in alcohol policy enforcement and bar staff practices, and significant reductions in violence in the bar environment. Following the intervention, the number of incidents per 100 hours of observation dropped from 9.8 at pretest to 4.7 in Surfers Paradise and from 12.2 at pretest to 3.0 in the replication sites. However, the initial impact of the project was not sustained. Two years following the intervention in Surfers Paradise, the rate of violent incidents had increased to 8.3. This reversion in the rate highlighted the need to find ways to maintain gains achieved from community action projects—a need that was addressed by the longer timeframe of the STAD project (described in Box 10.4).

The Rhode Island Community Alcohol Abuse/Injury Prevention Project (Putnam *et al.* 1993) used a community mobilization approach to reduce alcohol-related injuries related to both off-premises and on-premises alcohol sales. One community was randomly selected for the intervention, whereas two others served as controls. The intervention included a 5-hour RBS training programme, policy development for on- and off-premises alcohol sales, enhanced enforcement of liquor and DWI laws, training of police, and mass media campaigns. The RBS programme trained 61% of servers in the intervention community. A high rate of adoption of house policies was achieved for both on-premises (79%) and off-premises (100%) establishments. Following the training there were significant improvements in knowledge and self-reported serving behaviour, with effects mostly sustained over a four-year period (Buka and Birdthistle 1999). Emergency department visits declined 9% for injuries, 21% for assaults, and 10% for motor vehicle crashes, compared with no declines in the control community. The 27% *increase* in alcohol-related assault arrest rates in the intervention community (despite the reductions in emergency department admissions) suggested that the enhanced enforcement may have played a critical role in the reduction of injuries. As with the Surfers Paradise project, however, follow-up data indicated that the increased enforcement stimulated by the project was not maintained after the project ended (Stout *et al.* 1993).

A more recent project, known as the Sacramento Neighborhood Alcohol Prevention Project (SNAPP), evaluated the effectiveness of the community approach when delivered at the neighbourhood level (Treno *et al.* 2007a). The overall goal of the project was to reduce alcohol access and related problems among persons aged 15–29 years in two low-income neighbourhoods that had high rates of assaults. The project included community mobilization, enhanced community awareness, RBS training and enhanced enforcement of laws prohibiting service to minor and intoxicated persons.

Box 10.4 The Alcohol-Linking project

The Alcohol-Linking project, implemented in New South Wales, Australia, involved (a) documenting the location of last drink for persons who had been drinking prior to involvement in an incident attended by police and (b) using this information to target enforcement toward high-risk commercial drinking establishments (Wiggers *et al.* 2004). The enforcement aspect of the project, which had been designed in collaboration with the police, included:

◆ delivery to licensees of a tailored 'feedback' report from police describing those incidents reported to have occurred following consumption of alcohol on their premises;

◆ a visit by police to high-risk premises during which an audit of the premises' responsible service and management practices was undertaken;

◆ a follow-up visit by police during which the results of the audit were presented to licensees, together with recommendations for service and management improvements (Wiggers *et al.* 2004, p. 358).

A randomized control evaluation of the programme showed a greater reduction in alcohol-related incidents in the experimental group than in the control condition. The outcome fell just short of the conventional cut-off for statistical significance ($p = 0.08$).

An important goal of the project from its inception was to make the last-drink protocol a permanent part of policing (Daly *et al.* 2002; Wiggers *et al.* 2004). Key aspects of this nine-year process included: an active role of an advisory committee comprised of representatives from police, industry and local establishments; developing an evidence base that could demonstrate the efficacy and acceptability of the alcohol-linking protocol; demonstrating that it was feasible to adopt the protocol as part of routine policing; demonstrating an impact on alcohol-related crime; and collaboration with other agencies to ensure that sufficient resources were available (Wiggers *et al.* 2004).

The study design used a phased approach so that the second neighbourhood served as a comparison and replication site. The findings showed significant reductions in service to apparent minors but no impact on service to apparently intoxicated persons when the two intervention areas were compared. The evaluation compared the two intervention sites to Sacramento at large. Both intervention neighbourhoods showed significant reductions in assaults reported by police and on emergency medical services outcomes, assaults and motor vehicle accidents. However, these findings are not easy to interpret because the intervention sites were selected for their high problem rates and were therefore not comparable to the community at large.

10.4.2 Voluntary 'accords'

Voluntary accords comprise a less comprehensive type of community approach than community action projects like STAD and Surfers Paradise. These involve voluntary

Box 10.5 The Geelong Accord

The Geelong Accord was initiated by local police in one Australian community to reduce pub-hopping (i.e. moving from one drinking place to another) and associated problems. The Accord also aimed to minimize heavy drinking by underage patrons. Stipulations within the accord included cover charges to enter bars after 11 p.m., removal of cover charge exemptions for women, prohibition of unlimited re-entry with cover charge, banning of drink promotions that lead to intoxication, consistent serving policies among bars, and increased enforcement of laws regarding underage drinking and drinking in the streets. Bar owners reported a positive impact of the Accord, which is consistent with an observed decline in the assault rate from 0.8 to 0.5 per day (Felson *et al.* 1997). The Geelong Accord appeared to have a substantial and sustained impact on the local crime rate, although the lack of a controlled evaluation makes this conclusion tentative. Support from the local police seemed to be a key factor in the success of the voluntary code.

agreements or 'Codes of Practice' between the local hospitality industry and among owners of licensed premises to limit activities and promotions associated with alcohol-related harms. For example, Box 10.5 describes the Geelong Accord in Australia that addressed problems resulting from patrons going from one premises to another. It imposed minimum entry charges after 11 p.m. and eliminated passes for patrons to leave and re-enter the premises without paying the entry fee again (Lang and Rumbold 1997). The idea of Community Accords began in Australia where they have become increasingly popular (McCarthy 2007). Similar approaches have been adopted in New Zealand as well as other countries. Despite their popularity and evidence from the Geelong Accord suggestive of effectiveness, rigorous evaluations have found that strictly voluntary accords are unlikely to result in reductions in alcohol consumption and related harms (Hawks *et al.* 1999; see also review by Graham and Homel 2008).

The TASC project in Cardiff, Wales was a police-led multi-agency programme that included targeted policing, attempts to influence community policy, RBS training, licensing of security staff, cognitive behavioural therapy, and school education programmes. TASC was developed as a community project, but we have included it under 'accords' because the cornerstone of the project was the accord among licensees, and many of the other components were not fully implemented prior to the evaluation. Although there was some evidence of a decrease in violence, the findings were mixed and the weak pre–post design precluded conclusions about the programme's effectiveness (Maguire and Nettleton 2003).

Overall, the evidence suggests that community action approaches can be effective, but the effects are not sustained unless implemented over a long timeframe, as was done in the STAD project. Because community action approaches involve multiple components, research conducted has not been able to identify the specific components that contribute to their effectiveness. For the Rhode Island and the STAD projects, the role of enforcement appeared to be key. On the other hand, enforcement was judged as playing a lesser role in the Queensland projects (Graham and Homel 2008), suggesting that other aspects such as training of staff, social pressure on licensees, community involvement, and a combination of formal and informal regulation may also be effective strategies for changing the context of drinking to reduce harm. The evidence to date on voluntary accords, on the other hand, suggests that these are not likely to have an impact.

10.5 Other approaches

10.5.1 Reducing risks in the social and physical environment

Many of the strategies described above have included components designed to reduce risks in the physical and social environment of the drinking establishment. For example, risk assessments have been part of many RBS programmes (Graham 2000). The Safer Bars programme included an environmental risk assessment (Graham 1999) to assist bar owners and managers to reduce risks within their own premises related to physical layout, characteristics of servers and security staff, closing time, and other aspects of the bar environment. Risk assessments were also integral parts of the Queensland projects (Homel *et al.* 1997; Hauritz *et al.* 1998a,b) and the Alcohol-Linking project (Wiggers *et al.* 2004). These approaches to prevention reflect more systematic versions of strategies used in the past century to improve patron behaviour by changing the bar-room environment (Gutzke 2006; Graham and Bernards 2009).

The effectiveness of strategies to modify the physical and social environment of drinking establishments has never been evaluated directly. The evaluation of the Queensland projects found some evidence that the reduction in aggression may have been mediated through environmental changes (Homel *et al.* 2004). The Safer Bars evaluation, however, suggested that training was the key component (Graham and Homel 2008). Thus, while there is consistent evidence linking the environment to aggression in drinking establishments, there is as yet only weak evidence linking changes in these environments to reduced harm.

10.5.2 Glassware

Tempered glassware has been recommended as a harm reduction measure in order to prevent cuts and other serious injuries that occur when regular glass vessels are used as weapons in bar fights (Alcohol Concern 1996). However, a randomized controlled trial found that injuries to bar staff actually increased when toughened glassware was used (Warburton and Shepherd 2000), suggesting that metal, paper, or plastic drink containers may be the only safe alternative currently available. Recent research on the effect of glassware bans (Forsyth 2008), although preliminary in nature, suggests that such bans are feasible and may reduce injury.

10.5.3 'Lockouts'

Lockouts are a recent regulatory approach to late-night problems in Australia. Lockouts require drinking establishments to refuse further entry to patrons after a certain time, although they may continue to serve alcohol to those who are already present until closing time. While this approach is currently being implemented in various centres in Australia, there is no evidence to date of its effectiveness (Chikritzhs 2009). A three-month lockout trial was conducted in Melbourne, Australia in 2008, but its implementation was limited by exemptions granted to many late-trading premises and the evaluation by a commercial firm was inconclusive, finding mixed trends in the trial period (KPMG 2008a).

10.6 Approaches beyond commercial drinking establishments

Theoretically, at least some of the approaches used with commercial drinking establishments could be used to reduce harm in other drinking contexts. However, there is much less research on reducing harm in drinking contexts other than licensed premises and none has demonstrated clear evidence of effectiveness. Third parties often play a role in controlling aggressive and other problem behaviours in licensed premises (Wells and Graham 1999) at fiestas and other drinking occasions (Perez 2000), and among adults generally (Graham and Wells 2001). Therefore, in addition to prevention interventions focused on bar staff, there have been efforts to enlist friends as prevention agents (e.g. the 'friends don't let friends drive drunk' campaign: see Hawkins et al. 1977; McKilip et al. 1985; McKnight 1990). Although one study (Kennedy et al. 1997) reported that 55% of a sample of men aged 21–34 years reported having received such an intervention, the effect of these programmes on drink-driving has not been demonstrated. Similarly, De Crespigny et al. (1998) noted that female bar patrons rely on girlfriends to assist them with safety issues. While training potential victims or bystanders in methods of reducing the harm from someone else's intoxication appears to have some promise, there has been no systematic research on the effectiveness of this strategy.

10.7 Conclusion

Interventions focusing on minimizing the likelihood of harm occurring during the drinking event are being implemented with increasing frequency, especially in societies and settings where drinking is widely accepted. The evaluation literature on interventions in drinking contexts is based primarily on research conducted in a few developed countries. However, even in these countries, many of the interventions currently in practice have not been adequately evaluated. When a programme has been evaluated and shown to be effective, this does not necessarily mean that all versions of the programme will be effective in all contexts (Komro et al. 2008). Unlike more straightforward policy approaches such as taxation and pricing, programmes directed toward the drinking context typically involve a complex combination of content. For example, RBS programmes vary considerably in quality, intensity and implementation—which may account for the inconsistency in findings of effectiveness. Similarly, the effects of enhanced police enforcement may vary with the extent of enforcement and the quality and consistency of implementation. Community mobilization approaches are even more complex, with their impact depending not only on the nature, number and quality of components but also on the intensity with which each component is implemented. Finally, the context itself can partially determine the evaluation results, with programmes delivered in contexts that have high rates of problems having more room for improvement than do programmes delivered in contexts that have relatively low rates of problems (Ponicki *et al.* 2007).

Training programmes for bar staff both in RBS and in managing and preventing aggression has demonstrated that they may be effective, although these effects tend to be fairly modest and significant effects of server training have not been found in all evaluations. The evidence, especially for training in RBS, is that a sustained impact on actual intoxication levels of patrons may be limited to contexts where training is backed by enforcement.

The potential effectiveness of training programmes might be better understood by considering the theoretical frameworks described in the introduction to this chapter. In particular, the culture and history of the hospitality industry is such that education about RBS may be insufficient to counteract the rewards (e.g. financial rewards, feeling good about providing service) and the social pressure to provide service without the additional deterrents provided by law enforcement and the potential threat of legal liability. Training programmes to prevent aggression, on the other hand, may not necessarily need the added deterrence impact from enforcement and liability because aggression is not financially or socially rewarding for most establishments.

Enhanced enforcement of laws and regulations by police, liquor licensing, municipal authorities and others has been shown to be a powerful approach to reducing harms in the commercial drinking environment. Enhanced enforcement is likely to have impact through situational deterrents such as increasing risk of being caught and punished, removing excuses and so on. However, even enforcement approaches have shown mixed results, suggesting that their effectiveness will also depend on the quality, intensity and consistency of implementation. Further, there is little knowledge at present regarding how enforcement approaches could be strengthened by the use of high-quality training programmes, community mobilization and other strategies.

Community action focused on licensed premises has proven to be an effective strategy for reducing problem behaviour, and potentially injury, at least in some contexts; possibly because these broad multi-component approaches are able to expand the role of guardianship, implement numerous situational deterrents and eliminate some precipitators. However, these projects require extensive resources and long-term commitment, including enhanced and sustained enforcement. Moreover, although community approaches have been demonstrated to be effective, the essential ingredients or mix of ingredients remains unknown.

In sum, the focus on high-risk environments such as commercial drinking establishments has several advantages. First, it can have a broader impact than individual approaches would have on persons who are at high risk, especially young people and subcultures with risky drinking practices. Second, a variety of approaches can be applied at one time (e.g. training, enforcement, reduction of environmental risk factors).

Finally, most approaches targeting high-risk environments are generally perceived as acceptable in most cultures and may be easier to implement than less-accepted prevention strategies such as general alcohol control and tax measures. Measures to reduce the harm in the drinking situation are thus a useful element in the mix of strategies for preventing alcohol-related problems.

Chapter 11

Drinking-driving prevention
countermeasures

11.1 **Introduction**

Although there have been significant gains in road traffic safety, especially in high-income countries, motor vehicle crashes remain a major public health issue. In 2002, as many as 1.1 million people died worldwide from traffic injuries (Peden *et al.* 2004). Overall, road traffic injuries in that year accounted for 2.1% of all global deaths and ranked 11th as a cause of death. It has been estimated that traffic crashes may cost as much as US $500 billion annually, representing between 1% and 2% of the gross national product (Global Road Safety Partnership 2007). Traffic crashes disproportionately affect low- and middle-income countries. High-income countries in the WHO European Region have a road traffic fatality rate of about 11 per 100 000 and those of the Western Pacific Region have a rate of 12 per 100 000 (Peden *et al.* 2004). By contrast, the regional averages for low- and middle-income countries are much higher. The rate for the African Region, for example, is more than 28 per 100 000. In general, there has been a decrease in traffic fatality rates in high-income countries in recent decades, but not in low- and middle-income countries.

Alcohol is a major risk factor for traffic fatalities and injuries. In high-income countries about 20% of fatally injured drivers have a blood alcohol concentration above legal limits (Peden *et al.* 2004). Studies in low- and middle-income countries have shown that between 33% and 69% of fatally injured drivers and between 8% and 29% of non-fatally injured drivers had consumed alcohol. As with overall traffic crashes, alcohol-related crashes showed substantial declines in most high-income countries from the 1970s through the early 1990s and then began to level off or increase (Sweedler and Stewart 2009). In some cases, large increases in alcohol-related crashes have been observed in recent years. In Sweden, for example, alcohol-related fatal crash rates increased from about 20% of all fatal crashes in 2000 to 42% in 2006. Although reliable data are scarce, it appears that reductions have not been achieved in developing countries and that alcohol-related crashes and fatalities have increased in many of these countries (Davis *et al.* 2003).

This chapter describes the relationship between drinking and driving, and how an understanding of that association can be used to design countermeasures that prevent alcohol-related injuries and death. The chapter begins with a discussion of blood alcohol concentration as the key mechanism of alcohol-related harm. Current theories of harm-minimization are then described before reviewing the evidence supporting various legal and regulatory measures as well as rules and procedures designed to reduce driving under the influence of alcohol.

11.2 **Blood alcohol concentration (BAC) and driving performance**

BAC is typically defined as mass of alcohol per volume of blood or sometimes as mass of alcohol per mass of blood. For example, a BAC of 0.01% means 0.01 g of alcohol per 100 ml of an individual's blood. The amount of alcohol consumed is the most important influence on BAC, but it also depends on other factors such as an individual's weight, rate of drinking, and presence of food in the stomach (Mumenthaler *et al.* 1999; Ogden and Moskowitz 2004). Objective measurement of BAC has made it possible to study dose–response relationships between alcohol and impairment, and has also contributed to advancements in drink-driving policies.

At a BAC of 0.05% judgement and reaction times are impaired, and at a BAC of 0.10% voluntary motor control is substantially diminished (Davis *et al.* 2003). Studies indicate that the relative risk of a traffic crash is significantly elevated when BACs reach 0.04–0.05% (Moskowitz and Fiorentino 2000). For example, it has been estimated that drivers with BACs between 0.02% and 0.049% were 2.5–4.6 times more likely to be involved in a single vehicle fatal crash, depending upon age and gender (Zador *et al.* 2000). The risk of any crash involvement at a BAC of 0.04% is 1.18 times greater than at a BAC of 0.0% (Blomberg *et al.* 2005). At a BAC of 0.08% the relative risk is 2.7 and at a BAC of 0.15% the relative risk is 22.1. Overall, crash risk increases exponentially with BAC (see Figure 11.1). However, even at very low levels (e.g. BAC of 0.015%) a driver's ability to divide attention between two or more sources of visual information may be impaired (Ogden and Moskowitz 2004). Not only does alcohol increase risk of a crash, it can also increase crash severity. Thus, crashes in which at least one driver had been drinking are more likely to be fatal or result in severe injuries than are non-alcohol-involved crashes (e.g. Zador 1991; Zador *et al.* 2000; Moskowitz *et al.* 2002). Typically, male drivers are about 1.5 times more likely to be involved in alcohol-related fatal crashes than females and the contribution of alcohol to such

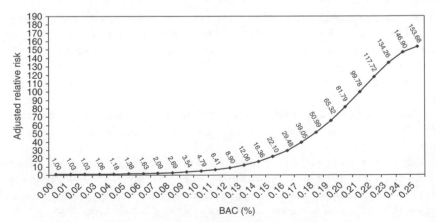

Fig. 11.1 Relative crash risk according to blood alcohol concentration (BAC).
Source: Blomberg *et al.* (2005), with permission.

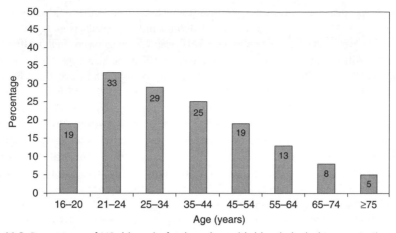

Fig. 11.2 Percentage of US drivers in fatal crashes with blood alcohol concentration ≥0.08% by age.

crashes peaks among US drivers in their early 20s (National Highway Traffic Safety Administration 2008).

Importantly, drinkers who consume relatively large amounts on some occasions may be at increased risk for involvement in alcohol-related crashes compared with other drinkers (Gruenewald *et al.* 1996; Treno *et al.* 1997; Valencia-Martin *et al.* 2008). In fact, evidence suggests that moderate drinkers who occasionally drink heavily may account for a substantial percentage of alcohol-impaired drivers (Flowers *et al.* 2008). Thus, at the individual level, drivers who qualify for a diagnosis of alcohol dependence or abuse are 1.8 times more likely to be involved in a fatal alcohol-related crash than current drinkers who never drank five drinks (for men; four for women) at a time (Voas *et al.* 2006). By contrast, drinkers who do not qualify for a dependence or abuse diagnosis but who sometimes drink five or more drinks (for men; four for women) were 2.6 times more likely to be involved in such crashes. Because of their relative numbers in the population, drinkers who qualify for a dependence or abuse diagnosis account for only 13% of fatal alcohol-related crashes compared with 25% for those who at least sometimes drink five or more drinks (for men; four for women) and 57% for those who always drink less than that.

It is clear that there are substantial differences among societies in the prevalence of drink-driving, as measured in studies carrying out breath tests from a random sample of motorists, usually during nights and weekends, when drink-drivers are more numerous. In the Scandinavian countries, there are relatively few drinking-drivers on the roads (Andenaes 1988; Ross 1993). Moderate to high BACs are found among less than 1% of drivers in these countries, even at peak driving times. Rates were higher in such studies in Australia, the USA, Canada, France, and The Netherlands, where between 5% and 10% of drivers have moderate to high BACs during night-time leisure hours (Smith *et al.* 1976); a recent roadside survey in the USA indicated that 15% of drivers had detectable alcohol in their breath and 6% had BACs above 0.05% (Lacey *et al.* 2007). Considerably higher drink-driving rates were found in a roadside survey in Diadema, Brazil using similar methodology (Duailibi *et al.* 2007a). This study found that 23.7% of drivers had consumed alcohol and that 19.4% were legally intoxicated with BACs >0.06%. In a second study (Campos *et al.* 2008) of high traffic density areas with a high concentration of bars, restaurants, and nightclubs in Belo Horizonte, Brazil, 38.0% of drivers had detectable alcohol in their breath and 19.6% were at or above the legal limit.

Societal differences in the prevalence of drink-driving also show up in surveys of drivers. Telephone survey data from the 2002–2003 Social Attitudes to Road Traffic Risk in Europe survey (SARTRE) indicated, on average, that 15% of European drivers reported driving at least once a week after drinking any alcohol (Cauzard 2004). Large regional differences were observed, with more than 20% of drivers in Cyprus, Italy, Spain, and Portugal reporting driving after drinking at least once a week. By contrast, fewer than 3% of drivers from Poland, Sweden, Hungary, the Czech Republic, Estonia, and Finland reported doing so. In general, driving after drinking any alcohol was relatively widespread in southern (43%) and Western European countries (19%), but less common in northern (8%) and eastern (11%) countries. Overall, 5% of drivers reported that they had driven while over the legal limit at least once in the previous week. The highest prevalence of such drivers was in Cyprus (22%), followed by Italy, Spain, Greece, and Croatia (7–8%). The lowest prevalence rates were observed in Sweden, Poland, Denmark, Finland, and the UK (<1%). Notable differences in drink-driving prevalence rates were found among southern European countries (13%), northern countries (0.2%), eastern countries (4%), and western countries (4%). In the USA, 23% of drivers report that they had driven at least once in the past year within two hours of consuming any alcohol and 19% reported having done so in the past month (Royal 2003).

11.3 Policy approaches to drink-driving

Drink-driving policy refers to legal and regulatory mechanisms as well as rules and procedures designed to reduce driving under the influence of alcohol. Such policies also include the enforcement of these measures (Grube and Stewart 2004; Grube 2007). The primary purposes of these policies are to deter drink-driving and to reduce the availability of alcohol. The deterrent effect of drink-driving policies is determined by their severity, the certainty of their imposition, and the swiftness with which they are imposed (Ross 1992). In general, severe penalties that are certain and swiftly administered will be most effective in deterring risky behaviour. However, the more severe the penalty, the less likely it may be that it will be applied and the more likely it will be that those who are caught will delay the process. Severity therefore often undermines certainty and swiftness; thus, the probability of being detected and having penalties swiftly imposed may be particularly important.

Penalties for drink-driving will certainly be ineffective if they are seldom enforced. Some research, in fact, suggests that policies that increase the probability of detection and arrest for drink-driving infractions may have greater effects on alcohol-related traffic fatalities than do policies that increase penalties (Benson *et al.* 1999). Overall, research strongly suggests that comprehensive approaches are related to lower rates of drink-driving and associated harms. A study in the USA found that individuals living in states receiving a poor rating on their drink-driving policies were 60% more likely to report alcohol-impaired driving during the past month than were those living in states receiving the highest rating (Shults *et al.* 2002). Similarly, the introduction of new comprehensive drink-driving legislation in Japan that included lower BACs, substantial fines, and jail sentences was associated with a 33–39% relative reduction in alcohol-related traffic fatalities (Desapriya *et al.* 2007; Nagata *et al.* 2008). The evidence for specific policies is summarized below.

11.4 Review of drink-driving policies

11.4.1 Lower legal BAC limits

Given the strong relationship between BAC and crash risk, countries have established *per se* **laws** concerning specific BACs at which a driver is presumed to be impaired and can be arrested. BAC can be measured by taking a blood sample from a driver but also via an analysis of the exhaled breath. The invention of portable devices for collecting samples of drivers' breath, combined with legislation establishing *per se* BACs defining impairment, have revolutionized law enforcement of drink-driving countermeasures in developed countries (Mann *et al.* 2001). BAC limits establish a legal definition of driving under the influence (i.e. the level at which a person is considered *per se* legally impaired). International BAC limits range from 0.0% (0.0 mg/ml) to 0.10% (0.1 mg/ml); 0.05% (0.5 mg/ml) is the standard in most countries (Desapriya *et al.* 2003).

An early review of the international evidence concluded that policies that lower BAC limits consistently reduce drink-driving crashes, and they also affect other indicators such as positive BACs among drivers and single vehicle night-time (SVN) crashes (Mann *et al.* 2001). The size of the effects, however, vary considerably between jurisdictions and in some cases appear to be temporary. Norström (1997) estimated that implementation of the 0.02% BAC law in Sweden in 1990 reduced fatal crashes by 6%. An analysis of daily crash data for four Australian states (Henstridge *et al.* 1997) between 1976 and 1992 concluded that the impact of a 0.05% BAC limit on fatal accidents ranged from a reduction of 8% in New South Wales to a reduction of 18% in Queensland. Using roadside survey data in South Australia, a 14% decline in drivers with a positive BAC was observed (Kloeden and McLean 1994).

A meta-analysis of data from the USA indicated that lowering the BAC limits from 0.10% to 0.08% was related to a 14.8% decrease in the number of drinking drivers in fatal crashes (Tippetts *et al.* 2005). The effects of these reduced BAC limits were greater in states that also had administrative license revocation laws (ALRs) and that implemented frequent sobriety checkpoints. Another US study found that reducing the BAC limits from 0.10% to 0.08% was associated with a 5.2% decrease in SVN crashes, after controlling for other possible confounders (Bernat *et al.* 2004). The effects of the 0.08% limit were found to be consistent across states. Another US **time-series** study of data from 1976 through 2002 estimated that lowering the legal BAC limit from 0.10% to 0.08% would prevent 360 deaths per year and that further lowering the BAC limit to 0.05% would save an additional 538 lives per year (Wagenaar *et al.* 2007b). Large variations were found across states in this study, although lowering the BAC limit affected drivers at all levels of impairment. That is, reducing the BAC affects not only lighter drinkers, but heavier drinkers as well. Similar reductions (7% to 10%) in alcohol-related fatal SVN crashes have been reported as a result of 0.08% BAC limits in the USA using a 15-year time series (Kaplan and Prato 2007). Lowering the BAC limits appeared to be less effective for men and younger drivers. Another time series study found a 9% reduction in fatal crashes involving drivers with BACs $\geq$ 0.08% and $\geq$ 0.01% for states that lowered BAC limits to 0.10% (Dang 2008). An additional reduction of 9% was found for states that further lowered BAC limits to 0.08%. Research in Europe suggests that lowered BAC limits may be ineffective unless accompanied by relatively strict enforcement (Albalate 2006). Thus, a 0.05% BAC limit, compared with the prior limit (typically set at 0.08%), was associated with a non-significant decrease in per-capita traffic fatalities, but with a significant 4.3% decrease when combined with sobriety checkpoints.

In summary, the evidence for the deterrent impact of establishing or lowering the legal BAC limit is strong (Asbridge *et al.* 2004; Fell and Voas 2009) in studies conducted in several countries. The effectiveness of these policies has led many countries to set increasingly stringent BACs. Introducing and lowering legal limits for driving can have enduring, long-term effects on drink-driving fatalities (Mann *et al.* 2001; Asbridge *et al.* 2004; Fell and Voas 2009). However, without consistent and visible enforcement the effects may be attenuated and may diminish over time. Ross (1982) hypothesized that the long-term deterrent impact of strict BAC limits may be undermined because drivers initially over-estimate the likelihood of apprehension but gradually come to realize that their chances of detection are, in fact, very low. To the extent that this is the case, rigorous and visible enforcement, combined with media attention, may be important for reinforcing the deterrent effects of lowered BACs.

11.4.2 Enforcement: selective and random breath testing

Certainty of punishment is central to deterrence. Unfortunately, the actual likelihood of being apprehended and convicted for drink-driving is quite low (Ross 1992). The traditional approach to increasing certainty of apprehension and punishment is to increase the frequency and visibility of drink-driving enforcement.

One approach to strengthening enforcement is to use **sobriety checkpoints** where law enforcement officials systematically stop every vehicle (or every *n*th vehicle) passing a predetermined fixed location on a public roadway to ascertain whether the driver might be impaired. The goal of sobriety checkpoints is to deter alcohol-impaired driving by increasing drivers' perceived risk of arrest. Sobriety checkpoints are often set up late at night or in the very early morning hours and on weekends when the proportion of impaired drivers tends to be the highest. A weakness of this approach, however, is that experienced offenders believe (with some justification) that they can avoid detection: there is evidence from the USA that police miss as many as 50% of drivers passing through sobriety checkpoints with a BAC >0.10% (McKnight and Voas 2001). Given this limitation, it is not surprising that drivers who have personally experienced a sobriety checkpoint, compared with those only indirectly exposed (e.g. through a friend, relative, or media), believe that the likelihood of arrest for drink-driving is relatively low (Beck and Moser 2006). Nevertheless, **meta-analyses** of available international studies found that sobriety checkpoints were associated with a 20–26% decrease in fatal crashes and a 20% decrease in total crashes (Shults *et al.* 2001; Elder *et al.* 2002). More recent studies have confirmed these effects. Thus, a reanalysis of the Charlottesville Sobriety Checkpoint Program found an 11.3% decrease in night-time crashes relative to the rest of the state of Virginia (Voas 2008). Notably, some failures have also been reported. The Maryland Checkpoint Strikeforce campaign had no discernible effects on self-reported drink-driving or on alcohol-related crashes (Beck 2009; Beck and Moser 2006). Perceptions of vulnerability to arrest for drink-driving actually declined during the campaign. Relatively few check-points were implemented and media efforts were insufficient to reach the majority of drivers. As a result, only about 30% of drivers were aware of the campaign and fewer than 10% were directly exposed to it. Although sobriety checkpoints can reduce drink-driving significantly, they are unlikely to be successful unless there is vigorous implementation, high visibility, and public awareness (Homel 1993).

Despite their promise, sobriety checkpoints are an under-used strategy to reduce drink-driving. In some cases, particularly in the USA, law enforcement agencies do not use checkpoints because of conflicts with state constitutions or laws. Other barri-ers to the use of checkpoints include the belief that they are difficult, expensive, and time consuming for enforcement personnel (Fell *et al.* 2003). However, studies indi-cate that cost-effective low-manpower checkpoints can have significant effects on self-reported drink-driving and on crashes (Lacey *et al.* 2006).

Random breath testing (RBT) or compulsory breath testing (CBT) is practiced in Australia, New Zealand, and some European countries. In this approach, motorists stopped at random by police are required to take a preliminary breath test, even if they are in no way suspected of any offence. The defining feature of RBT is that any motor-ist at any time may be stopped and required to take a breath test. To maximize its deterrent effects, RBT is generally conducted in such a way as to be highly visible and widely publicized. In many jurisdictions that implement RBT the chances of being tested are indeed high. In 1999, 82% of Australian motorists reported having been stopped at some time, compared with 16% in the UK and 29% in the USA (Williams *et al.* 2000). More recently in Queensland, Australia, police conducted the equivalent of one breath test per driver per year, with as many as 75% of motorists responding to a survey reporting having seen RBT within the past six months and 41% reporting having been breath tested themselves (Watson and Freeman 2007). Importantly, only a small percentage of drivers reported that they changed their driving habits to avoid RBT—fewer than 9% said they changed routes and fewer than 3% said they changed the times when they drove. Drivers who had seen an RBT or had been stopped and tested reported a somewhat greater perceived likelihood of apprehension for drink-driving, consistent with the programme's aim of having a deterrent effect. Those exposed to RBT, however, did not report more frequent use of alternatives to drink-driving (e.g. not drinking, using public transportation).

The available evidence suggests that RBT is an effective strategy to reduce alcohol-related traffic crashes. A review of early international studies of RBT and selective checkpoints (Peek-Asa 1999) suggested that RBT in Australia reduced alcohol-related fatalities by 33%, on average, alcohol-related injuries by 17%, and total fatalities by

35%. There was great variability, however, in the effects of programmes implemented in different jurisdictions or at different times, with reductions in total fatalities, for example, ranging from 20% to 76% and reductions in alcohol-related injuries from 0% to 24%. A later meta-analysis of 17 studies selected for soundness of research design found that RBT was related to a 22% decrease in crash fatalities, an 18% decrease in total crashes, and a 24% decrease in drivers with BACs > 0.08% (Shults *et al.* 2001). An evaluation of the New Zealand compulsory breath testing programme (CBT) using crash data from 1987 to 1997 found a 22% reduction in serious or fatal night-time crashes (Miller *et al.* 2004). Media publicity regarding the programme was related to an additional reduction of 14% in these crashes. Overall it was estimated that the CBT programme saved $1 billion in 1997 (1996 US dollars), far outweighing its costs.

In sum, the research evidence is quite strong that sobriety checkpoints and RBT can have sustained and significant effects in reducing drinking-driving and associated crashes, injuries and deaths. The effects of sobriety checkpoints and RBT appear to be comparable (Shults *et al.* 2001), with studies of sobriety checkpoints showing about a 20% decrease in crash rates and those of RBT showing about an 18% decrease. There is considerable variability in the effectiveness of different sobriety checkpoint and RBT programmes, however. A number of factors, including visibility, intensity of implementation, and public awareness seem to be important for the success of both sobriety checkpoints and RBT (Beck 2009). It has been suggested that checkpoint programmes and RBT are most likely to be effective when they (a) are highly visible, (b) include rigorous enforcement, (c) are sustained and consistent, and (d) are accompanied by extensive publicity, which reinforces or increases the perceived likelihood of being stopped by police and tested (Homel 1993).

11.4.3 Severity of punishment

A tenet of deterrence theory is that a punishment for a behaviour must be sufficiently severe if it is to reduce the likelihood of that behaviour occurring in the future. It is often assumed, all other things being equal, that more severe penalties are more effective than less severe penalties. However, as noted above, increased severity may reduce other factors that increase deterrence such as certainty or alacrity of punishment. Severity in the context of drink-driving has typically been addressed either by changing maximum penalties or by introducing mandatory minimum penalties.

A number of studies have investigated **mandatory jail sentences** for drink-driving. Overall the evidence for the effectiveness of mandatory jail sentences is mixed. A few studies find that they decrease alcohol-related fatalities or related outcomes (e.g. Stout *et al.* 2000), but most do not find such effects (e.g. Legge and Park 1994; Sloan *et al.* 1994a; Ross and Klette 1995; Ruhm 1996; Benson *et al.* 1999). A recent time series study of mandatory jail sentences across the USA found no discernible effect of the implementation or severity (length) of these sentences on SVN or alcohol-involved crashes (Wagenaar *et al.* 2007a). One study (McKnight and Voas 2001) observed that more severe penalties such as minimum imprisonment may have beneficial indirect effects when such punishments motivate repeat offenders to participate in programmes such as probation or treatment.

There is some evidence that mandatory fines may reduce drink-driving. Thus, in a US study, mandatory fines were associated with an 8% average reduction in fatal crash involvement by drivers with BAC $\geq$0.08 g/dl (Wagenaar *et al.* 2007a). The amount was not significantly related to fatal crash rates, although it was estimated that each dollar increase was associated with a decline of 0.023 driver involvements in SVN crashes per state per year. The results, however, varied widely from state to state and overall the implementation of mandatory fines did not affect SVNs. Another study using data from the 1984–1995 US Behavioral Risk Factor Survey showed that the size of the minimum fine for a first drink-driving offence was inversely related to self-reported drink-driving among moderate drinkers, but not heavy drinkers (Stout *et al.* 2000). Other studies, however, have found no effect of increased fines on alcohol-related crashes (e.g. Benson *et al.* 1999).

Overall, there is limited evidence that increased sanctions by themselves reduce drink-driving or alcohol-related crashes (Ross and Voas 1989; Mann *et al.* 1991). Indeed, they may be counterproductive if the judicial system is overburdened, causing delays in punishment, or if prosecutors fail to pursue these cases (Little 1975; Ross and Voas 1989). In many cases the implementation of more severe sanctions such as increased fines or jail sentences is confounded with other policy changes, making it difficult to ascertain unique effects. It may be more reasonable to consider the totality of sanctions when evaluating effects on drink-driving. In this regard, it has been found that people living in US states with stricter and more comprehensive drink-driving policies (including criminal and administrative sanctions and fines) are about 60% less likely to report drink-driving compared with those from states with less restrictive policies (Shults *et al.* 2002). The introduction of strict sanctions in Japan was associated with a 39% relative reduction in alcohol-related fatal crash rates among 16- to 19-year-old drivers and a 33% reduction in such crash rates among adult drivers (Desapriya *et al.* 2007). The sanctions included a reduced BAC from 0.05% to 0.03%, a tenfold increase in the fine, a possible three-year jail sentence, and commercial host liability, Similarly, the Taipei criminal sanctions for drink-driving implemented in 1999 included a mandatory jail sentence, a substantial fine, and license suspension. The new policy was also accompanied by considerable media attention. An evaluation showed a 73% reduction in fatal alcohol-related crashes over 20 months following implementation (Chang and Yeh 2004). Interestingly, the effect of this policy package appeared to be greater initially and then declined, suggesting increased sanctions may have a natural 'life cycle'and lose their effectiveness over time unless accompanied by renewed enforcement or media attention to reinforce these efforts.

11.4.4 Swiftness of punishment

Celerity or swiftness of punishment refers to the proximity of punishment to the drink-driving event. Deterrence theory proposes that punishments that are administered quickly will have a greater deterrent effect than those that are delayed. Many sanctions for drink-driving are imposed only after long delays necessitated by administrative hearings or court proceedings. One exception is pre-conviction **administrative license revocation** (ALR) or suspension for drink-driving. With an administrative suspension, licensing authorities can suspend a driver's license without a court hearing, often at the time of or very shortly after the actual offence. Administrative suspension is permitted in 40 of the 50 states in the USA and in ten of Canada's 13 provinces and territories.

Enforcement of ALR may be problematic, with as many as 75% of offenders continuing to drive with a suspended license (Voas and DeYoung 2002). Nonetheless, recent evaluations of ALR interventions have found consistent effects on alcohol-related crashes. In a recent evaluation it was found that a 90-day ALR in Ontario was associated with a 14% reduction in total driver fatalities (Asbridge *et al.* 2009). McKnight and Voas (2001) reported an average reduction of 5% in alcohol-related crashes and a 26% reduction in fatal crashes associated with ALR in the USA. Similarly, a 5% reduction in alcohol-related fatal crashes for drivers of all ages was found in a long-term follow-up of ALR in 46 states (Wagenaar and Maldonado-Molina 2007). This study also found that the effects on crash involvement were greater for low- vs medium- or high-level BAC crashes, although consistent effects on the percent reduction in crashes was found at all BACs. Finally, a study of novice drivers concluded that the benefit-to-cost ratio was $11 per dollar invested when violators receive a six-month license suspension (Miller *et al.* 1998), suggesting that ALR is a cost-effective strategy.

11.5 Preventing recidivism: Treatment, enhanced sanctions, vehicle programmes, and victim impact panels

Some convicted offenders continue driving after drinking and are re-arrested or involved in further traffic crashes. In the USA, for example, between 10% and 16% of those arrested for driving under the influence (DUI) with BACs >0.15% have a prior offence within the previous three years (McCartt and Williams 2004). Overall, about one-third of drivers arrested for DUI in the USA have at least one prior conviction (Williams *et al.* 2007). Approaches to preventing drink-driving recidivism have included treatment, enhanced sanctions against repeat offenders, driving restrictions or vehicle immobilization, and victim impact panels. Preventing repeated drink-driving is difficult, in part, because many recidivists are alcohol dependent or suffer from other comorbid disorders. As many as 54% of repeat impaired-driving offenders may meet clinical criteria for alcohol dependence and 40% or more may meet criteria for lifetime drug abuse (Lapham *et al.* 2006a). As a result, recidivist drink-drivers may be less receptive to traditional deterrence and may need a more comprehensive approach (Simpson *et al.* 2004; Williams *et al.* 2007).

Although the research is inconclusive, remedial treatment that is either mandated or imposed as a condition for reduced sanctions may have modest effects on drink-driving recidivism (DeYoung 1997; Dill and Wells-Parker 2006). An early meta-analysis of 215 studies of drink-driving remediation programmes, for example, concluded that treatment alone had only modest effects (Wells-Parker *et al.* 1995). A more recent **Cochrane Review** concluded that there was insufficient evidence to determine whether treatment (primarily brief interventions in a clinical setting) alone reduced motor-vehicle crashes and related injuries (Dinh-Zarr *et al.* 2004). Other studies, however, have provided support for the effectiveness of treatment programmes in combination with other sanctions for preventing recidivism. An intervention in New Mexico mandating a 28-day treatment programme in conjunction with a jail sentence reduced the likelihood of re-arrest over five years by 22% relative to a jail-only group (Kunitz *et al.* 2002). The effects of this programme on re-arrest were consistent across gender and ethnic groups, but no effects were observed for alcohol-related crashes (Woodall *et al.* 2004). In another study in New Mexico, DUI offenders undergoing treatment in addition to serving a jail sentence had a lower probability of re-arrest than those simply convicted but not sentenced and those convicted and sentenced to jail without treatment (Delaney *et al.* 2005). Length of jail sentence did not affect recidivism. Similarly, a treatment programme in Spain (Gómez-Talegón and Alvarez 2006) indicated that DUI offenders were substantially less likely to re-offend (4.3%) after treatment than before (15.9%), although there was no comparison group. In general, the more successful remedial programmes tend to be well structured, go beyond simply providing information to address alcohol abuse, are conducted for more than ten weeks, and have rules of attendance enforced by a court (Wells-Parker 2000; Dill and Wells-Parker 2006).

Enhanced sanctions may include fines and mandatory jail sentences. Although enhanced sanctions for high-BAC drivers have been strongly advocated by some, there is concern that large fines or severe jail sentences may increase BAC test refusals or lead to lower conviction rates because of plea bargaining or reluctance on the part of prosecutors and judges to impose such penalties. Interestingly, recidivist DUI offenders find drink-driving penalties to be fair although severe, but not swift and certain (Freeman *et al.* 2006).

Little research has been conducted in this policy area. An evaluation of the Minnesota enhanced sanctions law for high-BAC drivers indicated that the stricter penalties for high BAC were enforced on a majority of those arrested with high BACs, although enforcement for first-time offenders declined somewhat with the passage of time (McCartt and Northrup 2004). The stricter sanctions appeared to have reduced recidivism rates by about 19% in the first year of implementation, but was less effective in later years. The Oregon DUI Intensive Supervision Program (DISP) includes a short jail sentence, mandated treatment, weekly attendance at Alcoholics Anonymous meetings, electronic monitoring, breath testing by telephone, mandated sale of any vehicles owned by the offender, frequent contact with probation officers, regular court appearances, and periodic polygraph testing. A five-year evaluation indicated that drink-driving offenders undergoing the programme, compared with matched controls, were 51% less likely to re-offend, 48% less likely to drive while suspended, and 62% less likely to get other traffic convictions (Lapham *et al.* 2006b). A follow-up study to determine which of the components contributed to the effectiveness of the programme led to somewhat equivocal findings (Lapham *et al.* 2007). Compared with those receiving the complete DISP, the risk of re-offending during the first 90 days was four times higher among those not undergoing electronic monitoring, nearly twice as high among those not required to sell their vehicles, and 3.4 times higher among those who were required to do neither. The effects of monitoring appeared to dissipate after 90 days.

Many jurisdictions attempt to prevent drink-driving recidivism by limiting or eliminating a repeat offender's access to, or use of, a motor vehicle through vehicle immobilization, impoundment, and license plate confiscation or registration cancellation. Very few evaluations of these programmes have been conducted, although the available research suggests that some (e.g. impoundment) may reduce recidivism (Voas and DeYoung 2002; Voas et al. 2004). These sanctions, however, are rarely enforced even where allowed by law.

Ignition interlock devices are a relatively new innovation that prevent a vehicle from being started until the driver passes a breath test using special equipment installed in the automobile. Interlock programmes are in place or are being introduced in a large number of jurisdictions in North America, Europe, and Australia. Interlock programmes range from those that are mandatory and require offenders to have interlock devices installed on their vehicles, to voluntary programmes that allow offenders to have a shortened period of license suspension if they have these devices installed. Well-implemented interlock programmes may reduce recidivism by 65% or more (Roth et al. 2007; Marques 2009). An evaluation of the Swedish alcohol ignition interlock programme (Bjerre and Thorsson 2008) found a greater reduction in arrests for drink-driving among drivers in the programme (60%) compared with drivers not offered the programme, but indicating an interest (19%) and drivers refusing participation in the programme (0%). Those in the programme, however, had a higher rate of drink-driving offences during the five years prior to the study, making the results difficult to interpret. In general, self-selection of drinking drivers into interlock programmes is a problem for many evaluations. Nonetheless, a Cochrane review of the best available studies concluded that drink-driving offenders with interlocks installed are about 36% as likely to recidivate as drivers without interlocks (Willis et al. 2004). However, the effects of interlock programmes seem to be limited to the period of time that the interlock is actually installed on the vehicle (Marques and Voas 1995, 1998, 2005; DeYoung et al. 2005; Marques 2009). At present, there is no consistent evidence that interlock programmes reduce alcohol-related crashes overall (Marques 2009), perhaps because only a small proportion of eligible offenders (typically around 10%) have the devices installed (DeYoung 2002; Voas and Marques 2003; Bjerre 2005). This may be particularly problematic when programmes are voluntary or discretionary. Options for increasing use of interlock devices to prevent drink-driving include linking interlock programmes more closely to remedial treatment programmes, providing incentives for participation, or making their use mandatory (Marques 2009). Using interlock devices and related technologies as primary prevention measures may also be effective. A study with commercial drivers in Sweden found a reduction in drink-driving incidents from 5% per year to nearly zero (Bjerre 2005). Bjerre and Kostela (2008) estimated that installing interlock devices on all commercial vehicles in Sweden would prevent about half a million drink-driving events per year.

Another intervention to reduce drink-driving recidivism is the victim impact panel (VIP) or restorative justice conferences, where people representing victims of drink-driving incidents meet with the offender in a structured situation with a trained facilitator (Shinar and Compton 1995). The panel members collectively determine a penalty or level of restitution. VIP programmes are based on the assumption that offenders will be motivated to reduce their future drink-driving behaviour if they are made to understand the impact that an alcohol-related collision has on victims

(Wheeler *et al.* 2004). Empirical support for the effectiveness of VIP programmes is mixed. Although a meta-analysis of 35 randomized studies of VIPs (Latimer *et al.* 2001) found that this process decreased recidivism (72% of 32 studies yielded a reduction in recidivism), most of the studies in this review did not involve drink-driving offenders. In fact, with some exceptions (Fors and Rojek 1999), evidence from studies on VIPs does not support the effectiveness of this approach in reducing drink-driving (C'de Baca *et al.* 2001; Polacsek *et al.* 2001; Wheeler *et al.* 2004). For example, a study of first-time offenders who were randomly assigned to attend or not attend a VIP found no significant differences between the two groups on alcohol consumption, drink-driving behaviour, or recidivism over two years (Wheeler *et al.* 2004). In another study, increased recidivism was reported for female drink-driving offenders participating in a VIP programme (C'de Baca *et al.* 2001). Similarly, a large-scale randomized experiment in the Australian Capital Territory showed a slight increase in recidivism for drivers in the programme compared with those assigned to court (Sherman *et al.* 2000). The findings from these studies are consistent with earlier reviews reporting mixed, but mostly null, results for the effects of VIP on drink-driving recidivism (Shinar and Compton 1995).

Overall, evidence supports the effectiveness of treatment for reducing recidivism when combined with other sanctions for drink-driving. There is no evidence for the effectiveness of VIPs. Vehicle programmes that prevent access to cars or restrict driving appear to be effective while the restrictions are in place. In this regard, interlock programmes appear to be particularly promising. Comprehensive approaches to drink-driving recidivism, combining treatment with licence suspension, vehicle impoundment, interlocks, and other sanctions may be most effective in preventing recidivism. This comprehensive approach, however, has not been widely tested.

11.6 Restrictions on young or novice drivers

Young drivers (adolescents between 16 and 20 years) are at elevated risk for traffic crashes, especially alcohol-involved crashes, as a result of their limited driving experience and their tendency to experiment with heavy or binge drinking. Data from the New Zealand's Land Transport Safety Authority show risk increasing from around 0.05 g/100 ml blood alcohol for adults, and a much earlier, sharper rise for those aged <20 years (Land Transport Safety Authority 2003). Special policy strategies have been formulated to prevent drink-driving among this age group.

11.6.1 Low BAC limits for young or novice drivers

Zero tolerance laws for young or novice drivers set the BAC limits at the minimum that can be reliably detected by breath testing equipment (i.e. 0.01–0.02%). Zero tolerance laws also commonly invoke other penalties such as automatic loss of the driving license for drink-driving. An analysis of the effect of zero tolerance laws in the first twelve US states to enact them found a 20% relative reduction in SVN fatal crashes among drivers aged <21 years, compared with nearby states that did not pass zero tolerance laws (Hingson *et al.* 1994; Martin *et al.* 1996). A review of six studies on the effects of zero tolerance concluded that all of the studies showed a reduction in injuries and crashes, although the differences were not statistically significant in three of the smaller studies (Zwerling and Jones 1999). A national study of US states found a net decrease of 24% in the number of young drivers with positive BACs as a result of zero tolerance laws (Voas *et al.* 2003). Similarly, a 19% reduction in self-reported driving after any drinking, and a 24% reduction in driving after five or more drinks, was found using survey data from 30 states (Wagenaar *et al.* 2001). A time-series analysis of data from 1982 to 2005 in the USA indicated that implementing zero tolerance laws resulted in a 15% reduction in fatal crashes for young drivers with BACs ≥0.08% and an 18% reduction in these crashes for young drivers with BACs ≥0.01% (Dang 2008). Although evidence of the effectiveness of lower BAC limits for young drivers is quite strong, all of these studies were conducted in the USA. A review of both US and Australian studies (Shults *et al.* 2001) found reductions between 9% and 24% in fatal crashes associated with the implementation of zero tolerance laws. Similarly, a review of Canadian studies concluded that lower BACs for young drivers were related to a 25% reduction in reported drink-driving among young males in Ontario and an 8.9% reduction in SVN crashes in Quebec (Chamberlain and Solomon 2008). Recent research, however, indicates that although zero tolerance laws can significantly increase the chances of a young drinker being arrested and sanctioned for drink-driving, recidivism may be a serious issue, with as many as 25% of those arrested being re-arrested at a later time (McCartt *et al.* 2007).

11.6.2 Licensing restrictions and graduated licensing

Although the minimum driving age for automobiles in Canada, Japan, and most European countries is 18 years, the minimum age for drivers' licenses has traditionally been lower in other countries, sometimes as low as 14 years. In the USA, unsupervised driving has been allowed at 14, 15, 16, and 17 years of age, with most states opting for 16. A comparison of US states with differing ages for licensing (McCartt *et al.* 2008; Williams 2008) concluded that substantial reductions in 16-year-old driver fatal crash involvement could be achieved by raising the legal age of driving to 17 years. However, such laws may be unpopular. As an alternative to raising the driving age, some countries have implemented **graduated driver licensing** (GDL), which places restrictions on young or novice drivers (e.g. prohibits night-time driving, driving with other young people in the vehicle, driving without an adult in the car) in order to achieve some of the benefits of delayed licensing. A review of early programmes in the USA concluded that GDL reduced the risk of fatal or injury crashes among young drivers by 11–24% and the risk of any crash by 25–27% (Shope and Molnar 2003). A review of more recent GDL programmes found a 20–40% reduction in crash risk (Shope 2007). A Cochrane Review of studies from the USA, Canada, New Zealand, and Australia similarly concluded that GDL reduced crashes among first-year drivers by as much as 26–41% (Hartling *et al.* 2004). This same review found that GDL programmes reduced alcohol-related crashes and night-time crashes (a surrogate for alcohol crashes) among youth affected by the licensing restrictions by as much as 9–12% relative to other age groups. Other recent studies confirm that graduated licensing is related to reduced overall, night-time, and injury crash rates and reduced hospitalization rates among young drivers (Margolis *et al.* 2007; O'Connor *et al.* 2007).

By contrast, a few studies (e.g. Masten and Hagge 2004) have found no effects of GDL on teenage crash rates. There is also evidence that graduated licensing may adversely affect older teenage drivers, increasing crash rates and alcohol-related crash rates among these drivers when they obtain an unrestricted driver license (Hartling *et al.* 2004; Males 2007). Large variations in how graduated driver licensing programmes are implemented across jurisdictions may account for the mixed findings. An analysis of US graduated licensing programmes suggested that good and fair programmes reduced night-time driver fatalities among 15–17-year-olds by 10% and 13%, respectively, vs <2% for marginal programmes (Morrisey *et al.* 2006). In addition, some GDL programmes incorporate zero tolerance provisions, making it difficult to evaluate the unique contributions of delayed licensing and other restrictions to reductions in crash rates among young people.

In short, the evidence shows that lower BAC limits, delayed access to a full licence, and other driving restrictions for young drivers can be effective strategies for reducing drink-driving among the young and, more importantly, driving fatalities. Graduated licensing can incorporate all of these strategies within one system by imposing zero-tolerance measures and controlling the rate and manner in which young drivers gain access to full driving privileges. GDL has been well accepted where implemented, and the available evaluations as a whole demonstrate benefits.

11.7 **Designated driver and safe ride programmes**

Many drink-driving incidents originate in locations other than the home, such as licensed establishments, parties, and other social events (Morrison *et al.* 2002; Usdan *et al.* 2005; Tin *et al.* 2008). Interventions in these settings are thus important for preventing driving after drinking.

Designated driver programmes were developed to decrease driving after drinking by encouraging groups of drinkers in public or social settings to select a member of the group to serve as the designated sober driver. The use of a designated driver has shown tremendous gains in popularity since it was first introduced in North America with some form of use common around the world (Derweduwen *et al.* 2003; Valde and Fitch 2004; Pan-European Designated Driver Campaign 2006: 2007; Rivara *et al.* 2007; Watson and Nielson 2008).

A systematic review (Ditter *et al.* 2005) concluded that the evidence for the effectiveness of designated driver programmes was marginal, at best. Overall, population-based campaigns to encourage use of designated drivers resulted in an average 13% increase in drinkers saying they used a designated driver, but no significant change in self-reported drink-driving or riding with alcohol-impaired drivers. This review found some evidence that designated driver programmes implemented in drinking establishments modestly increased the number of patrons who reported being a designated driver, and one study found a decrease in self-reported driving after drinking or riding in a car with an intoxicated driver.

Drinking groups sometimes run into problems using a designated driver, including pressure to drink despite being the driver, the lack of incentive to serve as the sober driver and other issues (Rothe 2005). In some cases, the designated driver is the person in a group who has consumed the least alcohol (rather than no alcohol) or has consumed less alcohol than usual (Rivara *et al.* 2007), even if this amount is considerable (Nygaard *et al.* 2003). For instance, a survey of college students in Australia indicated that 26% of those who served as a designated driver reported doing so while feeling the effects of alcohol (Stevenson *et al.* 2001). Males may be particularly likely to drink when serving as designated drivers (Timmerman *et al.* 2003). Furthermore, there is some evidence that those who serve as designated drivers are often heavier drinkers and more likely to report drink-driving and riding with drinking drivers than are drinkers who never serve as designated drivers (e.g. Caudill *et al.* 2000a). On the other hand, encouraging drinking groups to plan ahead regarding who will serve in the designated driver role and reinforcing the person taking that role may be an effective strategy in reducing the amount that designated drivers drink. In a study of one programme that (i) induced groups to designate drivers in advance of drinking, (ii) clearly identified designated drivers (e.g. with a bracelet), and (iii) rewarded them for not drinking, Lange *et al.* (2006) found substantial increases in the number who reported moderating their drinking or refraining from consuming alcohol. An evaluation of the 'Skipper' programme in Queensland, Australia (Watson and Nielson 2008), whereby licensed premises provide free non-alcoholic beverages to designated drivers, found significant increases in past three-month use of a designated driver in the intervention area, whereas there were no significant changes in the comparison area. However, there was no significant change in serving as a designated driver or in use of a designated driver on the night of the survey, suggesting a modest effect at best.

Despite evidence of increased use of designated drivers, the effectiveness of this approach is likely to be limited, in that it applies only to those drinking as part of a social group (i.e. a lone drinker will not have easy access to a designated driver), requires planning prior to the drinking occasion, and depends on the designated person not drinking rather than just drinking less than the rest of the group. In addition, research suggests that some drinkers may consume more alcohol than usual on occasions when they use a designated driver (Harding *et al.* 2001; Rivara *et al.* 2007) and that bartenders are more likely to serve an intoxicated customer if the customer is accompanied by a designated driver (Reiling and Nusbaumer 2007).

Ride service or safe ride programmes are the quintessential harm-reduction approach to drink-driving in that they allow people to drink as much as they want with the idea that some of the harms will be reduced by providing transportation to drinkers who would otherwise drive. Unlike designated driver programmes, safe ride programmes apply to all drinkers who are potential drivers, not just to pre-existing social groups, and they do not require planning prior to the social event.

There is evidence that ride services are popular in some countries. For example, in one US study of college students using safe rides programmes, 44% reported that they would otherwise have driven after drinking (Sarkar *et al.* 2005). On average, they consumed 7.8 drinks during the evening, indicating a high rate of impairment among drinkers who presumably would have driven except for the programme. Similarly, a survey of past users of the 'Operation Nez Rouge' (Operation Red Nose) programme in Quebec, Canada, involving volunteer drivers providing transportation home for drinkers during the Christmas season, found that while about half planned on using the service before they began drinking, the other half decided to use the service after they had been drinking (Ayer *et al.* 1994). Almost 75% of those using the programme thought that it was a good prevention programme, while 7.5% thought that it encouraged people to drink. About two-thirds reported that the programme made them more aware of possible impairment due to alcohol. A survey of a representative sample of 544 young adults in Quebec, Canada (Lavoie *et al.* 1999) found that 17% had telephoned for the ride service when they were the driver and 36% had telephoned as passengers. More than half of respondents intended to use the service or to recommend it to a friend.

Evaluations (Molof *et al.* 1995) of two longstanding, well-functioning US-based ride service programmes, one serving primarily bar patrons and persons attending corporate or social host parties (providing 2500 free rides per year) and the other operating over the Christmas and New Year season (providing 700 free taxi rides home) found no discernible impact of either programme on annual crash rates, although the programmes were well established and popular. Other research on US safe rides programmes, however, suggested that they are used relatively infrequently by drinkers (Caudill *et al.* 2000b; Harding *et al.* 2001).

In summary, designated drivers and ride services can be popular among people who presumably would otherwise drive while intoxicated, reach high-risk groups for drink-driving (young, male, heavier drinkers), and may generally increase awareness of the risks of drink-driving. However, because these services account for a relatively small percentage of drivers, no overall impact on alcohol-involved accidents or other drink-driving outcomes has been demonstrated.

11.8 **Conclusion**

One of the most important public health and alcohol policy successes in the twentieth century has been the reduction in alcohol-involved traffic crashes, particularly in higher-income nations. The international evidence suggests that drink-driving countermeasures can consistently produce population-wide long-term reductions in drink-driving and in alcohol-related crashes and mortality. Recognition of the problems remaining, such as the persistent recidivism among high-risk impaired drivers, should not detract from the enormous achievements of recent decades. It is also clear, however, that many countries, especially those in the lower-income parts of the world, have not benefited equally from these advances. As such countries become able to purchase and operate automobiles, problems associated with impaired driving will become even more acute.

Developing countries face special challenges in preventing alcohol-related crashes and fatalities, including poorer road conditions; higher density and diversity of vehicles; greater intermingling of pedestrian, non-motorized, and motor vehicle traffic; and limitations on resources that can be devoted to improving traffic safety (Mohan 2002; O'Neill and Mohan 2002). In particular, lack of funding, manpower, equipment, and political support may be serious barriers to effective drink-driving policy implementation and enforcement (Davis *et al.* 2003). Enforcement of legal BAC limits, for example, may be impossible where police do not have breath-testing equipment.

Cultural factors such as traditional heavy use of alcohol in the context of social activities (e.g. weddings, funerals) may both increase risk in an increasingly motorized environment and make some interventions unacceptable or more difficult to implement.

Because of these and other differences it cannot be assumed that strategies that are effective for preventing and reducing drink-driving in developed countries will be equally effective or feasible in developing countries. Some may be applicable, some may not. Obtaining adequate evaluation data is also an issue. In many developing countries there is a lack of road safety data in general and impaired driving in particular. Although there is much to be learned from research on what is effective in developed countries, it must be recognized that policies and other interventions must be developed, adapted to, and evaluated within the unique cultural contexts of developing and non-western countries. Finally, providing technical assistance and support to developing countries in addressing impaired driving has been identified as an important issue (Davis *et al.* 2003).

Much can be accomplished through new laws or more imaginative enforcement of existing laws. Sweedler (2000) observed that evidence-based strategies adapted to local conditions will differ from country to country, but the overall results of the mixture of countermeasures may ultimately be similar. To decrease alcohol-related fatal crashes, communities need to enforce strategies that are known to be effective, such as random breath testing to enforce BAC laws, minimum legal drinking age laws, and lower BAC limits and 'zero tolerance laws' for young drivers. GDL may also be effective in reducing drink-driving among younger or novice drivers. Finally, a consistent finding is that sustained governmental support of enforcement is needed for preventive countermeasures to result in long-term positive effects.

In general, the research evidence supports the following strategies as potentially effective drink-driving countermeasures:

1) Random breath testing. The consistent and high-profile enforcement of drink-driving has demonstrated evidence of effectiveness, especially as it achieves deterrence of drivers from drinking before or while driving.

2) Sobriety checkpoints are a less intensive enforcement to RBT. They are potentially effective, but effectiveness is proportional to the frequency of implementation and the programme's visibility as a means to achieve deterrence.

3) Severe sanctions/punishment. The evidence is mixed concerning mandatory or tougher sanctions for conviction for drink-driving. In cases where these strategies are shown to be effective, the effects appear to decay over time, which suggests that severe sanctions may lose their effectiveness unless accompanied by renewed enforcement or media efforts.

4) Low or lowered BAC limits. In general, the lower the BAC legal limit, the more effective the policy. Whereas very low BAC limits have been shown to be effective for youth, they can be also be effective for adult drivers. But low BAC limits (e.g. lower than BAC <0.02%) can become difficult to enforce properly.

5) Low BAC for youth. Even if the legal BAC limit for adult drivers is relatively higher, there is clear evidence that lower BAC limits for youth, especially those who are below the legal drinking or alcohol purchase age, can be effective. This strategy becomes particularly useful when adult BAC >0.03%.

6) Administrative licence suspension. In general, when punishment for drink-driving is swift, the effectiveness of the punishments (at any level of severity) is increased. Administrative licence suspension is most effective in those countries that consistently apply this strategy and bring enforcement and sanctions closer in time, as when legal or judicial authorities remove a driver's licence within a short time following arrest for drink-driving.

7) Licensing restrictions and graduated licenses for youth drivers. Policies to delay youth access to a full licence and other driving restrictions can be effective strategies for reducing drink-driving problems among this population. Graduated licensing can be used to incorporate lower BAC limits and licensing restrictions within one strategy.

8) Designated driver, and safe ride programmes. Such programmes may have some effect for people who presumably would otherwise drive while intoxicated, i.e. high-risk groups for drink-driving (young, male heavier drinkers). However, because these services account for a relatively small percentage of drivers, no overall impact on alcohol-related accidents has been demonstrated to date.

Chapter 12

Restrictions on marketing

12.1 Introduction

The extent and the nature of alcohol marketing have changed globally in the last decade, and the research has also expanded considerably to better understand its effects. Most of the new research is directed to the measurement of the impact of marketing on youth. More is now known about the effects of marketing on younger people's beliefs and intentions to drink as well as on their drinking behaviour. Research has investigated the impact of marketing other than the broadcast and print media advertising, although some of the new media and marketing approaches being used by the alcohol industry remain unmeasured and under-researched (e.g. sponsorship of music and sports events).

In this chapter we first provide an introduction to the current state of alcohol marketing and what is known about the way in which marketing has its impact. Second, two different policy approaches—codes of content and restrictions to reduce exposure—are assessed for their likely impact on consumption and harm. Interventions that change exposure to advertising have often been limited and evaluations have mixed findings. More effort has gone into the establishment of codes aimed to affect the content of the advertising. Conclusions regarding the likely effects of these approaches can be made based on theoretical understanding and empirical evidence about the way in which marketing has its effects and its measured impacts. Conclusions may also be informed by research on tobacco advertising where the impacts are established and widely accepted (Lovato *et al.* 2004; Henriksen *et al.* 2008).

12.2 Alcohol marketing practices

As discussed in Chapter 5, commodity chain analysis highlights the importance of advertising, sponsorship and other forms of marketing to a globalized alcohol industry (Jernigan 2006). The marketing of the products and brand(s) produced is essential for the profit-making enterprise. Marketing now involves much more than advertising using traditional media outlets such as print, television, and radio. Marketing exploits the possibilities provided by the design of products (e.g. sweetened beverages), the place of sale, and price promotions (Hastings and Haywood 1991). It utilizes a range of new media opportunities including electronic means, and a key element is the sponsorship of sporting and cultural events. The measured media (usually broadcast and print) is known to be an underestimation of the marketing effort by a factor of two to four (Anderson *et al.* 2009b).

New products and packaging have been developed to meet the needs and wants of different sectors of the market (Brain 2000). Premixed drinks in which spirits or beer are made more palatable by the addition of a soft drink base or fruit flavourings have expanded in sales very rapidly and have become associated in some contexts, but not all, with heavier consumption (Huckle *et al.* 2008b). Packaging has increased acceptability and palatability of alcoholic beverages among young people (Copeland *et al.* 2007; Gates *et al.* 2007).

Marketing at the place of sale has become increasingly important with an expansion of alcohol sales into more retail outlets. This often goes hand in hand with pricing promotions. Point-of-sale promotions documented in Australia included free gifts with purchase, competitions, and buy-some-get-some-free (Jones and Lynch 2007). A study of US college students found that participation in 'all you can drink' bar promotions resulted in higher levels of intoxication, although not all promotions had a significant impact (Thombs *et al.* 2009). In Asian countries promotional activity includes encouragement of consumption by 'beer girls' who are employed by the alcohol producer and paid on a commission basis (Lubek 2005).

Promotion of alcohol brands in electronic media is a major part of marketing. Advertising is also shown in cinemas and this is increasingly supplemented by product placement in movies and television. Newer forms of electronic communication such as internet networking sites, e-mail and cell phones have also provided new opportunities for alcohol promotion which are popular with young people (Jernigan and O'Hara 2004). They provide opportunities for **viral marketing** in which young people transmit marketing material on to peer networks.

Sports and cultural events, particularly those with appeal to young people, are widely sponsored by alcohol brands. Branded sports events, for example, provide the opportunity to build the brand into the name of the event through mention in sports commentaries; signage on clothing and sports grounds; and products retailed to fans. They also provide opportunities for direct marketing through free gifts and exclusive 'pourage' rights (Hill and Casswell 2004). Carlsberg's sponsorship of the EURO 2004 football/soccer championship was reported to grow the brand by about 6% worldwide; Carlsberg told shareholders that its signage had appeared in the background of television sport coverage for an average of 16 minutes per game (Carlsberg 2006). Much marketing, including that based on sponsorship, crosses national boundaries. For example, in Ireland, which has some national level restrictions on alcohol advertising on television, more than half of the advertisements seen come from outside Ireland (Breen 2008). Box 12.1 provides an example of a multi-media promotion targeted at young people.

12.3 Research on marketing and public health

Much current research on alcohol marketing emphasizes the impact of marketing on children and teenagers. This reflects an understanding of the role of marketing in recruitment of new consumers as well as concern over the harm experienced by younger drinkers. In emerging markets, the recruitment of non-drinking adults to become drinkers may also be affected by marketing (Benegal 2005); in both mature

Box 12.1 The best weekend you'll never remember!

A campaign for a beer brand in New Zealand in 2004 illustrated an integrated multi-media campaign and the way in which such promotions work to produce and naturalize drinking to intoxication. It took the form of a brand-based competition with the prize of an all-expenses-paid weekend in a luxury ski resort to which the winner would fly with three friends to take part in extreme sports. The winner and his or her friends were hosted by a radio announcer who was an acknowledged youth advocate and were guests of honour at a performance by a popular band where they had access to an unlimited beer supply. The promotion was run for several weeks through youth radio stations, music television, and websites that encouraged people to enter the contest by text, cell phone, or email. The e-mail promotion read: 'the best weekend you'll never remember!' (McCreanor *et al.* 2008).

and emerging markets women are an unsaturated sector for which marketing can play an important role (Beccaria 1999). In the USA, minority groups with below-average levels of drinking have also been targeted (Alaniz 1998; Center on Alcohol Marketing and Youth 2006). Another issue from a public health perspective, although less researched, is the possibility that marketing reduces people's ability to cut back or stop drinking when there is a desire to do so (Thomson *et al.* 1997).

Research has also suggested that the effects of marketing on beliefs about alcohol counteract any possible effect from health promotion activities (Wallack 1983; Center on Alcohol Marketing and Youth 2003). Recipients, who bring their own cultural and social experiences to their interpretation of the marketing, may perceive heavy drinking or intoxication as represented within the advertising even when it is not shown directly (Duff 2003; McCreanor *et al.* 2008). This is particularly likely to have an impact on efforts to reduce heavier drinking as a cultural norm.

Direct effect on exposed individuals is not the only concern which underpins restrictions on marketing, however. It is possible that widespread marketing, which promotes alcohol as a positive and commonplace element of everyday life, has an impact on social norms around alcohol which may, in turn, affect the acceptability of more restrictive policies and practice. In effect, marketing is a force for ensuring that alcohol is dealt with as if it were an ordinary commodity (Casswell 1997).

12.4 Impact of marketing on total population consumption

One strand of research in this field has used econometric methods to look for an impact on total population consumption using expenditure on measured media as a proxy for changing levels of exposure to advertising, covering the time period 1950–1990 mainly in North America and in the UK. These studies have produced mixed results. Some found no impact of advertising [e.g. Bourgeois and Barnes 1979 (Canada 1951–1974); Duffy 2001 (UK 1964–1996); Lee and Tremblay 1992 (USA 1953–1983); and Nelson and Moran 1995 (USA 1964–1990)]. Others have reported small effects on total consumption [e.g. Blake and Nied 1997 (UK 1952–1991)] or, more commonly, positive effects in relation to specific beverages [e.g. Franke and Wilcox 1987 (USA 1964–1984, small positive effect of beer and wine advertising); McGuiness 1980 (UK 1956–1975, small positive effect of spirits advertising); and Selvanathan 1989 (UK 1955–1975, small positive effect of beer advertising)]. In addition to the **time-series analysis**, a cross-sectional study in the USA showed an effect on highway fatalities (Saffer 1997). A recent **meta-analysis** of 132 econometric studies that included 322 estimated advertising elasticities found a small positive elasticity between advertising and alcohol consumption that was significant, however, only in relation to spirits (Gallet 2007).

The use of expenditure on alcohol advertising as a proxy for exposure has been critiqued on a number of grounds. Expenditure on the measured media (usually broadcast and print) is known to have been an underestimation of the marketing effort even prior to the development of the new marketing techniques (Stewart and Rice 1995). The limited impacts of alcohol advertising shown in econometric studies may reflect the diminishing marginal effect of additional advertising expenditure in markets already saturated with both alcohol products and marketing (Saffer 1998). Impacts may be very different in emerging markets. In addition, given the known sensitivity of young people to marketing, and the focus of most econometric studies on the total population, it is likely that important effects of advertising have been missed by econometric studies (Hastings *et al.* 2005). Similar critiques have been made and similar inconsistencies found in econometric analyses in relation to tobacco advertising (Hoek 2004).

12.5 Impact of marketing on beliefs and behaviour among young people

Analysis of advertising by the beer and spirits industries, and the way in which young people interact with it, has suggested that it works as predicted by communications theory and research on tobacco advertising (Pierce 2007). Research has documented a progression through different stages of the young person's development. The first stage is liking alcohol advertisements, followed by a desire to emulate the featured characters (including those that depict the lifestyle of young adults), and then the belief expressed that acting this way will result in positive benefits (Austin *et al.* 2006). Much of the marketing that targets young people is driven by an understanding of the importance of alcohol consumption for identity formation. The advertising is designed to provide humour, attractive ideas, images, phrases, and other resources that are used in the process of peer-to-peer interaction as identity is formed and communicated (McCreanor *et al.* 2005).

Awareness of and liking for such alcohol advertising has been shown to have an effect on intentions to drink (Grube 1993, 1995) and intentions to purchase (Chen *et al.* 2005). Associated with the changes in beliefs are also changes in self-reported behaviour (e.g. Wyllie *et al.* 1998b). Such effects of marketing on children and young people have also been shown with tobacco and food research (Hastings *et al.* 2003; Lovato *et al.* 2003).

Research has investigated the effect of both short- and long-term exposure. Brief exposure to alcohol advertisements has been found to affect university students' beliefs about the social benefits of alcohol and also the amounts consumed in an experimental, but realistic, context (Wilks *et al.* 1992; Zwarun *et al.* 2006). However, the full effect of exposure to advertisements with consistent messages is likely to be cumulative (Abrams and Niaura 1987, cited in Zwarun *et al.* 2006; Gerbner 1995), and there is a substantial body of research that investigates the effect of longer-term exposure to advertising on self-reported drinking behaviour by young people. Cross-sectional studies of the relationships among young people's exposure to alcohol advertisements, their response to advertising and their alcohol consumption have consistently shown an effect on self-reported drinking behaviour (Casswell 2004). Structural equation modelling has demonstrated that the cross-sectional data fit a model in which advertising increases consumption rather than the reverse (Grube and Wallack 1994; Wyllie *et al.* 1998a,b). Longitudinal studies, which provide an added methodological strength, have also found evidence of effects (Casswell and Zhang 1998; Stacy *et al.* 2004; Ellickson *et al.* 2005; Snyder *et al.* 2006).

Many of the earlier studies of young people's responses used measures of recalled exposure to all advertising or specifically exposure to advertising in broadcast media. More recently other media and marketing approaches have been researched. Longitudinal analysis has shown the effect on subsequent drinking of exposure of children to both in-store beer promotions (Ellickson *et al.* 2005) and outdoor advertising (Pasch *et al.* 2007). A longitudinal study in Germany found that young people who watched more movies in which there were considerable amounts of alcohol product placement were more likely to drink alcohol without parental consent (Hanewinkel *et al.* 2007).

The longitudinal studies have been subjected to systematic reviews. The strength of the association, the consistency of the findings, the temporal relationship, the dose–response relationship and the theoretical plausibility of the effect have led to the conclusion that alcohol advertising increases the likelihood that young people will start to use alcohol and will drink more if they are already using alcohol (Jernigan 2006; Smith and Foxcroft 2009; Anderson *et al.* 2009b).

Broader aspects of marketing, such as price promotions, have been found to increase heavier drinking among college students (Kuo *et al.* 2003b). A study of ownership of branded items found that one-fifth of US teenagers owned at least one such item, and ownership was shown to be related to drinking and to intentions to drink (Hurtz *et al.* 2007; Henriksen *et al.* 2008).

Some US studies have taken advantage of natural experiments provided by different media markets with different levels of exposure. Young people who lived in US markets with greater alcohol advertising expenditures drank more, and each additional dollar spent per capita raised the number of drinks consumed by 3%. Importantly, the duration of increasing consumption seemed also to be affected by the level of advertising: young people in higher-exposure areas in their mid-20s increased their drinking, whereas this was not found in lower-exposure markets (Snyder *et al.* 2006). Another US survey of youth drinking in conjunction with measures of advertising in five media suggested that a 28% reduction in alcohol advertising from 1996 to 1997 would have reduced the rate of binge drinking among adolescents from 12% to between 11% and

8% (Saffer and Dave 2006). On the basis of Saffer and Dave's findings on the effects of variations in advertising expenditure, largely determined by commercial marketing decisions, Hollingworth *et al.* (2006) estimated that a total ban on alcohol advertising would result in a 16% reduction in alcohol-related life-years lost. Estimates like this based on essentially cross-sectional data should, however, be treated with caution.

12.6 Current approaches to limiting harm

Experience with policies to restrict the negative impacts of marketing is less well developed than with other areas of alcohol policy. In part this reflects the rapid developments in marketing and media over the last four decades and a failure of policy developments to keep abreast of marketing practices. Most policy has focused on advertising rather than broader approaches to marketing such as sports sponsorship.

Legislated restrictions on alcohol advertising in the traditional media (often beverage- or media-specific) are common, although few countries prohibit all forms of alcohol advertising. Nearly a third of non-Muslim WHO member states have implemented partial restrictions. Around 15% relied on industry voluntary codes alone, and a significant number of countries have no policy or code in place (Österberg and Karlsson 2003; WHO 2004b). Industry voluntary codes focus primarily on the content of alcohol advertisements, whereas legislation by governments typically aims to reduce the amount of alcohol advertising to which the public, particularly children and young people, are exposed (Hill and Casswell 2004).

12.7 Voluntary efforts by the alcohol industry

Voluntary codes on alcohol advertising adopted by the advertising, media and alcohol industries typically address advertising content but not the amount of advertising or other forms of marketing. In Europe, voluntary code content reflects the EU's Audiovisual Media Services Directive Article 15. A number of the global corporations now have a company policy on responsible marketing, but much of the industry focus is on encouraging responsibility by the drinkers themselves, rather than controls on marketing, selling or the product itself.

Many companies have messages on websites and, in some cases, on brand advertisements telling their customers to 'drink responsibly'. There is, however, evidence to suggest that these responsibility messages are not effective in reducing alcohol-related harm. Their placement and nature means that, in the context of commercial advertising, they are rarely if ever more dominant than the positive appeals in the advertisements (Austin and Hurst 2005). Such messages have also been found to be interpreted differently by different viewers. Generally, both the messages and the alcohol companies involved were evaluated positively and the authors of one study concluded that the research demonstrated how seemingly pro-health messages can serve to subtly advance alcohol sales and public relations interests (Smith *et al.* 2006). Similar sentiments have been reported in relation to sponsorship. In Thailand following the sponsorship of the 2004 [football/soccer] World Cup by Thai Bev, a major beer producer, a survey found that the majority of young people wished to repay the sponsor (Thamarangsi 2008).

A common approach promoted by the industry as the 'gold standard' (International Center for Alcohol Policies 2001, 2005) is that of voluntary codes, put in place by the vested interests concerned (often including advertising industry, media interests, and the alcohol industry), and addressing the content of advertisements. In general there is a focus on measured, established media such as television and print advertising, with some expansion more recently to satellite and channel television and the Internet and promotions in licensed premises. The emerging media and sponsorship and branded events are seldom covered by these codes.

Research has suggested that voluntary codes are subject to under-interpretation and under-enforcement (Rearck Research 1991; Saunders and Yap 1991; Sheldon 2000; Dring and Hope 2001; Jones *et al.* 2008), including a bias in favour of the corporations represented on the decision-making board (Marin Institute 2008a). There are also documented cases of the instability of such voluntary codes in response to changing market conditions (Martin *et al.* 2002; Hill and Casswell 2004) and trends towards the liberalization of codes (Babor *et al.* in press). These findings of poor compliance and inherent instability have been found to be characteristic of self-regulation in a range of industries (Baggott 1989; Ayres and Braithwaite 1992). A recent analysis of self-regulation by the alcohol industry in the UK concluded it was not an effective driver of change towards good practice (KPMG 2008b). Overall there is no evidence to support the effectiveness of industry self-regulatory codes, either as a means of limiting advertisements deemed unacceptable or as a way of limiting alcohol consumption (Booth *et al.* 2008).

12.8 The effect of codes on advertising content

Codes on alcohol advertising usually develop as part of advertising industry efforts to maintain advertising standards through self-regulation. Public concerns give rise to particular issues in regard to advertising alcohol products, such as associations with alcohol that are considered unsafe or culturally inappropriate and the risk that advertisements will appeal to and encourage drinking by those below the minimum legal age. Codes of content are similar across the world, whether they are voluntary on the part of the industry or set by regulation. They commonly include some or all of the following: must not be aimed at young people or depict young people in the advertisement; must not link consumption of alcohol to sexual or social success, to enhanced physical performance, or to driving; must not make therapeutic claims for alcohol; must not encourage immoderate consumption or present abstinence in a negative light; and must not portray intoxication and risky behaviour in conjunction with alcohol (e.g. Babor *et al.* 2008d; Österberg and Karlsson 2003; European Commission 2007; Ofcom 2007).

Research has shown that the codes as commonly framed and implemented do not have marked effects on the appeal and nature of the content. Content analyses of the advertisements have shown the way in which codes are circumvented using approaches such as 'plot ambiguity'. For example, US advertisements that show both alcohol and risky behaviour are not explicit about when consumption occurs relative to the activity and are therefore not in contravention of the code (Zwarun and Farrar 2005).

Research in other cultures with codes of content operating has also shown the presence of 'artful circumvention' of the codes (Haustein *et al.* 2004). Computer imagery, the use of humour and irony, and the use of colours and music that signify the brand without specifically showing the brand are ways in which the advertisements breach the intention of the codes while remaining technically within their guidelines. Children and adolescents are responsive to advertising elements such as humour, attractive and animated characters, youth-oriented music, and lifestyle/image advertising (Waiters *et al.* 2001; Kelly *et al.* 2002; Martin *et al.* 2002; Collins *et al.* 2003). Humour appears to be an important aspect of many highly appreciated advertisements and is not generally covered by codes (McCreanor *et al.* 2005).

Research has demonstrated that televised advertising that has been approved by systems relying on codes of content retains its appeal to young people. In Australia advertising that has been judged by the self-regulatory system to be compliant with the code of content has been judged by teenagers and young adults as showing alcohol contributing to social and sexual success and to produce stress reduction and relaxation (Jones and Donovan 2001). Analysis of recent television advertisements in relation to the US voluntary codes of content has shown that, although advertisements are in line with the codes when a literal interpretation is taken, compliance does not mean that the codes are effective in terms of their ostensible goal of reducing influence on young people's beliefs and behaviour (Zwarun and Farrar 2005). Following the introduction of a 'co-regulatory'approach in the UK, in which a government agency was delegated the handling of broadcast complaints to the Advertising Standards Authority (funded by the industry), a code change was introduced. Research demonstrated that advertisements continued to contain attributes that appealed to young people and the data showed a link between exposure to advertisements and consumption of specific beverages (Gunter *et al.* 2008).

The studies of liking for and exposure to alcohol advertising and the impacts on attitudes and behaviours of young people described above have been carried out in countries with industry codes of content in place. Most of this research comes from the USA, with some studies from New Zealand, and more recently Belgium and Germany. This substantial body of research has shown that, even if alcohol marketing remains in line with codes on alcohol advertising content, it nevertheless encourages drinking and has an impact on younger people's beliefs and alcohol consumption levels.

There are some examples, in a regulatory context, in which more stringent controls on the content of alcohol promotions have occurred. For example, in the media in which advertising of alcohol is currently permitted in France (print media with little appeal to young people, some radio channels, and on billboards), the advertising material must be confined to showing only the product, with reference only to product characteristics such as composition and provenance. It is no longer permitted to show drinkers and drinking contexts, and no reference to lifestyle is allowed (Rigaud and Craplet 2004). Research has shown that advertisements without reference to image or lifestyle are less attractive (and therefore likely to be less effective) with young people (Kelly *et al.* 2002). However, there are limited studies on the effect of this level of restriction of content.

12.9 **Controls to reduce exposure**

In some jurisdictions there are restrictions, typically by regulation, on exposure to alcohol marketing by media type, beverage type, time of broadcast or composition of media audiences (particularly relating to exposure of younger people). Most research has focused on exposure of young people to the measured media. This varies by country. In the USA, young people aged 15–26 years on average reported seeing the equivalent of almost 360 advertisments per year, the majority on television (Martin *et al.* 2002). CAMY monitoring indicated a rise in annual exposure among 12–20-year-olds from about 200 in 2001 to about 300 in 2007 (Center on Alcohol Marketing and Youth 2008). In New Zealand levels were higher with 12–17-year-olds, who were exposed to about 500 TV advertisements in 2005, than with older teenagers (Huckle and Huakau 2006).

12.9.1 **Voluntary restrictions**

In response to concern and advocacy in the USA over youth drinking, the trade associations for beer, wine and spirits production have adopted voluntary codes which prevent advertising where young people comprise more than 30% of the audience. This has reduced exposure somewhat, but young people, who are 16% of the US population, are still disproportionately exposed compared with adults (Jernigan *et al.* 2005). A restriction framed in terms of the percentage of young people in the audience does not prevent exposure of a significant number of young people. For example, advertising in television sports programming, which has been shown to have themes that appeal to young people and which are likely to increase their perception of the social benefits of alcohol, is likely to reach many young people even if they are a small fraction of the audience, due to the sizeable adult audience (Zwarun and Farrar 2005).

Restrictions imposed by agreement among industry actors are inherently unstable. In the context of the EU and other trade agreements, they may be subject to legal attack as an illegal restraint of trade. They may also be easily breached or dropped. Thus, a voluntary ban on advertising of spirits on television and radio in the USA, originally adopted under the threat of congressional legislation, was eventually abandoned when one major producer broke the code and other industry actors considered that the ban was no longer feasible.

12.9.2 **Restrictions by law or regulation**

While few examples can be found except in Islamic countries of a complete ban on alcohol advertising and promotion, there are many jurisdictions in which legislation restricts advertising in specific media and/or of particular beverages. For example, in Austria, broadcasting legislation prohibits advertising of spirits on radio and television, and also advertising and infomercials for alcohol on cable and satellite. A number of East European countries, now part of the EU, prohibit spirits advertisements or all alcohol advertisements in most media. Bans on alcohol advertising in some Scandinavian countries have become more partial as they have entered into various trade arrangements with the EU, sometimes as a result of challenges on market access. France's legislation, the Loi Évin (see Box 12.2), is an often-cited example of relatively

Box 12.2 Loi Évin: France's regulation of alcohol marketing

Following a period of unregulated marketing of alcohol in France, a high level of community and medical concern led to the adoption of legislation to prohibit advertising on television, in cinemas and all sponsorship. The advertising that is allowed, in print media for adults and on some radio channels and billboards, is restricted to information about the product, such as where it was produced and its strength. A real change in alcohol advertising has been observed since 1991. The law has resulted in the language of advertising losing most of its seductive character. It is no longer allowed to depict drinkers and drinking environments. There has been a complete disappearance of the drinker from the images in favour of highlighting the product itself (Rigaud and Craplet 2004).

In the law a clear definition of alcoholic drinks is given: all drinks of more than 1.2% alcohol by volume are considered to be alcoholic beverages.

Places and types of media where authorized advertising can be conducted are defined as follows: no advertising should be targeted at young people, no advertising is allowed on television and in cinemas, and no sponsorship of cultural or sport events is permitted.

Advertising is permitted only in the press for adults, on billboards,[a] on radio channels (under precise conditions), and at special events or places such as wine fairs and wine museums.

When advertising is permitted, its content is controlled. Messages and images should refer only to the qualities of the products such as degree, origin, composition, means of production, and patterns of consumption.

A health message must be included on each advertisement to the effect that 'l'abus d'alcool' est dangereux pour la santé' (alcohol abuse is dangerous to health).

[a] The text limited billboard advertising to the places of production and selling. Later, another law permitted billboard advertising anywhere that alcohol is served or sold.

comprehensive regulation of alcohol marketing, and one which has maintained political support for more than a decade. One of the key elements of the Loi Évin (relevant to the need to control the current ongoing proliferation of marketing approaches) is that advertising of alcohol is prohibited in all media unless the law provides for an exemption; there is a complete ban on sponsorship and on advertising in many media, including television and cinema. Such advertising regulation has been challenged. However, restrictions on alcohol advertising to meet public health goals have been upheld by the courts (see Box 12.3), although sometimes with some modification.

12.10 Research on effects of partial bans

Although bans on some aspects of advertising are not uncommon, there is a limited amount of evaluation research on their effectiveness. In many of the countries where

Box 12.3 The European Court of Justice defends a challenge to the Loi Évin

The French ban on alcohol advertising in bi-national broadcasts was upheld by the European Court of Justice in 2004. The court stated:

1. 'It is for Member States to decide on the degree of protection which they wish to afford to public health and on the way in which that protection is to be achieved.'

2. 'The law [reduces] the occasions on which television viewers might be encouraged to consume alcoholic beverages.'

3. 'The French rules on television advertising are appropriate to ensure their aim of protecting public health.'

4. The laws 'do not go beyond what is necessary to achieve such an objective.'

Source: C-262/02 and C-429/02.

most alcohol research is done, recent changes have tended towards a liberalized marketing environment. Three studies were performed to evaluate the lifting of restrictions in Canadian provinces. Two of these found no effect of lifting of partial bans in Manitoba and British Columbia (Smart and Cutler 1976; Ogborne and Smart 1980). The changes in Saskatchewan in 1983 allowed beer and wine advertising on the broadcast media and spirits advertising only in the print media. The study found no effect on total consumption but did find a significant increase in beer consumption at the expense of spirits (Makowsky and Whitehead 1991). This might reflect the greater impact of the broadcast media (Viser 1999).

Other studies have used multivariate/cross-sectional designs to compare jurisdictions with different restrictions and have produced mixed effects. A positive effect of price advertising was reported in the USA between 1974 and 1978 (Ornstein and Hanssens 1985) but no effect of state bans of price advertising of spirits (Nelson 2003). A number of analyses comparing countries have been carried out with conflicting results. Saffer and Dave have shown small significant effects of bans (Saffer 1991; Saffer and Dave 2002), with a pooled time-series analysis of data from 20 countries over a period of 26 years indicating that an increase of one ban (of media or beverage type) could reduce alcohol consumption by 5–8%; they argue that the more comprehensive the restrictions the greater this effect would be (Saffer and Dave 2002). However, other analysts have reported mixed (Young 1993) and even a positive effect of bans (Nelson and Young 2001). The effect of partial bans was also reported not to have affected consumption in seventeen countries over 26 years (Nelson 2008a), in a study with material that included at least fifteen consequential changes in bans.

A recent systematic review included ten heterogeneous studies of bans and concluded that the variation in the use of advertising restrictions and the methodological challenges meant that the findings were inconclusive, and that any positive effects were likely to be modest. There was some evidence to suggest that bans have an additive effect when accompanied by other measures within a general environment of restrictive measures (Booth *et al.* 2008).

The tobacco field has had the advantage of the implementation of more restrictive policies in a number of countries, particularly in the lead up to the Framework Convention on Tobacco Control, adopted in 2003. The empirical literature, while not consistent (e.g. Nelson 2003), suggests that comprehensive bans have played a role in reducing tobacco consumption in developed countries, whereas limited policies have not (Saffer and Chaloupka 2000; Blecher, 2008). Recent comparisons across 18 European countries found that the intensity of tobacco control policies predicted smoking cessation and that advertising bans followed taxation in showing the strongest association (Schaap *et al.* 2008). Analysis of developing countries has suggested that tobacco advertising bans are even more effective in the developing world than they are in the developed world (Blecher 2008). Unfortunately there are no comparable studies related to alcohol advertising in developing countries, and there has been less comprehensive policy change to evaluate.

12.11 Conclusions and policy implications

There has been a marked increase in alcohol marketing using an expanding repertoire of media and communication technologies with considerable appeal and utility for young people. There are unprecedented levels of exposure to sophisticated marketing. Attempts to control the content of the marketing messages using voluntary codes of content have not decreased their appeal to young people sufficiently to reduce their impact.

The evidence reviewed has suggested that exposure of young people to alcohol marketing speeds up the onset of drinking and increases the amount consumed by those already drinking. The extent and breadth of research available is considerable, utilizes a range of methodologies, and is consistent in showing effects with young people. Marketing to young people undoubtedly contributes to the ongoing recruitment of young people to replace drinkers lost to the industry by attrition in mature markets and to expand the drinking population in emerging markets.

The lack of conclusive evidence from the studies of restrictions of alcohol advertising to date is likely to reflect the limited experiences of the imposition of comprehensive restrictions and methodological difficulties. However, the findings of an effect of exposure to marketing put the question of controls on advertising high on the policy agenda. The extent to which effective restrictions would reduce consumption and related harm in younger age groups must remain somewhat of an open question. The most probable scenario, based on the theoretical and empirical evidence available, is that extensive restriction of marketing would have an impact.

There is a continued expansion in extent and modes of marketing and increasing use of media that cross national boundaries in an internationally unregulated environment. Much marketing occurs in movies, television programmes, and Internet sites that transcend national boundaries. Unlike tobacco, there is as yet no international or regional agreement to restrict alcohol marketing. The evidence demonstrating the impact of current levels of marketing on the recruitment of heavier-drinking young people suggests the need for urgent policy action. Such action would require establishing a regulatory framework incorporating monitoring and enforcement, independent of industry interests, that is able to cross national boundaries.

Chapter 13

Education and persuasion strategies

13.1 Introduction

Education and persuasion strategies are among the most popular approaches to the prevention of alcohol-related problems. In this chapter, these strategies are examined in several contexts and settings, including schools, colleges, and communities and the general population. The chapter is organized into three main sections: initiatives involving the media, school-based programmes, and college programmes.

Both individual-level and population-level orientations are evident in these strategies, which usually involve one or more of the following objectives: (i) changing knowledge about alcohol and risks related to drinking; (ii) changing intentions to drink in order to lower risks; (iii) changing drinking behaviour itself (e.g. delaying onset of drinking among youth); (iv) lowering the frequency or seriousness of problems related to drinking; and (v) changing public attitudes to increase support for alcohol policies (see Casswell *et al.* 1989; Cuijpers 2003). In the analysis that follows, a specific intervention was considered to have a positive impact if evidence demonstrated that it was able to delay the onset of drinking or to reduce the prevalence of high-risk drinking and alcohol-related harm.

Some school-based programmes focused on alcohol and illicit drugs, or alcohol, illicit drugs, and tobacco. This chapter focuses on outcomes that pertain to alcohol. A distinction between approaches that is often used pertains to the foci of the intervention. 'Universal' approaches are directed at the entire population, 'selective' approaches focus on those considered at risk, and 'indicated'approaches deal with persons considered to be at the early stages of use or related problem behaviour (Shamblen and Derzon 2009).

As with other chapters in this book, the goal is to derive policy-relevant conclusions from an objective review of the research evidence; however, this chapter differs from the others in that, on balance, the research generally leads to negative conclusions. These conclusions were also evident in earlier reviews (Edwards *et al.* 1994; Babor *et al.* 2003). For the most part, the three behaviour change criteria listed above have not been realized. There are some exceptions. However, given the extent of initiatives in this area, and the diversity of interventions that have been implemented, there are relatively few that point to long-term impact on drinking behaviour or alcohol-related problems.

13.2 Initiatives involving the media

13.2.1 Social marketing, mass media, health campaigns, and information campaigns

Social marketing has been defined as the application of commercial marketing technologies to the analysis, planning, execution, and evaluation of programmes designed to influence the voluntary behaviour of target audiences in order to improve their personal welfare and that of society (Gordon *et al.* 2006). Gordon *et al.* concluded that social marketing can positively affect alcohol abuse, but this conclusion was tempered by the following limitations in the studies they reviewed: imperfect research designs, difficulties in identifying whether the effects are attributable to individual intervention components or a combination of activities, differences at baseline between the intervention and comparison communities, and participant attrition (Gordon *et al.* 2006).

In response to the extensive promotion of alcoholic beverages in many countries, governments and private organizations have sponsored information campaigns. These have taken several forms, including social advertising, also called **public service announcements** (PSAs), and placement of warning messages on actual advertisements. These social advertising messages are prepared by governments, non-governmental organizations, health agencies, and media organizations for the purpose of providing important information for the benefit of a particular audience. In some cases PSAs depend upon donated time or space for distribution to the public. When applied to alcohol, PSAs often deal with **responsible drinking**, the hazards of drink-driving, and related topics.

Counter-advertising involves disseminating information about a product, its effects, and the industry that promotes it, in order to decrease its appeal and use. It is distinct from other types of informational campaigns in that it directly addresses the fact that the particular commodity is promoted through advertising (Agostinelli and Grube 2002).

Social advertising or PSAs use a number of media vehicles—television or radio, paid counter-advertisements, billboards, magazine and newspaper pieces, and news or feature stories on television and radio—in order to provide information about the risks and complications associated with drinking. Although it is expected that these messages will have a direct effect on the behaviour of the target audience, this is seldom the case. Tactics include health-warning labels on product packaging and **media literacy** efforts to raise public awareness of the advertising tactics of an industry as well as prevention messages in magazines and on television (see Barlow and Wogalter 1993). Information messages may also be included in community or school prevention programmes (e.g. Giesbrecht *et al.* 1990; Greenfield and Zimmerman 1993), or used as part of government liquor board retail systems (Goodstadt and Flynn 1993).

In most countries, the number of PSAs and counter-advertisements concerning alcohol are at best a small fraction of the total volume of alcohol advertisements (see Fedler *et al.* 1994; Wyllie *et al.* 1996) and are rarely seen on television. Moreover, the content of information campaigns cannot easily challenge the other persuasive influences supportive of drinking. For example, a study of French high-school students (Pissochet *et al.* 1999) found that respondents considered alcohol risk prevention advertising to be less effective than alcohol advertising. Furthermore, those who might be seen as the primary targets—daily drinkers—were more critical than intermittent drinkers and non-drinkers.

Although public acceptance of information campaigns is high (e.g. Giesbrecht and Greenfield 1999), legislative initiatives to place warnings directly on alcohol advertisements, particularly electronic messages, have not succeeded in the USA (Greenfield *et al.* 1999; Giesbrecht 2000). In some countries, however, such warnings are required. Billboard advertisements in Mexico, for instance, carry general warnings to use alcohol with caution. Newspaper advertisements in Sweden are required to carry one of 11 rotating warnings in sufficiently large type to occupy one-eighth of the advertisement (Wilkinson and Room 2009).

Other developments related to information campaigns include media literacy efforts to teach young people to resist the persuasive appeals of alcohol advertising. Some small positive effects have been observed in media literacy programmes with children (Austin and Johnson 1997). Slater *et al.* (1996) found that recency of exposure to alcohol education classes and discussion of alcohol advertising predicted cognitive resistance to such advertising. Canzer (1996) exposed college students to educational videos about the alcohol industry, its advertising efforts, and health-related information. A general reduction in drinking was observed. Nearly two-thirds of the participants reduced the number of times they entered social environments where risky alcohol consumption was likely.

From a public health perspective, counter-advertising has intuitive appeal and may be a more realistic political option than seeking a ban on alcohol advertising (Saffer 2002). But counter-advertising typically does not offer powerful outcomes within realistically available budgets. Although the US tobacco experience suggests that a hard-hitting counter-advertising programme can be effective as part of a comprehensive prevention strategy (Rohrbach *et al.* 2002), it is unlikely that intensive alcohol counter-advertising programmes will be politically feasible in many jurisdictions. Thus there are limitations on the extent to which this dimension of the tobacco control experience can be transferred to the alcohol context.

Drink-driving has commonly been the focus of mass media campaigns. A systematic review of eight studies (Elder *et al.* 2004) concluded that carefully planned, well-executed mass media campaigns are effective in reducing alcohol-impaired driving and alcohol-related crashes, if they attain adequate audience exposure and are implemented in conjunction with other prevention activities. However, they noted that decision-making based on the success or failure of such campaigns is complicated by the 'efficacy paradox', that is, it was difficult to generalize about the potential utility of an initiative if the campaigns studied had been poorly implemented. For example, Ditter *et al.* (2005) reviewed nine campaigns to encourage designated driver programmes. They found insufficient evidence to determine the effectiveness of these programmes due to small magnitudes of effects and the limitations of the outcome measures.

In many cases information campaigns are intended to be particularly relevant to drinking by youth (Connolly *et al.* 1994; Holder 1994a). Gorman (1995) pointed out the limited impact that mass media interventions using a **universal strategy** have on alcohol use and alcohol-related problems. Despite their good intentions, PSAs are not an effective antidote to the high-quality pro-drinking messages that appear much more frequently as paid advertisements in the mass media and involve much more extensive exposure (see Ludwig 1994; Murray *et al.* 1996).

13.2.2 Warning labels

A fairly extensive amount of research has been conducted on US-mandated alcoholic beverage container **warning labels**, which were introduced in 1989 (Kaskutas 1995). Emphasis has been placed on the potential for birth defects when alcohol is consumed during pregnancy, the danger of alcohol impairment when driving or operating machinery, and general health risks. Some states require posted warnings of alcohol risks in establishments that serve or sell alcohol.

There is evidence that warning labels impact knowledge, awareness, intentions, and perceptions, but evidence on drinking behaviour is at best equivocal. Surveys indicate that a significant proportion of the population has seen these warning labels (Kaskutas and Greenfield 1992; Graves 1993; Greenfield *et al.* 1993). There is some evidence (Kaskutas and Greenfield 1992; Greenfield 1997; Greenfield and Kaskutas 1998; Greenfield *et al.* 1999) that warning labels increase knowledge regarding the risks of drink-driving and drinking during pregnancy among some groups (e.g. light drinkers) and result in more conversations about risks among frequent drinkers, including young adults (Kaskutas and Greenfield 1997a; Greenfield and Kaskustas 1998). One US national survey examined recall of warning messages on alcohol container labels, signs at point-of-sale, and warning messages in media advertisements. Recall was good for all three types of messages; for warning labels, recall was especially high among young people, males, and heavy drinkers (Kaskutas and Greenfield 1997b). There was a dose–response relationship between pregnancy-related conversations about drinking while pregnant and the number of types of messages seen (e.g. point-of-sale signage, advertisements, magazine stores, and warning labels: Kaskutas *et al.* 1998).

Several warning label studies have focused on youth. The first year after warning labels were introduced, MacKinnon *et al.* (1993) found that 12th-graders (about 17 years old) reported increases in awareness of, exposure to, and recognition of warning labels. However, there were no substantial changes in alcohol use or beliefs about the risks contained in the labels. An experimental study by Snyder and Blood (1992) involved a sample of 159 college students who viewed six different advertisements for alcohol products, some with the official warning and some without. The warnings did not increase perceptions of alcohol risk, and may even have made products more attractive to both drinkers and non-drinkers.

Another experimental study involved 274 college age students in two universities, one in the USA and one in Australia (Creyer *et al.* 2002). The authors noted that the warning 'alcohol is a drug' resulted in greater perceived risk than the standard US warning label on alcoholic beverage containers. They concluded that there is evidence to suggest that the incremental benefits of the current US labels with regard to pregnancy are declining and that other rotating warnings might be desirable.

Systematic reviews support the main conclusions of specific studies. Argo and Main (2004) reported on a **meta-analysis** of 48 studies of warning labels, seven of which pertained to alcohol. They noted that consumers are less likely to notice a warning label on alcohol because it is considered a 'convenience' good as opposed to a 'shopping' good; the latter typically requires comparison shopping and therefore provides more opportunity to notice a warning label. They note some impact from warning labels on consumers' attention, reading and comprehension, and recall. There was a weak relationship between warnings and consumers' judgements of a product's hazards and risks. In their analysis, reaction to the labels was assessed on several dimensions: attention, readability/comprehension, recall, judgements, and behavioural compliance. Alcohol warning labels, on the basis of the studies reviewed, were considered to impact attention or awareness, recall, and judgement about danger or perceived risk, but not behavioural compliance.

A review by MacKinnon and Nohre (2006) concludes that there is no convincing evidence of an effect of general alcohol warning labels on behaviour, such as alcohol consumption and driving after drinking, and across studies little evidence that alcohol use has decreased as a result of warning labels. **Natural experiments** provide evidence that persons are aware of the alcohol warning label and have seen it, and the effect of the alcohol label is stronger among alcohol users. MacKinnon and Nohre (2006) also note that a change in the design of the US label could improve recognition.

There is evidence that some intervening variables are affected, such as intention to change drinking patterns (in relation to situations of heightened risk such as drink-driving), having conversations about drinking, and willingness to intervene with others who are seen as hazardous drinkers. Considering the small size and relative obscurity of the typical US warning label, it is surprising that any impacts have been observed. The potential impact of warning labels may be enhanced by combining it with other strategies, such as community-based campaigns to change alcohol policies or enforce alcohol-related regulations, but these types of intervention studies (e.g. combining warning labels with alcohol policies) have not yet been undertaken.

In summary, the warning label research does not demonstrate that exposure produces a change in drinking behaviour *per se*. Andrews (1995) concludes that warning labels are not significantly effective in preventing alcohol consumption by heavy drinkers. Other reviews (Grube and Nygaard 2001; Agostinelli and Grube 2002; Giesbrecht and Hammond 2005) conclude that there is little evidence that alcohol warning labels have measurable effects on drinking behaviours.

13.2.3 Low-risk drinking guidelines

A number of jurisdictions have disseminated low-risk drinking guidelines. These initiatives are motivated by evidence of relative risk of alcohol in trauma and chronic disease (Rehm *et al.* 2004) and by epidemiological research on the effects of moderate drinking on cardiovascular problems (e.g. Marmot 2001). The discussion of the health benefits in the media has created political pressures in some countries to provide the public with promotional and educational material about the benefits of moderate alcohol use. Surveys in several countries have noted an increase in the number of adults who are aware of these putative health benefits. For example, in New South Wales, Australia, the proportion identifying health benefits increased from 28% in 1990 to 46% in 1994, with relaxation (54%) and cardiovascular benefits (39%) most often mentioned (Hall 1995).

Official or semi-official guidelines have been adopted in a number of countries on 'moderate' drinking or 'low-risk drinking' in recent decades (Bondy *et al.* 1999). Given the complex considerations that underlie any such guidelines, it is not surprising that the guidelines vary considerably from one country to another (Stockwell 2001b), although there are signs of convergence towards relatively low limits (e.g. National Health and Medical Research Council 2009). Walsh *et al.* (1998) reported that there is little research on the impact of these messages, and this has not changed substantially in the past decade. One study by Dawson *et al.* (2004) examined US consumption data from two large national surveys during a period of declining alcohol sales (1992–2003). They found that the proportion of US adults classified as regular drinkers whose intake exceeded recommended daily or weekly limits declined from 32.1% to 29.3% in that period. By contrast, the percentage drinking at or above the current low-risk drinking guidelines in Ontario, Canada (Adlaf and Ialomiteanu 2007) has been increasing in recent years, concurrent with increased dissemination of these guidelines. Increases in drinking above the guidelines were also seen in the UK over the time period when information campaigns promoting the low-risk levels was the major strategy to reduce harm.

It is unclear whether such messages should be expected to lead to an overall decrease in alcohol consumption and related problems (Casswell 1993). For example, guidelines may be misinterpreted by the public and could lead some abstainers to take up drinking, and influence moderate drinkers to drink more. It may be argued that disseminating low-risk guidelines is an appropriate consumer information action, but there is no evidence that they have any effect on consumption or problems.

13.3 **School-based programmes**

Prevention initiatives focusing on adolescents and school-based **alcohol education programmes** have one or more goals: to increase knowledge about alcohol in adolescents (Cuijpers 2003); to change the adolescent's drinking beliefs, attitudes, and behaviours; to modify factors such as general social skills and self-esteem that are assumed to underlie adolescent drinking (Paglia and Room 1999); to delay the onset of first use of alcohol; to reduce the use of alcohol; to reduce high-risk drinking; and to minimize the harm caused by drinking (see Cuijpers 2003). Over the past 50 years there have been three main phases in the development of school-based prevention programmes that focus on alcohol (Cuijpers 2003). During the 1960s to early 1970s they mainly focused on the provision of knowledge of alcohol use and associated risks. School-based interventions popular during the 1970s and 1980s relied solely on informational approaches and often taught students about the dangers of drug use as well. Such programmes have been found ineffective in changing behaviour (Tobler 1992; Hansen 1994; Botvin *et al.* 1995). Although they can increase knowledge and change attitudes toward alcohol, tobacco, and drug use, actual substance use remains largely unaffected.

The second phase involved the so-called **affective education** programmes that focused not on alcohol or other drugs, but on 'broader issues of personal development such as decision making, values clarification and stress management' (Cuijpers 2003, p. 10). Approaches that address values clarification, self-esteem, general social skills, and **alternatives to drinking** approaches that provide activities assumed to be inconsistent with alcohol use (e.g. sports) are also assessed to be ineffective (Moskowitz 1989).

During the third phase, from the early 1980s onward, the social influence model has dominated school-based prevention programmes (Cuijpers 2003). This was sometimes combined with broader personal and social skills training and sometimes included an emphasis on community-based aspects or family-based interventions (Spoth *et al.* 1999; Murray and Belenko 2005; Petrie *et al.* 2007).

13.3.1 Social influence programmes

Social-influence programmes were developed partly in response to the ineffectiveness of informational, affective, and alternative approaches. Drawing from contemporary social psychological theory, these programmes were based on the assumption that most adolescents are negatively predisposed toward alcohol and drug use, but rarely have to justify their unfavourable attitudes toward these behaviours. As a result, when challenged, their beliefs were easily undermined. These new programmes attempted to 'inoculate' young people against such challenges to their beliefs by addressing resistance to social pressures to use drugs and by focusing on short-term and immediate social consequences (Evans *et al.* 1978). Early evaluations of these programmes seemed promising, particularly for tobacco, and they form the basis for many current school-based alcohol prevention efforts. However, it has been recognized that adolescent alcohol use results not so much from direct pressures to drink but from more subtle social influences (Hansen 1993). It has been suggested that **resistance skills training** may be counterproductive because it leads young people to conclude that drinking is prevalent among, and approved by, their peers (Hansen and Graham 1991; Donaldson *et al.* 1997). In the 1990s there was a shift toward providing **normative education** that corrects adolescents' tendency to overestimate the number of their peers who drink and approve of drinking (Hansen 1992, 1993, 1994). Many school-based programmes now include both resistance skills training and normative education.

Tobler *et al.* (2000) conducted a meta-analysis of 207 universal school-based drug prevention programmes with many including alcohol as a focus. They found little effect from non-interactive programmes such as lectures that stress knowledge or affective development. However, interactive programmes that fostered the development of interpersonal skills showed some effects.

Scientific evaluations of school-based resistance and normative education interventions have produced mixed results with regard to alcohol. On the one hand, some researchers believe that these interventions are effective in reducing drinking and alcohol-related problems (e.g. Botvin and Botvin 1992; Hansen 1993, 1994; Dielman 1995; Botvin and Griffin 2007). On the other hand, others are critical of the research evidence, noting that better-designed studies typically do not find an impact on behaviour (e.g. Gorman 1996, 1998; Foxcroft *et al.* 1997; Brown and Kreft 1998; Paglia and Room 1999).

The Alcohol Misuse and Prevention Study (AMPS) is typical of a generation of US school-based education programmes focusing on pressures to use alcohol, risks of alcohol misuse, and ways to resist pressures to drink (Shope *et al.* 1996a,b). The AMPS programme had positive effects on alcohol and resistance skills knowledge that persisted up to 26 months (Shope *et al.* 1992). Overall, there were few effects on actual drinking behaviour, except for some short-term changes for students in several grades (Shope *et al.* 1996a). Other school-based alcohol resistance skills programmes have produced similarly modest results (Botvin *et al.* 1995; Klepp *et al.* 1995).

Normative education programmes have two goals: (i) to correct the tendency for students to overestimate the amount of drinking in their peer group and (ii) to change what is considered to be the acceptable level of peer drinking. Within these programmes, teachers provide information from survey data showing actual drinking prevalence rates, and guide class discussions about appropriate and inappropriate alcohol use. Initial evaluations of normative education programmes seemed promising. Hansen and Graham (1991) found an 8% decrease in reported drunkenness by eighth-graders in these programmes compared with comparable students in information-only programmes. Similar results have been reported for other normative education interventions (Graham *et al.* 1991; Hansen 1993), although some investigators have been critical of the research on these programmes (e.g. Kreft 1997).

School-based educational interventions, even when using normative education and resistance-skill training innovations, generally produce modest effects with regard to knowledge and attitudes that are short-lived unless accompanied by ongoing booster sessions. Although some evaluations have measured heavy drinking and self-reported problems, very few have demonstrated substantive effects on rates of intoxication, drink-driving, injury, and alcohol-related crashes. In most cases such outcomes are not even reported. There is some evidence that certain subgroups may be more affected by school-based interventions. For example, youth with previously unsupervised drinking experience may be more responsive to resistance skills training (Shope *et al.* 1994; Dielman 1995), while those who are more rebellious may be less responsive to normative education (Kreft 1997). However, there are methodological flaws, as indicated in a **Cochrane Review** (Foxcroft *et al.* 2002).

One study focusing on a **harm reduction** goal, rather than abstinence, reported some impact on behaviour. The School Health and Alcohol Harm Reduction Project (SHAHRP study) (McBride *et al.* 2004) was a longitudinal intervention research study that used alcohol education lessons to reduce alcohol-related harm in young people. The critical features of the SHAHRP intervention were drawn from a range of health and drug education programmes and from the research literature. The SHAHRP study delivered 13 harm minimization classroom lessons over a two-year period. The lessons were designed to enhance students' ability to use strategies that would reduce the potential for harm in drinking situations and that would assist in reducing the impact of harm once it has occurred. Students who participated in the SHAHRP programme had a 10% greater alcohol-related knowledge, consumed 20% less alcohol, experienced 33% less harm associated with their own use of alcohol, and experienced

10% less harm associated with other people's use of alcohol than did the control group (McBride *et al.* 2004). These findings are important given that school-based drug education is often criticized for not impacting on young people's behaviour. In addition, the behavioural effect was maintained and in some cases even increased up to one year after the final phase of the programme. This suggests a latency effect of the programme rather than a decaying effect over time.

These results (McBride *et al.* 2004) indicate that a relatively brief classroom alcohol intervention that is based on prior evidence of effectiveness can produce a change in young people's alcohol-related behaviours, particularly the harm associated with their own use of alcohol. Some of the key components are ensuring that lesson content and scenarios are based on the experiences of young people, testing the intervention prior to implementation, offering booster sessions in subsequent years, providing interactive activities and teacher training, and adopting a harm minimization approach. However, in a critical assessment, Foxcroft (2006) notes that the SHAHRP programme did not demonstrate a significant effect on the measures of risky consumption, and recommends interpreting the results with caution.

13.3.2 Comprehensive and community-based programmes

Some programmes include both individual-level education and family-level or community-level interventions. Project Northland was a school and community intervention designed to prevent or delay the onset of drinking among young adolescents in ten communities in north-eastern Minnesota (Perry *et al.* 1993, 1996). The primary school-based intervention comprised a series of sessions devoted to resistance skills, media literacy, and normative education. The programme also provided parents with information on adolescent alcohol use. Task forces in some communities were involved in local policy actions such as the passage of ordinances requiring responsible beverage service training. Other activities included the enlistment of local businesses to sponsor alcohol-free activities for youth and to give discounts to students who promised to remain alcohol-free and drug-free. The evaluation of Project Northland indicated that the programme had a positive influence on alcohol knowledge and family communication about alcohol. Alcohol use, however, was not significantly reduced at the end of the sixth grade (Williams *et al.* 1995) or the seventh grade, with the programme having no overall effect on drinking (Perry *et al.* 1996). Other analyses showed that those who were actively involved in the peer-planned social activities were less likely to report using alcohol in the past month than those who attended the alcohol-free activities but were not involved in activity planning, and those who were non-participants (Komro *et al.* 1996). Participation in the parents' programme in seventh grade was related to increases in parent communication about alcohol, especially in terms of family rules and the consequences of breaking those rules (Toomey *et al.* 1996). By eighth grade, additional differences emerged on programme-related attitudes and beliefs (Perry *et al.* 1996). Students in the intervention schools scored lower on a measure of tendency to use alcohol than students in comparison schools. They also reported significantly less alcohol use in the past month. All of these differences dissipated after the project ended (Perry *et al.* 1998).

Another comprehensive programme, the Midwestern Prevention Project, was implemented in 50 public schools in 15 communities in the state of Kansas, USA. A replication was conducted in 57 schools and 11 communities in another state. The intervention consisted of five components: (i) a 10–13-session school-based programme with five booster sessions; (ii) a mass media programme; (iii) a parent education and organization programme; (iv) training of community leaders; and (v) local policy changes initiated by the community organization. Monthly drinking was significantly lower in the intervention than in the comparison schools after one year (Pentz *et al.* 1989; MacKinnon *et al.* 1991), but it did not differ (34% vs 33%) after three years (Johnson *et al.* 1990). Effects on monthly intoxication were significant through the end of high school.

In sum, these well-designed evaluations suggest that even comprehensive school-based prevention programmes may not be sufficient to delay the initiation of drinking, or to sustain a small reduction in drinking beyond the operation of the programme. Reduced drinking was found when coupled with community interventions, especially those that were successful in reducing alcohol sales and provision of alcohol to youth. Community-based prevention trials are effective in curtailing drinking and alcohol-related problems (Hingson *et al.* 1996; Holder *et al.* 2000; Wagenaar *et al.* 2000a). These initiatives primarily involve a combination of policy or regulatory changes, enforcement, information campaigns, media advocacy, and community organizing. When educational and persuasion techniques are combined with community action, policy changes, regulation, and enforcement account for most of the observed effects. However, this research is typically not designed to isolate and measure the relative impact of educational strategies, particularly when the educational strategies are implemented concurrently with more potent interventions underway in these community-based trials.

13.3.3 Outcomes by length of follow-up

Several assessments of the scientific literature (Foxcroft *et al.* 2002, 2003; Foxcroft 2006) involved an assessment of the preventive impact of educational programmes according to the length of follow-up. Whereas some programmes focusing on adolescents show some initial impact, this typically does not last. Of particular relevance is the 2006 rapid review conducted by Foxcroft (2006) for the **World Health Organization (WHO)**, building on his prior Cochrane Review (Foxcroft *et al.* 2002). Findings from 23 evaluations of the most common youth-oriented prevention programmes indicate that a number of studies showed no effect of the intervention compared with a control group. In three studies, increased alcohol consumption was evident in the intervention group compared with that of the control. Seven showed some statistically significant positive effects but with a number of caveats. The results were compromised by poor methods, high attrition, inappropriate analysis, or small effect sizes.

Foxcroft (2006) highlighted two programmes as worthy of further consideration and implementation. One was a social marketing media-based intervention (supported by Slater *et al.* 2006) and the other the Strengthening Families Program 10–14, supported by three studies (Spoth *et al.* 2004, 2005; Brody *et al.* 2006). However, it is noteworthy that the Strengthening Families Program has been used with high-risk children and involves an approach that is closer to family therapy than the typical classroom-based primary prevention programme.

13.3.4 Foci: universal, selective, and indicated

The findings reported by Foxcroft are generally convergent with a meta-analysis by Shamblen and Derzon (2009) that focused on 43 studies of 25 programmes. They compared substance abuse prevention programmes that were targeted at the entire population (universal), those at risk (selective), or persons exhibiting the early stages of use or related problem behaviour (indicated). The analysis focused on US-based initiatives recognized as model programmes by the Substance Abuse and Mental Health Administration of the US government. A key finding was that at the population level, universal programmes were more successful in reducing tobacco and marijuana use whereas selective and indicated programmes were more successful in reducing alcohol use.

13.3.5 Limitations and challenges

A number of meta-analyses as well as narrative and systematic reviews have been published in the past decade, representing dozens of evaluated programmes where alcohol was a primary focus or among the substances examined. Several themes emerge from this literature. First, while the adolescent population is the central focus of the original studies and the reviews, a number of the interventions extend their scope beyond the classroom to include community-based settings and institutions (Skara and Sussman 2003), and involve families and parents in the intervention programmes (e.g. Spoth *et al.* 2001, 2002). This expanded programmatic scope might reflect frustration with the disappointing results from school-based interventions (e.g. Botvin *et al.* 1995), and, as noted by Foxcroft *et al.* (2002), evidence of positive impact from community-based policies and interventions that reach beyond information dissemination strategies (e.g. Hingson *et al.* 1996; Holder *et al.* 2000; Wagenaar *et al.* 2000a).

Second, some analysts have noted that the promotion, marketing and dissemination of some interventions appear to be unrelated to the evaluation findings. For example, two reviews of the US Drug Abuse Resistance Education (DARE) programme, conducted 10 years apart (Ennett *et al.* 1994; West and O'Neal 2004), concluded that the impact of DARE's core curriculum was not significant. Others have noted that despite the evidence of ineffectiveness, the programme continued to be widely popular and was taking the place of potentially more effective drug education programmes (Lindstrom and Svensson 1998). Similarly, the Life Education programme in Australia had the dubious honour of being very popular and receiving substantial government support without evidence of effectiveness. Furthermore it possibly contributed to drinking among adolescent boys (Hawthorne 1996; Midford and McBride 2004).

Third, reviewers of the literature initially tend to cast their nets widely, and then quickly narrow their focus to those publications that meet more stringent methodological criteria, typically experimental or quasi-experimental designs, using standardized measures of either drinking behaviour or alcohol-related problems. From this select group of studies the majority typically report no evidence of positive impact on reducing drinking behaviour or alcohol-related harm (e.g. Cuijpers 2003; Skara and Sussman 2003; Petrie *et al.* 2007; Skager 2007).

Fourth, despite innovations in selective and indicated programmes, most evaluations are based on universal programmes (Shamblen and Derzon 2009). An underlying but often unstated theme is that even the more elaborate interventions may not deliver a sufficient 'dose' to have an impact. Limitations with regard to design issues have also been noted: lack of rigorous evaluation (Botvin and Griffin 2007), lack of suitable control groups (Foxcroft *et al.* 2002), not enough randomized controlled trials (Wood *et al.* 2006), and threats to internal validity.

Fifth, most of the studies are based in the USA, with little research being conducted on European interventions and those in other jurisdictions (Cuipers 2003). Midford and McBride (2004), writing from Australia, noted that the abstinence goal of US-based studies meant that the literature tended to overlook benefits of reduced drinking among adolescents, as illustrated in the study by McBride *et al.* (2004).

Based on the reviews noted above (e.g. Foxcroft *et al.* 2003), it would appear that many programmes without demonstrated effectiveness continue to be implemented, apparently based on the assumption that providing information will somehow change behaviour and maintain the change. On the other hand, programmes with multiple interactive components and dimensions and those that reach beyond the classroom seem to have some potential. Education is not necessarily the best description of the adolescent-focused or school-based programmes that have some potential for positive impact. These dimensions may be part of such programmes, but their 'selective' or 'indicated' foci combined with components that resemble family therapy or screening and brief intervention may be the most potent components. The reviews typically show that information is not sufficient on its own to delay initiation of alcohol use or to prevent alcohol-related problems. In general, prevention programmes seem more successful when they maintain intervention activities over several years and incorporate more than one strategy.

13.4 **College and university programmes**

Interventions directed at alcohol use in college and university settings have been developed in response to concerns about the extent of heavy drinking (Engs *et al.* 1994; Wechsler 1996), its relation to sexual assaults (Meilman *et al.* 1993; Meilman and Haygood-Jackson 1996; Schwartz and Kennedy 1997), and its impact on school performance, drink-driving (Hingson *et al.* 2002), and other alcohol-related problems such as disorderly conduct. Large-scale surveys of college students in the USA (Wechsler 1996) and Canada (Gliksman *et al.* 2000) have documented the extent of drinking and alcohol-related risks. Both abstinence and harm-reduction goals are reflected in college intervention programmes.

Recent prevention efforts in the USA have been oriented to local and state authorities, university administrators, heavy drinkers, their peers, and alcohol retailers and producers (DeJong and Langford 2002; Larimer and Cronce 2002; Perkins 2002). Typically, a combination of strategies is used, including persuasive measures, staff training, guidelines and regulations, voluntary arrangements pertaining to alcohol marketing, restrictions on location of outlets, and campus alcohol policies. Interventions that rely primarily on educational and informational strategies are influenced by several theoretical approaches (Gonzalez and Clement 1994; Werch *et al.* 1994), such as the **health belief model** (Broughton 1997), the **empowerment model** (Cummings 1997), and by social marketing strategies (Zimmerman 1997). The social marketing approach, as discussed earlier, uses research to plan communications and is intended to change the environment as well as individual behaviour. More recently, there has been increasing attention to interventions that rely on providing information on group norms, feedback on drinking, motivational techniques and others.

13.4.1 Specific programmes

Normative education is the organizing principle in several interventions (Cameron *et al.* 1993; Robinson *et al.* 1993; Steffian 1999). Some evaluations have found short-term impact in the intervention group compared with the comparison group (Robinson *et al.* 1993). A similar approach compared a 'Health Enhancement Led by Peers' (HELP) group with an academic control group (Turner 1997). There were significant improvements in knowledge following exposure to the programme, but no changes were found in attitudes or behaviour.

More recent assessments (Wechsler and Nelson 2008) have not found substantial behaviour change impact from a social-norms marketing approach in college environments. There was no significant decrease in any measure of drinking observed in colleges that used a social-norms approach. Indeed, a significant increase in alcohol use was observed in these colleges, and they were less likely to implement policies that restrict alcohol on campus compared with those who did not use a social-norms intervention (Wechsler *et al.* 2003, 2004).

Until recently, there has been no convincing scientific support for the effectiveness of campus-wide educational programmes or awareness campaigns (Larimer and Cronce 2002) in reducing heavy drinking or alcohol-related problems. However, several studies have shown some promise in achieving at least short-term positive changes in drinking behaviour. Table 13.1 highlights the programmes that were perceived to have some positive effect by reviewers covering a period from 1987 to 2006. Fager and Melnyk (2004) and Larimer and Cronce (2007) had the most restrictive criteria for inclusion and are the most recent of the reviews. Both assessments identified a number of studies that were considered to have shown some short-term impact. In the latter case, 18 of the 42 studies were considered to illustrate some short-term impact. Nevertheless, Larimer and Cronce (2007) point to a number of limitations in this evaluation literature: small sample sizes, high attrition rates, lack of appropriate control groups, short follow-up periods, and randomization failures.

Carey *et al.* (2007) undertook a meta-analytical review of 62 studies published between 1985 and 2007 that focused on individual level interventions to reduce college student drinking. Three major findings emerged: (1) individual-level alcohol interventions for college drinkers reduce alcohol use; (2) these interventions also reduce alcohol-related problems, and reductions in problems vary by sample and intervention characteristics; and (3) the differences between students who receive

Table 13.1 Education/persuasion programmes directed at college students considered to have a positive effect with regard to alcohol use or drinking-related problems

Perceived norms

Participants randomly assigned to two conditions: those introduced to actual and perceived norms of student body drank significantly less alcohol in on a weekly basis up to 4–6 months later (Schroeder and Prentice 1998).

Significant reduction in high-risk or heavy episodic drinking rates (as much as 20%) in relatively short time periods from programmes that have intensity and persistently communicated accurate norms about the healthy majority of students (Haines 1996, 1998; Haines and Spear 1996; Berkowitz 1997; Johannessen *et al.* 1999; Jeffrey 2000; Perkins and Craig 2003).

Expectancy challenge

Expectancy challenge (EC) and information: short-term effectiveness (Darkes and Goldman 1993).

Reductions in consumption for men in the EC group at follow-up (Wiers *et al.* 2005).

EC, personalized feedback (PF). Significant reductions in past 30-day consumption at 1 and 3 months in EC condition (Wood, in Wiers *et al.* 2005).

Personalized normative feedback

Gender-neutral computerized personalized normative feedback (PNF) and protective behavioural tips. Gender-specific PNF. Both PNF conditions reduced drinking norms, overall alcohol use, typical weekly drinking, and drinks per drinking occasion (Lewis and Neighbors 2006).

Reduction in alcohol in PNF group mediated by reductions in perception of drinking norms (Neighbors *et al.* 2006).

Computer-based PNF. Reductions in weekly drinking in PNF group mediated by reductions in perceived drinking norms (Neighbors *et al.* 2006).

Web-based PNF. Reduction in drinking quantity, peak blood alcohol concentration (BAC), and negative consequences in both groups at 8-week and 16-week follow-ups, with significantly greater drinking reductions in the PNF group at 8 weeks (Walters *et al.* 2007).

Brief motivational intervention

Randomly assigned to two groups: Brief motivational intervention (BMI) showed reductions in heavy drinkers (Agostinelli *et al.* 1995).

BMI: Longest trial, reported on 4 years of follow-up data: significant difference in associated problems from alcohol use was evident between the experimental and control groups, but not alcohol intake (Baer *et al.* 2001).

BMI with cognitive component and multi-component skills intervention: short-term success at six months (Borsari and Carey 2000).

Timeline follow-back (TLFB) and BMI and decision balance: reduction in alcohol use at 1-month follow-up. At 12 months maintained for BMI, but not TLFB (Carey *et al.* 2006).

Normative discrepancies, BMI and motivational feedback (MF). Significant reductions in drinks per heaviest week and frequency of heavy drinking episodes at 6-week follow-up (trend at 6-month follow-up) in MF early success but lack of positive outcomes at follow-up (Collins *et al.* 2002).

Table 13.1 (Continued) Education/persuasion programmes directed at college students considered to have a positive effect with regard to alcohol use or drinking-related problems

BMI feedback skills group: Decreased alcohol-related problems in two- and three-session group. No significant decreases in drinking (Gregory 2001).

Computer-generated personalized BMI feedback; leaflet on alcohol information: significantly lower total consumption, frequency of heavy consumption, and personal problems in feedback group at 6 weeks. Lower personal and academic problems at 6 months (Kypri *et al.* 2004).

Group motivational feedback (BMI). Multi-component skills intervention. Decrease in problematic alcohol use in BMI group. Reduction in negative consequences in BMI and skills group (LaChance 2004).

Mailed personalized BMI feedback. Significant reductions in high-risk drinking (composite variable) and consequences for women by 3 months, maintained throughout 12 months. (LaForge in Saunders *et al.* 2004).

BMI, with 1-hour individual tailored feedback; short-term success (Larimer *et al.* 2001).

BMI, cognitive behavioral skills strategies, normative: significant reductions in heavy drinking among at-risk drinkers, reduced alcohol problems in both groups (McNally and Palfai 2003).

Cognitive BMI, evaluation of efficacy of Brief Alcohol Screening and Intervention of College Students (BASICS); reduction in weekly alcohol consumption among heavy drinkers (Murphy *et al.* 2001).

Preventing drink-driving

Group exposed to peer theatre intervention had more accurate perceptions of campus drinking norms and reported more frequent use of drinking drivers. No data provided on outcomes (Cimini *et al.* 2002).

Minimal effects on combined measure of drinking and driving and riding with drinking drivers (D'Amico and Fromme 2002).

Reduction in alcohol consumption; regarding lower BAC, percentage of drivers with positive BACs also declined (Foss *et al.* 2001).

Peer-led multi-component skills group (lifestyle management class; LMC). Professionally-led LMC. Reduction in driving after drinking in LMC group (Fromme and Corbin 2004).

Diminishing effects on reducing drink-driving over the 4-year follow-up (Klepp *et al.* 1995).

School-based instructional programme about riding with drinking drivers; included random assignment to control group (Newman *et al.* 1992).

Project Northland: community-wide alcohol use prevention programme (Perry *et al.* 1996).

Exposure to films and discussion led to a decrease in drinking and driving intent (Singh 1993).

Other interventions

Alcohol 101 CD-ROM, cognitive-behavioural skills training: greater reduction in quantity and frequency of consumption by high-risk students in skills training group (Donohue *et al.* 2004).

Social-norms marketing: reduction in binge drinking, media campaign changed norm perceptions, traditional prevention strategies not successful (Haines and Spear 1996).

(continued)

Table 13.1 (Continued) Education/persuasion programmes directed at college students considered to have a positive effect with regard to alcohol use or drinking-related problems

Pub intervention with skills training for bartenders; short-term outcome effectiveness (Johnson and Berglund 2003).

Alcohol-reduction decision balance. Reductions in quantity and frequency of consumption at 1-month follow-up (Labrie 2002).

Mailed personalized BASICS feedback and protective behavioural tips. Significant reductions in alcohol use (composite) and likelihood of heavy drinking compared with controls, and increased likelihood of maintaining abstinence for baseline abstainers in feedback condition (Larimer et al. 2007).

[a] Several documents are not summarized in this table, but discussed in the text of this chapter. Lewis and Neighbors (2006) provide an evaluation of social norms approaches. Carey et al. (2007) report on a meta-analytic review of 62 studies published between 1985 and 2007.

[b] Criteria for inclusion varied by reviewer. Perkins (2002): theoretical and empirical studies of social norms; some may have had design problems.

Elder et al. 2005: Evaluation of school-based programmes for reducing drink-driving and riding with drink-drivers, including those focusing on adolescents and on college students.

Fager and Melnyk (2004): Exhaustive search of all experimental studies between 1993 and January 2004 that met the following criteria: (1) intervention studies involving college students; (2) quasi-experimental or experimental designs that included a control group that did not receive the experimental intervention specifically targeting a decrease in alcohol use; and (3) at least one outcome measure focused on behavioural change in drinking or the consequences of drinking, such as injury, assault, aggressive behaviour.

Larimer and Cronce (2007): Studies had to meet all four criteria: '(1) include at least one active individual-focused alcohol prevention/intervention condition; (2) assess at least one behavioral outcome (such as reduction in total drinks per week, peak consumption, heavy episodic or "binge" drinking, blood alcohol concentration (BAC), and/or alcohol-related negative consequences); (3) include at least one control or comparison condition (assessment only, wait-list, attention, or alternative intervention); and (4) utilize some method of prospective randomization to condition (at the level of the individual or the group/class)' (Larimer and Cronce 2007, p. 2441).

interventions and those in control conditions diminish over time. Carey et al. (2007) also noted several characteristics that appear to be associated with successfully moderating alcohol-related problems:

* Interventions were less successful in reducing problems (compared with controls) when they targeted heavy drinkers or other high-risk groups.

* Interventions were more successful when they were delivered to individuals rather than groups, used motivational interviewing, provided feedback on expectancies or motives, and included normative comparisons.

* Interventions that included skills training or expectancy challenge components were less successful at reducing alcohol-related problems, relative to control interventions.

* Interventions reduced consumption within one month, but between-group differences ceased to be significant after 6 months.

Finally, Larimer and Cronce (2007) offered several observations about the impact of specific intervention techniques. They found strong support for the brief motivational interventions (BMIs), particularly when combined with other components. They concluded that campuses interested in implementing individual-focused prevention programmes should consider BMI or skills-based programmes, preferably incorporating personalized normative feedback, BAC training, and protective behavioural strategies for risk reduction, as well as other personalized feedback components.

A common thread in college-based programmes with some short-term impact is that the intervention goes beyond the conveying of information, education, or offering persuasive-oriented advice. For example, the brief motivational intervention and personalized normative feedback interventions are not broadly dissimilar from essential components of screening and brief interventions discussed in Chapter 14. As with the numerous school-based programmes discussed above, the few with intensive features, not unlike family therapy and focusing on 'selected' or 'indicated' adolescents, are more likely to have some impact.

13.5 Building support for health-oriented policies

Education campaigns can be used as a tool to build support for public-health-oriented policies as indicated by studies conducted in New Zealand (Casswell *et al.* 1989) and Norway (Rise *et al.* 2005). The New Zealand study concluded that a mass media campaign focusing on alcohol advertising and availability created a climate in support of policies likely to shape appropriate drinking behaviours in the community (Casswell *et al.* 1989). The goals of the Norwegian information campaign (Rise *et al.* 2005) were to increase knowledge of the harm related to alcohol consumption, increase awareness of the utility of restrictive alcohol policies, and provide advice on how to communicate about alcohol with one's children. Changes in three areas were found following the campaign: more positive attitudes towards the use of effective alcohol policy measures, more positive attitudes toward parental monitoring of children's alcohol consumption, and more restrictive parental behaviour in relation to their children. As these examples illustrate, the role and aims of school-based alcohol education could be redefined and refocused (Giesbrecht 2007) with an orientation to alcohol policy and increased awareness of the influence of social forces that influence drinking, including the role of the alcohol industry in marketing of alcohol, the responsibility of policymakers and parents, and the potency of environmental and other alcohol control strategies.

13.6 Conclusion

In recent years, the number of informational and educational programmes has grown exponentially (see Foxcroft *et al.* 1997; Foxcroft 2006). Many of these educational campaigns have not been evaluated. Where evaluations have been conducted, they often do not meet the criteria of 'methodological soundness' (Foxcroft *et al.* 1997, 2002; White and Pitts 1998, p. 1477). Compared with other interventions and strategies, educational programmes are expensive and appear to have little long-term effect on alcohol consumption levels and drinking-related problems. On the other hand, other strategies such as law enforcement initiatives, outlet zoning, pricing policies, and responsible serving practices have all been shown to have some impact on college campuses (Wechsler and Nelson 2008).

On balance, their hegemony and popularity seem not to be a function of either their demonstrated long-term impact or their potential for reducing alcohol-related harms.

It is tempting to qualify this conclusion by emphasizing the few positive findings emerging from several studies that have been reviewed above. In some instances where the interventions go far beyond providing information and include different components—focusing on families, links with community-based policies, or motivational interventions for college students—there is some evidence of impact. However, these are not examples of the bulk of the universal education programmes that are so popular but without evidence of effectiveness.

There is also the temptation to keep on trying—the triumph of hope over experience. Let us try one more education campaign, mount yet another school-based educational programme, fund another college social-norms initiative, and perhaps our pessimism will be confounded. Sadly, on the basis of the previous experience, our prognostication must be otherwise. It is likely that even with adequate resources, strategies that try to use education to prevent alcohol-related harm are unlikely to deliver large or sustained benefits. Education alone is too weak a strategy to counteract other forces that pervade the environment. An unanswered question, beyond the scope of this book, is why significant resources continue to be devoted to initiatives with limited potential for reducing or preventing alcohol-related problems.

Chapter 14

Treatment and early intervention services

14.1 Introduction

Alcohol policies are primarily the concern of local, regional, and national governments, which often view the provision of treatment as part of a comprehensive approach to alcohol-related problems. In addition to its value in the reduction of human suffering, treatment can be considered as a form of prevention. When it occurs soon after the onset of alcohol problems, it is called secondary prevention; when it is initiated to control the damage associated with chronic drinking, it is called tertiary prevention. As one of the first societal responses to alcohol problems, treatment interventions have not been critically examined as policy options, despite the resources they consume and the scientific evidence that is available concerning their effectiveness and costs. This chapter examines the scientific basis of alcohol treatment policies in terms of research on the effectiveness and costs of a wide range of treatment interventions. By treatment policy we mean governmental actions that affect the nature of treatment services, the allocation of resources, and the optimal mix of services for the management of alcohol use disorders (AUDs).

During the past 50 years, there has been a steady growth in the provision of specialized medical, psychiatric and social services to individuals with AUDs. The number and variety of services has in parts of the industrialized world increased enormously after World War II, when many countries with a high prevalence of alcohol problems invested in treatment services as part of a larger public health approach to reduce the burden of disease, disability, and social problems that accompany substance use (Klingemann *et al.* 1992; Klingemann and Hunt 1998). For example, in The Netherlands, admissions to Consultation Bureaus for Alcohol and Drugs increased from 45 000 in 1988 to 55 000 in 1995 and residential treatment admissions almost doubled between 1980 and 1990 (Derks *et al.* 1998). In other countries, such as Peru and Colombia, treatment resources are scarce and scattered despite increasing demand (Madrigal 1998). As a consequence, treatment is obtained in primary health care settings or through private practitioners. In the USA, it is estimated that alcohol and drug treatment services are delivered in more than 5000 specialized facilities, such as hospitals, residential settings, methadone clinics, therapeutic communities, and outpatient programmes (Hunt and Dong Sun 1998). These services employ more than 250 000 workers and serve more than 1 million substance users per day.

Within the context of expanding services, and the likelihood of expanded services in the developing countries, questions arise regarding the allocation of resources and the optimal mix of services for the management of AUDs. For example, the question central to this book's frame is: To what extent are alcohol treatment and early intervention services effective in reducing population rates of alcohol-related harm? Other questions relevant to treatment policy include the following: Should people with these conditions be managed within the general health care system, specialized addiction services, social welfare agencies, psychiatric facilities, the criminal justice system, or a combination of these entities? What is the optimal amount and best combination of services needed to serve the needs of a country or a geographic area? What kinds of treatment systems are best suited to prevent the marginalization of people with chronic alcohol problems? How can treatment services best be organized to provide the most effective treatment at the lowest cost?

14.2 Treatment services and systems of care

Treatment for alcohol problems typically involves a set of services, ranging from diagnostic assessment to therapeutic interventions and continuing care. Researchers have identified more than 40 therapeutic approaches, called treatment modalities, which have been evaluated by means of randomized clinical trials (Miller *et al.* 1995). Examples include motivational counselling, marital and family therapy, cognitive-behavioural therapy, relapse prevention training, aversion therapy, pharmacotherapy, and interventions based on the Twelve Steps of Alcoholics Anonymous. These modalities are delivered in a variety of settings, including freestanding residential facilities, psychiatric and general hospital settings, outpatient programmes, and primary care. More recently, treatment services in some countries have been organized into systems that are defined by linkages between different facilities and levels of care, and by the extent of integration with other types of services, such as mental health, drug dependence treatment, and mutual help organizations (Klingemann *et al.* 1993; Klingemann and Klingemann 1999).

Most treatment research and the scientific evidence derived from it are component-based, focusing on a single intervention or episode of care. In general, the research evidence can be organized according to three types of intervention within the emerging treatment systems of countries where information on efficacy and effectiveness is available: (i) interventions for nondependent high-risk drinkers, (ii) formal treatment for problem drinking and alcohol dependence, and (iii) mutual help interventions.

14.3 Interventions designed for non-dependent high-risk drinkers

Harmful drinking typically precedes the development of alcohol dependence, and by definition it can cause serious medical and psychological problems in the absence of dependence. With the increased interest in clinical preventive services in both developed and developing countries, early intervention programmes have been developed by the **World Health Organization (WHO)** and national agencies to facilitate the management of harmful drinking in primary health care and other settings. Following an initial screening to identify risk levels, the patient is referred either to a brief intervention or to more intensive specialized treatment. Brief interventions are characterized by their low intensity and short duration, consisting of one to three sessions of counselling and education. The aim is to motivate high-risk drinkers to moderate their alcohol consumption rather than promote total abstinence.

During the past two decades, more than 100 randomized controlled trials have been conducted to evaluate the efficacy of brief interventions. The cumulative evidence (Whitlock *et al.* 2004) shows that clinically significant reductions in drinking and alcohol-related problems can follow from brief interventions. Nurses are as effective as doctors in producing behaviour change and the positive effects have been observed with adolescents, adults, older adults, and pregnant women. Despite the evidence for benefit from this kind of intervention as applied in many different settings, difficulties are often encountered in persuading practitioners to deliver such care (Babor *et al.* 2007).

14.4 Specialized treatment for persons with alcohol dependence

In countries with well-developed health care systems, the range of agencies and professional service providers involved in specialist treatment of alcohol-related problems is extensive. Some of the key issues that treatment research has addressed with increasing scientific rigor include the most effective detoxification measures, the impact of different treatment settings, whether some therapeutic modalities are better than others, the effects of treatment intensity, and factors that influence long-term outcomes.

Detoxification services are mainly directed at patients with a history of chronic drinking (especially those with poor nutrition) who are at risk of experiencing withdrawal symptoms as part of a well-documented alcohol withdrawal syndrome. Administration of thiamine and multivitamins is a low-cost, low-risk intervention that prevents alcohol-related neurological disturbances, and is typically combined with supportive care and treatment of concurrent illness. Various medications have been used for the treatment of alcohol withdrawal, but the benzodiazepines, especially diazepam and chlordiazepoxide, have largely supplanted all other medications because of their favourable side-effect profiles. There can be no doubt that treatment that obviates development of the most severe withdrawal symptoms can be life-saving.

Following detoxification, various therapeutic modalities have been incorporated into different service settings to treat the patient's drinking problems, promote abstinence from alcohol, and prevent relapse. Alcohol treatment is typically provided in outpatient and inpatient hospital settings, but it can also be delivered in psychiatric clinics, social service agencies, and health care settings. In most comparative studies, outpatient programmes have been found to produce outcomes comparable to those of residential programmes, although some patients may benefit more from residential treatment because of their medical and psychiatric problems (Finney *et al.* 1996). In general, the research evidence on the cost-effectiveness of different treatment modalities has consistently found that the more expensive modalities do not necessarily produce better treatment outcomes.

A variety of therapeutic modalities are used within the context of outpatient and residential treatment services. The approaches with the greatest amount of supporting evidence are behaviour therapy, group therapy, family treatment, and motivational enhancement (Edwards *et al.* 2003). One example of behaviour therapy is 'relapse prevention', which focuses on coping with situations that represent high risk for heavy drinking. Research also indicates that Twelve Step Facilitation, which is designed to introduce problem drinkers to the principles of Alcoholics Anonymous, is as effective as more theory-based therapies (Ouimette *et al.* 1999; Babor *et al.* 2008a). Another treatment approach, often combined with behaviour therapy and group therapy, is the use of alcohol-sensitizing drugs, medications to directly reduce drinking, and medications to treat comorbid psychopathology (Kranzler and Van Kirk 2001). Alcohol-sensitizing drugs such as disulfiram and calcium carbimide cause an unpleasant physical reaction when alcohol is consumed. Although these drugs may help alcohol-dependent persons when special efforts are made to ensure compliance, their efficacy in the prevention or limitation of relapse has been limited. Another class of medications operates on the specific brain neurotransmitter systems implicated in the control of alcohol consumption, including endogenous opioids, catecholamines (especially dopamine), and serotonin. In general, opioid antagonists like naltrexone have been found in some but not all studies to be superior to placebo in delaying the time to relapse and reducing the rate of relapse to heavy drinking among patients (Kranzler and Van Kirk 2001; Anton *et al.* 2006). Another focus of medications research has been acamprosate, an amino acid derivative, which has been reported as having significant advantages over placebo, but other large-scale studies have been negative (Kranzler and Van Kirk 2001; Anton *et al.* 2006). Despite advances in the search for a pharmacological intervention that could reduce craving and other precipitants of relapse, the additive effects of pharmacotherapies have been marginal beyond standard counselling and behaviour therapies.

Because some people with alcohol dependence relapse repeatedly in spite of multiple treatment episodes, long-term residential treatment is used in some countries for alcoholics who do not respond to more limited efforts at rehabilitation. The effectiveness of these programmes has not been evaluated systematically, although continuing care by means of aftercare groups and other mutual help organizations is associated with better long-term outcomes (Timko *et al.* 2000).

Although mutual help societies composed of recovering alcoholics are not considered a formal treatment, they are often used as a substitute or as an adjunct to treatment. With an estimated 2.2 million members affiliated with more than 100 000 groups in 150 countries, Alcoholics Anonymous (AA) is by far the most widely used source of help for persons with drinking problems. Related organizations have been developed in a number of countries, such as Danshukai in Japan, Kreuzbund in Germany, Croix d'Or and Vie Libre in France, Abstainers Clubs in Poland, Family Clubs in Italy and Links in the Scandinavian countries (Humphreys 2004). Several large-scale, well-designed studies (Walsh *et al.* 1991; Ouimette *et al.* 1999; Babor and Del Boca 2003) suggest that AA can have an incremental effect when combined with formal treatment, and AA attendance alone may be better than no intervention.

Whatever the treatment approach under consideration, the difficulty in establishing convincing evidence on effectiveness needs to be kept in awareness. Excessive drinking is a behaviour which over time often regresses to the mean, and at least a portion of outcome variance in uncontrolled studies may reflect spontaneous recovery. Controlled studies face the difficulty that an untreated control group may be impossible for ethical reasons. And the research participants who are involved in treatment trials may be biased toward good outcomes by the selection criteria. Caution is therefore needed in interpreting any observed improvement and in estimating effect size.

14.5 Mediators and moderators of treatment effectiveness

The investigation of mediators and moderators of treatment effectiveness helps to answer questions about how and why treatment works (mediating effects) and for whom certain treatments work best (moderators). This kind of research has taken place within the clinical 'technology model' of treatment efficacy and treatment matching, which postulates that patient attributes and treatment process elements, respectively, constitute mediators and moderators of change in drinking following treatment. Studies show that matching patient attributes to what might be considered a particularly appropriate therapeutic orientation (e.g. matching patients with low motivation to motivational enhancement therapy) does not substantially enhance outcomes, as previously believed (Babor and Del Boca 2003). They also indicate that the mediational mechanisms underlying several of the most popular therapies are different from what is suggested by their proponents. In general, the technology model of treatment effectiveness may be flawed as it applies to alcohol dependence. Instead of distinct, non-overlapping elements, therapy may work through common mechanisms such as empathy, an effective therapist–client alliance, a desire to change, inner resources, a supportive social network, and the provision of a culturally appropriate solution to a socially defined problem (Cooney et al. 2003).

14.6 Cost considerations

A major policy issue with regard to the feasibility and extent of specialist treatment is cost. Little research has been conducted on the cost-effectiveness of services for alcohol treatment, but in recent years there have been significant improvements in the methodological tools used and a better formulation of policy questions. One question is whether individuals who undergo treatment for alcohol dependence have lower health care expenditures afterwards (i.e. cost offsets). Another question is whether some settings or treatment modalities are more cost-effective than others, i.e. whether they deliver similar outcomes for lower costs. Still other questions concern whether shorter or longer periods of inpatient treatment are more cost-effective.

Cost-offset studies conducted primarily in the USA have shown that: (i) alcoholics and their family members are heavier users of health care services than are non-alcoholics of the same age and gender; (ii) prior to entering treatment, general medical care costs for those who eventually seek treatment tend to increase; and (iii) following treatment, the demand for health services by alcoholics and their families declines (Holder 1987; Goodman et al. 1997). In some cases these savings are large enough to compensate for the expense of treatment, but a causal relationship cannot be assumed.

Regarding cost-effective alternatives to inpatient alcoholism treatment, reviews of this literature (Finney *et al.* 1996; Babor 2008b) conclude that: (i) inpatient alcoholism programmes lasting from four weeks to several months do not have higher success rates than periods of brief hospitalization; (ii) some patients can be safely detoxified without pharmacotherapy and in non-hospital-based environments; (iii) partial hospitalization programmes ('day hospitalization' with no overnight stays) have results equal or superior to inpatient hospitalization, at one-half to one-third the cost; and (iv) in some populations, outpatient programmes produce results comparable to those of inpatient programmes.

An obvious question is whether some treatment modalities and treatment settings are more cost-effective than the others. In one analysis of treatment modalities used in the USA, the range of treatment costs across settings was enormous, with a high of US $585 per day for hospital-based care and a low of US $6 per visit at social model, non-residential programmes. Nevertheless, the research evidence did not show that more expensive treatment was more effective (Holder *et al.* 1991; Goodman *et al.* 1997).

14.7 Aggregate effects of treatment

Despite evidence of the effectiveness of some treatment interventions, little attention has been paid to the mechanisms of action that would translate individual benefits to the population. Treatment interventions are primarily designed to serve the needs of individual patients or clients, but there are a number of ways in which these interventions may have an impact at community and population levels: by raising public awareness of alcohol problems, influencing national and community agendas, involving health professionals in advocacy for prevention, and providing secondary benefits to families, employers, and those who otherwise meet a drinking driver on the road. The effect of treatment interventions can also be manifested more directly, not only by reducing the amount of alcohol consumed by the drinker (and his or her associated risks) but also by influencing the social milieu of the drinker (Skog 1985). By removing a source of reciprocal influence that is likely to contribute to the maintenance of heavy drinking subcultures, treatment might perhaps diminish the alcohol-related problem rates in a community.

Given the scarcity of specialized treatment services in most countries (Klingemann *et al.* 1992), they are not likely to have an impact on morbidity and mortality at the level of communities and nation states. Nevertheless, there is some evidence that treatment has the potential to produce aggregate impact in countries where the treatment system is relatively well developed (Smart and Mann 2000). Several researchers have identified associations between declining liver cirrhosis rates and the growth of specialized treatment. Mann *et al.* (1988) found that decreased hospital discharges for liver cirrhosis were associated with increased treatment in Ontario. Romelsjö (1987) suggested that in addition to decreased per-capita consumption, outpatient treatment may have accounted for the reduction in liver cirrhosis rates in Stockholm, Sweden. Holder and Parker (1992) found that increased alcohol treatment admissions (both in- and outpatient) over a 20-year period in North Carolina were related to a significant reduction in cirrhosis mortality.

Despite these findings, there is a dearth of research about the overall impact of treatment systems and multiple episodes of care on population health or welfare indicators, and there has been little research on whether different system designs are more efficient or effective than others. Some studies have attempted to evaluate the effects of different organizational models and treatment system qualities. A study of the national alcohol treatment system in Denmark (Pedersen *et al.* 2004) showed that certain internal characteristics of the treatment system (accessibility, relation to drug treatment, treatment for special groups, and structured treatment) were important for getting patients into treatment (catchment), whereas certain external factors were relevant for the rate of treatment (i.e. a referral guarantee and a general appreciation in surrounding systems of the nature of alcohol treatment).

In a study of almost 1900 clients and patients in different parts of the substance abuse treatment system in Stockholm county, Stenius *et al.* (2005) found that in contrast to an organizational model where residential treatment predominated, a system organized around outpatient services was better at recruiting vulnerable groups into treatment.

In addition to research on national or regional treatment services, several international studies have used historical and comparative perspectives to monitor developments in alcohol treatment systems. In a study of drug and alcohol treatment services in twenty-three countries, Gossop (1995) found that most countries have a scarcity of resources for these kinds of services, and many report an inadequate level of professional training. Another comparative study (Klingemann *et al.* 1992, 1993) conducted in sixteen countries showed that the size, extent, and character of the treatment system depended more on a given country's view of the importance of alcohol problems than on changes in alcohol consumption, the need for treatment, or economic resources.

14.8 Toward a conceptual model of treatment systems

Figure 14.1 presents a public health model of the structural resources and qualities of alcohol treatment systems that begins with the policy determinants of treatment services and ends with the population impact of treatment systems. Treatment policies may also affect system qualities, specifying not only where services are located but also how they are organized and integrated. System qualities include equity (the extent to which services are equally available and accessible to all population groups), efficiency (the most appropriate mix of services), and economy (the most cost-effective services). These qualities can be considered as mediators of system effectiveness, to the extent that they transmit the effects of system structures and programmes. In this conceptual model, it is postulated that structural resources and system qualities contribute significantly to the effectiveness of services (Babor *et al.* 2007). As suggested in Figure 14.1, the cumulative impact of these services should translate into population health benefits, such as reduced mortality and morbidity, as well as benefits to social welfare, such as reduced unemployment, disability, crime, suicide, and health care costs. The model also provides for the possibility that both the effectiveness and population impact of treatment systems are influenced by certain moderating factors, such

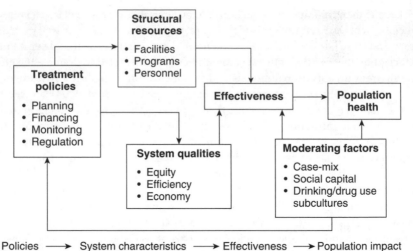

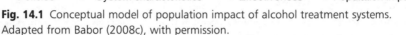

Policies ⟶ System characteristics ⟶ Effectiveness ⟶ Population impact

Fig. 14.1 Conceptual model of population impact of alcohol treatment systems. Adapted from Babor (2008c), with permission.

as the socio-demographic characteristics of the population with substance use disorders (i.e. the 'case-mix'), the social capital possessed by—or lacking in—these population groups (e.g. civic participation and community integration), and the cultural factors that determine patterns of substance use, as well as societal reactions to it. These moderating factors can contribute to the outcome of treatment regardless of system qualities and types of treatment, and should be taken into account in the design and evaluation of any treatment system. For this reason we have included a feedback loop from the moderating factors to the treatment policy box to emphasize that for optimal performance, treatment systems need to be designed to fit the characteristics of the population and its treatment needs.

14.9 **Treatment and the public's health**

Some progress has been made in the development of cost-effective treatments, including brief interventions and more intensive therapies, to manage persons whose drinking places them at risk (Institute of Medicine 1990). This is, however, not an area of research characterized as yet by large technical breakthrough: we advise as much against triumphalism as nihilism. To the extent that the prerequisites for a public health approach have been established, it is important to consider strategies designed to disseminate the potentially more cost-effective intervention strategies so that appropriate treatment will be available to those who need it. But the dissemination of individual-level interventions needs to be considered in the context of a population approach that goes beyond the traditional model of acute care focused on specific disease entities. If treatment is to be integrated into the overall policy response to alcohol, there are a number of requirements that treatment planning

Box 14.1 Conditions for a population approach to health services for alcohol-related problems

1) Attention to definition of cases

The national planning of any treatment response should start with a definition of suitable cases for treatment. The following behaviours and conditions must be included when defining the types of care with which alcohol treatment services should be concerned:

1. Personal alcohol consumption at a level likely to threaten or impair health
2. Alcohol dependence
3. Alcohol-related health or social impairments
4. Drink-driving, where drinking causes damage to others
5. Protection of families
6. Determination of the prevalence of cases within the population

2) Determination of the proportion of cases that will at any time seek and engage in treatment

In most developed countries survey data are available and can provide this kind of information about the extent of alcohol problems. Many people with drinking problems may be unwilling to become involved in treatment. Encouragement of help-seeking should be part of the strategy.

3) Treatment planning needs to take cognizance of natural history

Many seemingly troublesome alcohol-related problems are likely to remit spontaneously, while an individual who is a habitual heavy drinker may have much less likelihood of spontaneous remission. These considerations may speak to targeting of resources.

4) The treatment effectiveness question

This question relates not only to modality, but also to the duration and intensity of treatment and to the duration of any beneficial changes achieved. Alcohol problems are characterized by high relapse.

5) Economic benefits

Treatment policies need to be informed by awareness of costs and benefits in economic terms. In most countries the treatment response to alcohol problems has, up to now, more often developed from the compassionate effort to help individuals rather than from a consideration of the characteristics of a treatment system that would be needed to fit the kinds of criteria defined above. If in the future the treatment effort is more fully to achieve its public health potential, it will need to be based on objective performance criteria.

Source: adapted from World Health Organization (1993).

in the public health arena will need to meet. These requirements are identified in Box 14.1.

Treatment and prevention are traditionally conceived, implemented, and evaluated as largely unrelated activities. A more holistic vision is needed if alcohol policies are to address the complete spectrum of alcohol problems.

Chapter 15

The policy arena

15.1 Introduction

An arena is a place where contests, and at times conflicts, take place. When applied to policy, the word takes on the connotation of a sphere of action for opposing views, contending groups, and competing interests. Chapters 8–14 examined the evidence for a wide range of prevention and treatment strategies that could serve as instruments of alcohol policies. While there is now a growing scientific basis to support alcohol policy initiatives, there is much less understanding of the way in which governments, interest groups and communities operate within the policy arena to apply this information in the interests of public health.

In this chapter we consider the following question: Who makes alcohol policy? The answer is not simple and it differs across countries and between different levels of government within countries. The goal of this chapter is to describe the major players in the policymaking arena at the local, national and international levels. Implicit in our review is a model of the policymaking process that comprises the institutions, stakeholders, and the environment within which policy decisions are made. One model of the policy process forms a cycle, beginning with an assessment of alcohol-related problems, followed by implementation of evidence-based interventions, and concluding with systematic evaluation and corrective action if necessary. But the reality of the policymaking process is rarely that simple or straightforward.

In this chapter, policy formation in the area of alcohol is described as a process influenced by a combination of proximal and distal factors. Proximal factors begin with government institutions at the local and national levels. International agencies, such as the **World Health Organization** (WHO), can also play an important role. The next level of proximity includes public interest groups, particularly non-governmental organizations (NGOs), and commercial interests such as the alcohol industry, which attempt to influence the policymaking process directly through political lobbying or indirectly by changing public opinion. On the more distal side are found the mass media and health professionals, including alcohol scientists, medical practitioners, and public health advocates. The extent to which any interest group can influence alcohol policy depends on both the political power of a particular group and the governing images of alcohol problems to which the policymakers subscribe.

15.2 Governments

Alcohol policies can be developed and implemented at many different levels of government. Federal and national laws often establish the legislative framework, including state control over the production, export, and import of commercial alcohol products; control of wholesaling and retailing; legal minimum purchase ages for alcoholic beverages; apprehension of drivers with specified blood alcohol concentrations; alcohol marketing restrictions; and the support of treatment and prevention services. Furthermore, special taxes on alcoholic beverages are also subject to a regulatory framework that is enacted at a federal or national level.

Opportunities to influence the legal framework of alcohol polices are part of the democratic process in which many interested parties participate. The formal political process includes sector consultations, policy reviews and investigations by commissions. Draft legislation offers opportunities for various stakeholders to provide comments, meet with legislative committees, and make contact with representatives who will vote on the bill. Interested individuals, NGOs and industry representatives all participate in this way. All voices are formally equal in a democratic process, but not all parties have equal resources to support the time and effort needed to participate. This is also the case in regard to the many informal ways of participating in the policy process and influencing alcohol policy outcomes. These include ongoing lobbying of politicians and other policymakers and working through the mass media to influence both public opinion and the political climate (Casswell 1995). In many jurisdictions there has also been a long history of financial support by the alcohol industry for politicians and political parties who take a sympathetic position toward industry-favoured alcohol policies (Marin Institute 2008b).

Many different decision-making authorities are involved in the formulation, implementation, and enforcement of alcohol policy. Policy systems at the national level are rarely dominated by one decision-making authority, but tend rather to be decentralized, and different aspects of policy are delegated to a variety of different and sometimes competing decision-making entities such as the health ministry, the transportation authority, and the taxation agency. Countries vary tremendously, making it difficult to generalize about the policymaking process.

There are several important players in the public policy game. Civil servants tend to be relatively long-term players within government compared with elected representatives. Some of these individuals may be responsible for the process of alcohol policy development and implementation, although some policy development tasks can be contracted out to consultants. Ad-hoc committees and quasi-permanent advisory groups are sometimes appointed by governments to advise on alcohol policy, and independent research or policy institutes have sometimes become important sources of policy analysis and advice. In low-income countries, the WHO and a variety of development agencies may assist with this process. And in recent times, industry-funded organizations have attempted to influence national policy development.

Advocates of public health have had mixed results in their support of evidence-based alcohol policies. Recent policy development history in many countries has been one of public health advocates unsuccessfully opposing policy moves that were not supported by the research evidence (Mäkelä *et al.* 1981a; Casswell 1993; Hawks 1993; Moskalewicz 1993; Room 2004). But in a few nations, most noticeably France and the USA, the past decade has seen a policy debate driven by health sector stakeholders

(Dubois *et al.* 1989). This has resulted in a number of effective policies being introduced (Craplet 1997).

In some countries, the health and welfare sectors have attempted to establish broader national alcohol policies, which encompass a number of policy issues within an overall government philosophy and approach to alcohol issues (Room 1999). This was an approach strongly promoted by the WHO in the 1980s. A number of alcohol policy reviews have been published to provide a basis for such policy development (Farrell 1985), including the precursors to this book (Bruun *et al.* 1975a; Edwards *et al.* 1994; Babor *et al.* 2003).

Establishing a national policy sometimes entails the appointment of an organizational entity that represents the views of a number of sectors. Although the goal is to reach consensus, the diverse interests represented by these sectors makes agreement on any but the least contentious (and often least effective) policies very difficult (Christie and Bruun 1969). Add to this the strong positions of the vested interest groups, and national policy is not often a strong tool for public health advancement (Hawks 1990).

A national-level legislative and regulatory framework remains essential to the promotion of effective measures that curtail alcohol-related health and safety problems. Market liberalization and privatization have frequently been associated with increased regulation, albeit of a decentralized, less interventionist kind (Ayres and Braithwaite 1992). This offers the opportunity for 'responsive regulation', in which less prescriptive laws can enable a more negotiated process among commercial interests, regulators, and the community to increase both compliance and community satisfaction. **Liquor licensing**, particularly the conditions of sale pertaining to the licence, lends itself well to this model, but effectiveness nevertheless requires that this responsiveness at local levels operates within a firm national framework of evidence-based restrictions, laws, and sanctions.

Another approach to alcohol policy in federated jurisdictions (such as Australia, Canada, India, and the USA) is to delegate or share responsibility within a state-level framework. Alcohol policies and laws may be a matter for state governments, whereas alcohol taxation powers are retained at federal level. In the USA, for example, alcohol legislation is promulgated at the state level, with licensing controlled by Alcohol Beverage Control agencies. Local enforcement of controls on alcohol availability (shown by the extent of the budgets, the number of workers, and the citations issued) across different US states tends to be higher in states that have enacted formal laws and regulations controlling the marketplace, particularly with regard to price restrictions (Gruenewald *et al.* 1992).

National or state control and influence is paramount in the key alcohol policy area of taxation. Because of the relationship of the real price of alcohol with the levels of alcohol consumption and corresponding harms, taxation is central to alcohol policy (see Chapter 8). Taxation has a major influence on the real price of commercially produced alcohol in all jurisdictions. The alcohol industry is generally opposed to higher alcohol taxation levels because it is thought to affect sales revenues (Hawks 1990; Advocacy Institute 1992). However, in addition to reducing alcohol consumption and problems, alcohol taxation has the added benefit of providing an important revenue stream for both national and subnational governments, and it is relatively easy to collect. In industrialized countries such as the UK, governments obtain about 5% of their revenue from alcohol taxes (Raistrick *et al.* 1999). The proportion of alcohol tax revenue in some developing countries is even larger, as much as 20% (WHO 1999). In some countries (e.g. Botswana, New Zealand, Thailand), a hypothecated tax levy on alcohol sales is used to fund prevention and treatment programmes as well as the activities of NGOs.

15.3 Public interest groups

Public interest groups, often represented by NGOs, contribute to the policymaking process in many countries. Since the 1830s, **temperance societies** in the USA and other countries have been a major advocate for alcohol control policies, and they still contribute to the policy process in some countries (Sulkunen 1997). More recently, alcohol issues have increasingly become the concern of health professionals, mirrored by a change in the organization of health and welfare services as well as increasing professionalization in the 'caring' occupations (Raistrick *et al.* 1999). The public health policy developments in France in the 1980s, for example, were initiated by the efforts of a group of medical specialists, 'the five sages' (Craplet 1997), who employed traditional welfare state arguments (Sulkunen 1997). Professionals concerned with law and order have also played a role in the policymaking process in some countries (Baggott 1986).

In many nations there is a vacuum in advocacy for the public interest. It is difficult for state employees to engage in both political activity and policy advocacy, leaving members of NGOs to represent the public interest (Craplet 1997). These have occasionally involved interest groups representing victims of alcohol-related harm, Mothers Against Drunk Driving (MADD) being a notable example that originated in the USA (DeJong and Russell 1995). In recent years there has been a growth in NGOs taking an interest in alcohol policy in terms of both national and regional issues. The Global Alcohol Policy Alliance, for example, supports local NGOs in different countries in efforts to apply evidence-based measures to reduce alcohol-related harm.

Many alcohol policy approaches that have demonstrated evidence of effectiveness at the national or regional level require implementation at the community level. The community's readiness to support and encourage implementation may be increased by recognition that it is local communities that deal with much alcohol-related harm, such as injuries and deaths from crashes involving alcohol-impaired drivers. Hospital and emergency medical services, autopsies, and rehabilitation take place within communities. Alcohol problems are often personal experiences for community members who are motivated to take local action. Parent groups, for example, have been formed around a concern for underage drinking. Such groups can create public pressure against retail alcohol sales to underage persons and against access to alcohol at youth social events. The consequences of harmful drinking are experienced locally, meaning that communities can be a voice for advocacy in support of effective policies.

While it is relatively easy to introduce educational or informational campaigns locally, challenges are quick to emerge against the actual implementation of policies that are directed to law enforcement, drinking environments, access to alcohol, and regulation changes. Unless the citizens who support efforts to implement special policies are prepared for opposition, the enthusiasm and effectiveness of local groups can be reduced. Unfortunately, in some communities the prevailing local efforts are devoted to initiatives that have a high profile (e.g. providing free coffee to drivers on New Year's Eve) but little or no impact on alcohol-related problems. These programmes are popular and relatively uncontroversial, but may channel resources and public attention away from strategies with a much higher potential for impacting alcohol-related problems.

Another approach is to translate evidence-based strategies into local alcohol policies through community action projects that join local activists with public health professionals. Some of the earliest attempts to develop, implement, and evaluate local level strategies (Casswell and Gilmore 1989; Casswell et al. 1989; Casswell and Stewart 1989; Duignan et al. 1993) took place in New Zealand in the 1980s and 1990s following considerable liberalization of alcohol licensing laws (Stewart et al. 1993). Administration of licensing, monitoring and enforcement was delegated to the local level, while licensing decisions and appeals were retained at the national level. Community action projects conducted during this period assisted in the development of local partnerships, which included a public health perspective, as well as the increased compliance and responsible management of local licensed premises to reduce alcohol-related harm (Hill and Stewart 1996; Stewart et al. 1997). Despite some limitations, New Zealand's two-tier decision-making structure provided a model of increasing community control over alcohol outlets within a national level legislative framework. By contrast, alcohol licensing occurs entirely at the local level in many countries, so there is little national oversight. A disadvantage to the latter approach has been the absence of a clear framework of decision-making that takes into account health and safety issues. Licensing authorities vary in the extent to which they use their authority to prevent alcohol-related problems (Raistrick et al. 1999). Box 15.1 provides an example of research showing how community action can inform the policymaking process.

15.4 **Commercial interests**

As discussed in Chapter 5, alcohol is a commodity, and there are significant commercial interests involved in promoting its manufacture, distribution, pricing, and sale. Although the alcohol industry is not monolithic in terms of its motives, power, or operations, in many instances the industry's commercial imperative to make a profit for shareholders competes with public health interests. For example, the elimination of restrictions on hours of sale, often favoured by industry interests, can lead to an increase in alcohol consumption and related problems (Chapter 9). Media advertising and marketing in its many other forms is considered by health advocates to pose particular risk for vulnerable populations such as adolescents (see Chapter 12), but regulations on advertising are consistently opposed by the alcohol industry in favour of their own self-regulation approach. The introduction of new products and marketing schemes is considered a right of market access under international trade agreements, but some products, such as sweet-tasting alcoholic beverages variously called

---

Box 15.1 Community Trials Project: USA (1992–1996)

The Community Trials Project (Holder *et al.* 1997) was a five-component community-level intervention conducted in three experimental communities matched to three comparison communities selected for geographical and cultural diversity. The five interacting components included: (1) a 'Community Knowledge, Values, and Mobilization' component to develop community organization and support for the goals and strategies of the project; (2) a 'Responsible Beverage Service Practices' component to reduce the risk of intoxicated as well as underage customers in bars and restaurants; (3) a 'Reduction of Underage Drinking' component to reduce underage access; (4) a 'Risk of Drinking and Driving' component to increase enforcement of drink-driving; and (5) an 'Access to Alcohol' component to reduce overall availability of alcohol. The programme evaluation showed a statistically significant increase in coverage of alcohol issues in local newspapers and on local television in the experimental communities, a significant reduction in alcohol sales to minors, increased adoption of responsible alcohol serving policies, and a statistically significant reduction in alcohol-involved traffic crashes over the initial 28-month intervention period (see Voas *et al.* 1997), largely due to the introduction of special and highly visible drink-driving enforcement and support from increased news coverage.

'**alcopops**', 'coolers', 'malternatives', and premixed or 'designer' drinks, have been associated with heavier drinking by adolescents.

The relative scale of industry vested interests is illustrated by the situation in the UK, where the public expenditure on health education and the support of voluntary organizations in the alcohol field in 1984 represented less than 1% of the expenditure by the alcohol industry on advertising in the same year (Baggott 1986). The alcohol industry's combined wealth exceeds the gross national product of most non-industrialized countries, and its capacity to influence public policy is significant (Edwards 1998; Room 1998). In many countries, large sums of money are spent on marketing, thus making the advertising industry, the communications media, and even some parts of the sports industry interested in alcohol policies from a commercial perspective.

With these kinds of vested interests in alcohol policies, it is not surprising that the alcohol industry should be actively involved in the policy arena. Supported by free market values and concepts, the alcohol industry has become increasingly involved in the policymaking process in order to protect its commercial interests. In some countries, the industry is the dominant non-governmental presence at the policymaking table. A common claim among public health advocates is that industry representatives are influential in setting the policy agenda, shaping the perspectives of legislators on policy issues, and determining the outcome of policy debates (e.g. Hawks 1993; Baggott 1990; Babor 2004; Room 2004). As an example, in 1990, an attempt to increase the excise tax in California was successfully opposed by a media campaign funded by the alcohol industry costing in excess of US $30 million (Advocacy Institute 1992).

Similarly, excise taxation was opposed in Australia by industry interests during the drafting of a National Alcohol Policy (Hawks 1993). When France's Loi Évin introduced strong controls over sponsorship and advertising on television, in movies, and at sporting events, the alcohol industry opposed it both politically (Craplet 1997) and in the courts.

Another way that the large producers advance their policy interests is through philanthropic giving and corporate social responsibility activities (CSRs). By 2005, 13 out of 24 global alcohol corporations had CSR policies or social reports on their websites (Hill 2008). Some alcohol brand websites mention health risks as well as benefits of drinking and advocate responsible drinking as part of their CSRs. Because public relations activities aim to raise the profile and approval rating of a company or brand, CSRs may actually be an indirect form of marketing. SABMiller and Diageo reported funding responsible drinking campaigns aimed at teenagers and establishing partnerships on drink-driving with government and non-governmental agencies in both mature and emerging markets. The alcohol industry has widened its public relations repertoire beyond education, however, to branded disaster relief and the support of scientific research. Following Hurricane Katrina, Anheuser-Busch used branded beer cans to distribute water, and in Sri Lanka after the 2004 tsunami Carlsberg launched a new local beer by distributing water in branded bottles (IOGT International 2006). Despite the appearance of charitable giving, there is evidence that corporate philanthropy by some segments of the alcohol industry functions to support corporate marketing and lobbying activities that are inconsistent with the public health goals of effective alcohol control policy (Babor 2006; Jahiel and Babor 2007; Tesler and Malone 2008).

To promote their policy objectives, over the past 25 years the largest alcohol companies have set up more than 30 'social aspects' organizations, mostly in Europe, the USA, and more recently in the emerging markets of Asia and Africa (Anderson 2002, 2004; International Center for Alcohol Policies 2006). Figure 15.1 illustrates the growth in these organizations, which operate alongside more traditional (and more explicitly named) trade organizations representing the wider beer, spirits and wine industries. Social aspects organizations typically promote a set of key messages that align with industry interests (Anderson 2004), such as drinker responsibility, and support policies for harm reduction, typically those that will have least impact on total sales (Rae 1991; Sheldon 1996; McCreanor *et al.* 2000; Babor 2004; Room 2004). Social aspects organizations present a socially responsible face for the industry by involving themselves in campaigns against drink-driving or in support of alcohol education programmes for young people. One consequence of these prevention initiatives is that the industry perspective is present in the policy debates of many of the major producer and consumer nations (Hawks 1990; Casswell *et al.* 1993; Simpura 1995; Babor *et al.* 1996; Raistrick *et al.* 1999; Jernigan *et al.* 2000) as well as, increasingly, the emerging markets (Casswell and Thamarangsi 2009). For example, social aspects organizations and alcohol companies have sought to influence the policy process in a number of African countries by providing policy advice and by helping to draft national alcohol control strategies (Bakke 2009).

Organizations representing the hospitality and retail-trade sectors have similar interests on policy issues. The economic benefits from the night-time economy can

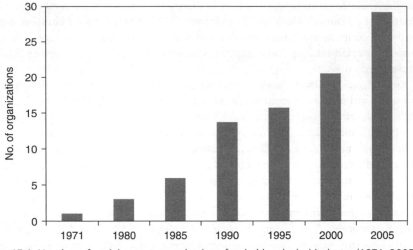

Fig. 15.1 Number of social aspect organizations funded by alcohol industry (1971–2005). Sources: Witheridge (2003), Anderson (2004), International Center for Alcohol Policies (2006), with permission.

deter successful policy setting and enforcement with regard to public drinking (Hobbs *et al.* 2000, 2003, 2005). The high sums spent by global producers on advertising and other marketing are vital to the alcohol retail sector and also to allies in industries such as advertising and broadcasting. The greater the concentration of ownership, the more likely that all these industry voices will align with the interests of the global companies. In summary, because of its vested interest, the alcohol industry has become a major player in the policy arena at both the national and international levels.

15.5 The mass media and public opinion

In many countries, public concern about alcohol-related problems only occasionally finds political expression. For example, concerns about drink-driving, drunken disorders in central cities, and the behaviour of intoxicated football supporters have periodically resulted in changes in public opinion about the need for a particular alcohol policy. In some countries there is public support for a number of effective alcohol policies, but more often the public is indifferent (Room *et al.* 1995b; Giesbrecht and Greenfield 1999; Giesbrecht and Kavanagh 1999). Rising popular concern reflects both a real increase in the rates of alcohol-related problems, and greater attention by the media and scientific community to alcohol-related issues. Unfortunately, the general public has relatively limited opportunities to influence alcohol policy in most countries. In Canada, for example, the general public is considerably more concerned and cautious about such issues as alcohol availability than those involved in the public discourse and political debate (Giesbrecht *et al.* 2001).

Because the mass media plays a dominant role in contemporary culture, it can have a significant influence on the policy debate at the national and local levels

(Milio 1988). Media coverage has an 'agenda-setting' function (McCombs and Shaw 1972; Erbring *et al.* 1980) by influencing whether policymakers perceive a problem as well as the importance they attach to it. For example, the media's coverage of alcohol issues in the UK has heightened interest in a series of governmental reports and has stimulated consideration of related parliamentary questions (Babor 2004, 2008a; Room 2004). The media further influence policy by framing the issue, defining the problem, and suggesting possible solutions. The media can also establish the credibility of commentators on current issues (Flora *et al.* 1989).

Although media coverage that brings attention to alcohol problems has a valuable place in the policy process, it is never sufficient. Campaigns such as an 'Alcohol Awareness Week' produce personally satisfying experiences for citizens and leaders, but there is no evidence that they have an impact on alcohol-related problems. Such programmes generate enthusiasm and public recognition, and may give the appearance that something is being done, without providing substantive and effective interventions.

The importance of the media in shaping the policy debate has led to an increasing use of media advocacy among public health advocates engaged in national and local policy debates (Wallack and Dorfman 1992; Chapman and Lupton 1994; Jernigan and Wright 1996). 'Media advocacy' refers to the strategic collaboration with the media to advance policy goals (Wallack 1990; Holder and Treno 1997). With regard to alcohol, one aim of media advocacy is to move public discourse from a focus on the individual person to an appreciation of the social, economic, and political influences on alcohol problems. Media advocacy is usually undertaken as a component of a multi-faceted community action initiative (Stewart and Casswell 1993) or in connection with regulatory changes, law enforcement, community mobilization, and monitoring of high-risk behaviour (Treno *et al.* 1996; Treno and Holder 1997; Holder and Treno 1997). As noted by Wallack and DeJong (1995), media advocacy is used to gain access to the media and to frame stories so that they focus on policy issues rather than on the unhealthy behaviour of individuals. By having newspaper or television reporters 'tell the story', alcohol policy supporters can avoid having to purchase media services for counter-advertising, and thus save valuable resources (Jernigan and Wright 1996). The results of the New Zealand Community Action Project (Stewart and Casswell 1993), for example, showed that media advocacy could produce a significant increase in media coverage of alcohol-related topics such as moderation in drinking and informed alcohol policy.

15.6 **The scientific community**

Policy debate increasingly relies on research findings to bolster a point of view (Moskalewicz 1993). However, there is no simple relationship between scientific findings and policymaking. Bruun's (1973) conclusion that research 'produces arguments rather than logical conclusions regarding policy and action' remains valid. Nevertheless, there has been exponential growth in scientific research on alcohol, with concomitant increases in articles published, specialized scientific journals and career scientists (Babor 1993; Babor *et al.* 2008b). Although biomedical research still takes precedence over alcohol policy research in many countries, there has also been significant growth in the policy area.

Researchers often provide the raw material for policy decisions, measuring trends in alcohol consumption and related harms by monitoring social indicator statistics and collecting social survey data. These data can play an important role in evaluating the need for alcohol policy. The absence of such data in Eastern Europe and most developing countries has made it difficult for public interest groups to challenge the view that alcohol should be treated as an ordinary commodity with no special controls on its marketing, price, or availability.

Researchers also play an important role evaluating the effectiveness of particular programmes or policies. For example, current knowledge of the effectiveness of brief interventions (Chapter 14) and alcohol taxation measures (Chapter 8), and of the general ineffectiveness of school-based alcohol education (Chapter 13), is based on the accumulation of evaluation studies in each of these areas.

One of the clearest examples of research contributing to an effective policy was the debate over random breath testing (RBT) legislation in New South Wales, Australia (Homel 1993). Research findings that suggested the effectiveness of RBT were disseminated widely in a context of high public concern over drink-driving statistics. Another policy initiative in which research played a key role was US federal and state legislation that raised the minimum alcohol purchasing age to 21 years, after it had been lowered in many states in the 1970s. The process of communicating key research findings to policymakers influenced the adoption of an effective policy (Wagenaar 1993), which was later confirmed by further research.

An important long-term contribution of research is to provide new ways of thinking about old issues. The broad perspective on 'alcohol-related problems' in which this book is written, for instance, can be seen as having first emerged in the course of epidemiological alcohol research (Room 1984b). The problem perspective eventually shifted the policy emphasis from a primary focus on **alcoholism** to a broader view that included harmful and hazardous drinking even in the absence of alcohol **dependence**. Research is not value-free, in the sense that the framing and choice of research topics inevitably reflects judgements and choices between competing priorities. However, investigators have a duty to be faithful to the research evidence, wherever it may lead. This inevitably means that the findings of researchers will sometimes conflict with conventional beliefs, commercial interests and fixed policy positions. In an applied field such as alcohol studies, scientific investigators should be attuned to the potential utility of their research. To be useful, research evidence must be simply communicated and given meaning in relation to current issues. To contribute constructively to policy debates, researchers need to ask policy-relevant research questions and generate the data to answer them (Bucuvalas and Weiss 1980). Such contributions may only be possible in the context of a long-term publicly funded research programme designed to engage members of the scientific community in each country in the collection, evaluation, and interpretation of research data that is relevant to a country's alcohol policy needs.

The need for an independent scientific community capable of contributing to the policy process is underscored by the increasing involvement of commercial interests in scientific research on alcohol, which has raised questions about the integrity of the science produced by such sponsorship (Stenius and Babor 2009). In one review of this issue (Babor 2008), the involvement of the alcohol industry in scientific research was identified in six areas: (i) sponsorship of research funding organizations; (ii) direct financing of research studies and university-based scientists and centres; (iii) research conducted by trade organizations and social aspects/public relations organizations; (iv) efforts to influence the public's and policymakers' perceptions of the implications of research findings for alcohol policies; (v) publication of scientific documents and support of scientific journals; and (vi) sponsorship of scientific conferences and presentations at conferences. While industry involvement in research activities is increasing, it presently constitutes a rather small direct investment that is unlikely to contribute to alcohol science, lead to scientific breakthroughs, or reduce the burden of alcohol-related illness. The industry's scientific activities can, however, confuse public discussion of health issues and policy options, and provide industry with a convenient way to demonstrate 'corporate responsibility' in its attempts to avoid taxation and regulation (Babor 2006; Tesler and Malone 2008). For these reasons alcohol scientists have become increasingly sceptical about accepting industry funding for their research (Casswell 2009; Miller *et al.* 2009; Stenius and Babor 2009).

15.7 **Conclusion**

Within each jurisdiction of the policy arena, there are parallel and competing processes as different interest groups attempt to influence the outcome. Groups involved in for-profit alcohol production and sales are increasingly becoming key players in policy debates. The media also play an important role, and those who communicate research findings are often drawn into the policy arena. Addiction professionals and non-governmental organizations are major voices on behalf of the public interest in many jurisdictions.

An appreciation of the various players in the alcohol policy arena can heighten our understanding of the following fundamental conclusion: alcohol policy is often the product of competing interests, values, and ideologies. Alcohol is like any other commodity in that it is a product that is exchanged for economic or social capital. However, it is not an ordinary commodity because it also requires an extraordinary amount of public policy attention in the form of regulation, taxation, and human services to address the damage it causes. As this chapter has suggested, industry interests diverge considerably from those of public health professionals and NGOs (Anderson and Baumberg 2006b). Experience suggests that working in partnership with the alcohol industry is likely to lead to ineffective or compromised policy by both government and NGOs (Room 2004; Munro 2004; Caetano and Laranjeira 2005; Anderson 2007).

The process of alcohol policy creation, in each country and internationally, needs to be better understood and made more transparent. It needs to be more responsive to the needs of the citizens who are the end-consumers of emerging policies. Too much of the action in the alcohol arena is conducted behind the scenes, and subject to political considerations or vested interests. Uninformed by science, and insufficiently monitored in its outcomes, alcohol policy is often neither evidence-based nor effective. If alcohol-related problems are to be minimized, mechanisms are needed at the international, national, and local levels to ensure that alcohol policies serve the public good.

Chapter 16

Alcohol policies: a consumer's guide

16.1 Introduction

The preceding chapters have provided detailed reviews of the relevant science base for a comprehensive consideration of how alcohol policy can better serve the public good. We will now try to make explicit the connection between the research and the practical needs of the policymaker who wants to implement evidence-based responses to the problems within society caused or exacerbated by alcohol. Our intention is to make science useful at the real-world front lines of policy. The difference between good and bad alcohol policy is not an abstraction, but very often a matter of life and death. We believe that it is right to ask for the science to be taken seriously. Research has the capacity to indicate which strategies are likely to succeed in their public health intentions, and which are likely to be less effective or even useless, diversionary, and a waste of resources. In this concluding chapter the evidence supporting the various strategies and interventions reviewed in earlier parts of the book is summarized.

16.2 Choosing effective strategies

With an ever-expanding research output, the need increases for a systematic procedure to evaluate the evidence, compare alternative interventions, and assess the benefits to society of different approaches. To that end, several attempts have been made in the addiction field to synthesize information from a wide variety of perspectives, using consensus panels, expert committee ratings, and objective decision models (Coffield *et al.* 2001; Shults *et al.* 2001; Karlsson and Österberg 2001; Babor and Caetano 2005; Stockwell *et al.* 2005; Anderson *et al.* 2009).

Building on previous work in this area, the authors developed a relatively simple method to synthesize the results of our review. Table 16.1 provides ratings for each of the forty-two strategies and interventions reviewed in Chapters 8–14. The ratings reflect the consensus views of the authors and are designed to serve as a guide for those who would like to evaluate the strengths and weaknesses of different policy options. The table is organized according to three major criteria: (i) evidence of effectiveness; (ii) amount of research support; and (iii) extent of testing across diverse countries and cultures.

16.2.1 Effectiveness

'Effectiveness' refers to the likely effectiveness of the intervention, reflecting the strength of scientific evidence establishing whether a particular strategy is effective in reducing alcohol consumption and/or alcohol-related problems. In some cases, an intervention may have the objective of changing an intermediate outcome, such as a young person's knowledge or attitudes about drinking, or preventing alcohol sales to young persons. Although we will document these outcomes, our focus remains on consumption and harm. In addition, these ratings generally reflect the consistency of findings rather than the size of the effect. We are concerned with the overall conclusion that a reasonable person can draw based on the quality of research and the consistency of the effect under both idealized research conditions (efficacy studies) and real-world settings (effectiveness studies, including 'natural experiments'). To be considered in this compendium, strategies had to be carefully investigated in at least one well-designed study, which was able to account for alternative and competing explanations. Only studies that met minimum scientific standards were used in these evaluations. Particular attention was given to the rules of evidence (Chapter 7) and the studies cited in Chapters 8–14. The following rating scale was used:

0	Evidence indicates a lack of effectiveness.
+	Evidence for limited effectiveness.
++	Evidence for moderate effectiveness.
+++	Evidence for a high degree of effectiveness.
?	No controlled studies have been undertaken or there is insufficient evidence upon which to make a judgement.

16.2.2 Breadth of research support

'Breadth of research support' goes beyond the quality of the science to look at the quantity and consistency of the available evidence, including conflicting evidence. Ratings were influenced by the conclusions of integrative reviews and meta-analyses. Here we are concerned with the number of scientific studies and the consistency of the results, whereas the effectiveness criterion is concerned with the direction of the evidence independent of the number of studies undertaken. The highest rating was influenced by the availability of integrative reviews and meta-analyses by experts in their respective fields of study. Breadth of research support was evaluated independent of the effectiveness rating (i.e. it is possible for a strategy to be rated low in effectiveness but to also have a high rating on the breadth of research support). We used the following scale:

0	No studies of effectiveness have been undertaken.
+	One or two well-designed effectiveness studies completed.
++	Several effectiveness studies have been completed, sometimes in different countries, but no integrative reviews were available.

+++ Enough studies of effectiveness have been completed to permit integrative literature reviews or meta-analyses.

16.2.3 Cross-national testing

'Cross-national testing' means that the evidence for a particular intervention was drawn from studies conducted in different countries, regions, subgroups, and social classes. In evaluating the evidence, we were particularly interested in the extent to which interventions developed for, and evaluated in, the established market economies can be transferred to developing societies. This criterion is thus concerned primarily with the diversity of geography and cultures within which each strategy has been applied and tested. It refers to the robustness of international or multi-national testing of a strategy as well as the extent to which a strategy applies to multiple countries and cultures. The following scale was used:

0 The strategy has been studied in only one country.

+ The strategy has been studied in at least two countries.

++ The strategy has been studied in several countries.

+++ The strategy has been studied in many countries.

16.2.4 Other considerations

Other policy-relevant considerations that are reported in the Comments section of the table include population reach, the target group for the intervention, feasibility, adverse side effects, and cost to implement and sustain.

The population reach refers to the number of people in the target group that can be served when an intervention is provided under real-world conditions. Target group refers to the population most likely to be affected by the strategy: 1) the general population of drinkers, 2) high-risk drinkers or groups considered to be particularly vulnerable to the adverse effects of alcohol (e.g., adolescents), and 3) persons already manifesting harmful drinking and alcohol dependence. Feasibility reflects the intervention's likelihood of being translated into effective policies. Feasibility can be assessed in terms of political considerations (leadership, opposition from industry, public support), economic implications (cost effectiveness and cost-benefit analysis), and the presence or absence of reactive effects, such as the increased use of informal market or illegal imports that may occur in response to high taxation. Adverse side effects include the tendency for some interventions to stimulate criminal activity such as tax evasion or illicit production of alcohol.

Cost to implement and sustain refers to the relative monetary cost to the state to implement, operate, and sustain a strategy, regardless of its effectiveness. Cost estimates can only be very rough guides to policymakers because the true costs of the strategy or intervention for the state may depend on a number of factors. For example, the initial costs of implementing a training program with licensed premises may be moderate for the state but ultimately these costs may be eliminated by passing them on to the consumer. Enhanced enforcement by police and regulatory authorities may involve substantial costs, but for effective programs these costs may be offset entirely by cost savings in health services due to the reduction in problems (e.g., Levy and Miller 1995).

True costs of an intervention will depend on the availability of existing resources and the size of the target population, among other things. In general, individual services are likely to be more costly to the state than policy measures that change the availability or price of alcohol for the entire population, but the effectiveness of these aggregate-level interventions may depend on enforcement and other costly resources. Although cost-oriented evaluations have been conducted in some areas of alcohol policy, the results differ by country and according to the intervention. For these reasons we have chosen not to rate the interventions presented in Table 16.1 according to their costs, cost-effectiveness, or cost benefits to society. Nevertheless, later in this chapter we do summarize the results of an extensive international study that illustrates the potential cost-effectiveness of several of the most popular policy options listed in Table 16.1.

16.3 Policy options considered

The left-hand column of Table 16.1 lists the wide array of possible policy choices that were reviewed in Chapters 8–14. Each strategy has at some point in the past been employed as an instrument of alcohol policy in some part of the world. The extensiveness of the list (forty-two options) shows that the policy solutions developed to deal with alcohol are not only numerous but are also extraordinarily diverse, ranging from individual therapeutic services to community and population level interventions designed to influence the affordability, availability and accessibility of alcohol. If two or more pluses on each of the three evaluation criteria (effectiveness, amount of research support, and cross-national testing) can be considered an indication of a consistently good performance, then nineteen options appear to be particularly good choices. In the following sections each of the major approaches to alcohol policy is discussed in terms of the ratings presented in Table 16.1.

16.3.1 The strong strategies: restrictions on affordability, availability, and accessibility, as well as drink-driving deterrence measures

Of all the policy options, alcohol taxes is rated as one of the strongest. Population reach is good as well. This may surprise many policymakers, but the research is extensive and the findings are convincing. As described in Chapter 8, increasing alcohol taxes not only reduces alcohol consumption and related harm but it also provides revenue to the state. Another advantage of pricing policies is that heavier drinkers appear to be as responsive to price as lighter drinkers, and these policies are effective with younger drinkers as well as with adults. One disadvantage of pricing policies is that the informal or illicit market for alcohol in some countries can complicate policy in this area by shifting consumption to less expensive and possibly more hazardous beverages. Under these circumstances, concomitant measures are needed to bring the informal and illicit market under government control.

Table 16.1 Ratings of policy-relevant strategies and interventions

Strategy or intervention	Effectiveness	Breadth of research support	Cross-national testing	Comments
Pricing and taxation				
Alcohol taxes	+++	+++	+++	Generally evaluated in terms of how price changes affect population-level alcohol consumption, alcohol-related problems and beverage preferences.
				Increased taxes reduce alcohol consumption and harm. Effectiveness depends on government oversight and control of the total alcohol supply.
Minimum price	?	+	0	Logic based on price theory, but there is very little evidence of effectiveness. Competition regulations and trade policies may restrict implementation unless achieved via taxation policy.
Bans on price discounts and promotions	?	+	0	Only weak studies in general populations of the effect of restrictions on consumption or harm; effectiveness depends on availability of alternative forms of cheap alcohol.
Differential price by beverage	+	+	+	Higher prices for distilled spirits shifts consumption to lower-alcohol content beverages resulting in less overall consumption. Evidence for the impact of tax breaks on low-alcohol products is suggestive.
Special or additional taxation on alcopops and youth-oriented beverages	+	+	+	Evidence that higher prices reduce consumption of alcopops by young drinkers without complete substitution; no studies of impact on harms.
Regulating physical availability				
				Generally evaluated in terms of how changes in availability affect population-level alcohol consumption and alcohol-related problems.
Ban on sales	+++	+++	++	Can reduce consumption and harm substantially, but often with adverse side-effects from black market, which is expensive to suppress. Ineffective without enforcement.
Bans on drinking in public places	?	+	+	Affects young or marginalized high-risk drinkers; may displace harm without necessarily reducing it.

(continued)

Table 16.1 (Continued) Ratings of policy-relevant strategies and interventions

Strategy or intervention	Effectiveness	Breadth of research support	Cross-national testing	Comments
Minimum legal purchase age	+++	+++	++	Effective in reducing traffic fatalities and other harms with minimal enforcement but enforcement substantially increases effectiveness and cost.
Rationing	++	++	++	Effects greater on heavy drinkers.
Government monopoly of retail sales	++	+++	++	Effective way to limit alcohol consumption and harm. Public health and public order goals by government monopolies increase beneficial effects.
Hours and days of sale restrictions	++	++	+++	Effective where changes in trading hours meaningfully reduce alcohol availability or where problems such as late-night violence are specifically related to hours of sale.
Restrictions on density of outlets	++	+++	++	Evidence for both consumption and problems. Changes to outlet numbers affect availability most in areas with low prior availability, but bunching of outlets into high-density entertainment districts may cause problems with public order and violence.
Different availability by alcohol strength	++	++	++	Mostly tested in terms of different strengths of beer and for broadened availability of wine.
Modifying the drinking environment				
Staff training and house policies relating to responsible beverage service (RBS)	0/+	+++	++	Generally evaluated in terms of how staff training, enforcement, and legal liability affect alcohol-related violence and other harms. Not all studies have found a significant effect of RBS training and house policies; needs to be backed by enforcement for sustained effects.
Staff and management training to better manage aggression	++	+	++	Evidence currently limited to one randomized controlled study and supportive results from multi-component programmes. Evidence is available from Australia, Canada, and Sweden.

Policy option				Comments
Enhanced enforcement of on-premises laws and legal requirements	++	++	++	Sustained effects depend on making enhanced enforcement part of ongoing police practices.
Server liability	++	++	+	Effect stronger where efforts made to publicize liability. Research limited to USA and Canada.
Voluntary codes of bar practice	0	+	+	Ineffective when strictly voluntary but may contribute to effects as part of community action projects.
Late-night lockouts of licensed premises	?	+	0	Limited research, and no studies have identified effective approaches.
Drink-driving countermeasures				Most research has focused on intervention effects on traffic accidents and recidivism after criminal sanctions.
Sobriety check points	++	+++	+++	Effects of police campaigns typically short term. Effectiveness as a deterrent is proportional to frequency of implementation and high visibility.
Random breath testing	+++	++	++	Effectiveness depends on number of drivers directly affected and the extent of consistent and high profile enforcement.
Lowered BAC limits	+++	+++	+++	The lower the BAC legal limit, the more effective the policy. Very low BAC levels ('zero tolerance') are effective for youth, and can be effective for adult drivers, but BAC limits <0.02 are difficult to enforce.
Administrative licence suspension	++	++	++	When punishment is swift, effectiveness is increased. Effective in countries where it is applied consistently.
Low BAC for young drivers ('zero tolerance')	+++	++	++	Clear evidence of effectiveness for those below the legal drinking or alcohol purchase age.

(continued)

Table 16.1 (Continued) Ratings of policy-relevant strategies and interventions

Strategy or intervention	Effectiveness	Breadth of research support	Cross-national testing	Comments
Graduated licensing for novice drivers	++	++	++	Can be used to incorporate lower BAC limits and licensing restrictions within one strategy. Some studies note that 'zero tolerance' provisions are responsible for this effect.
Designated drivers and ride services	0	+	+	May be effective in getting impaired drinkers not to drive, but can also encourage passengers to drink more. Does not affect alcohol-related crashes.
Severity of punishment	0/+	++	++	Mixed evidence concerning mandatory or tougher sanctions for drink-driving convictions. Effects decay over time unless accompanied by renewed enforcement or media publicity.
Restrictions on marketing				Draws on two separate literatures: effects of advertising and promotion on youth drinking and attitudes, and effects of initiating or removing advertising bans and other interventions.
Legal restrictions on exposure	+/++	+++	++	Strong evidence of dose-response effect of exposure on young people's drinking, but evidence of small or insignificant effects on per-capita consumption from partial advertising bans; advertising bans or restrictions may shift marketing activities into less-regulated media (e.g. Internet).
Legal restrictions on content	?	0	0	Evidence that advertising content affects consumption but no evidence of the impact of content restrictions as embodied in industry self-regulation codes.
Alcohol industry's voluntary self-regulation codes	0	++	++	Industry voluntary self-regulation codes of practice are ineffective in limiting exposure of young persons to alcohol marketing, nor do they prevent objectionable content from being aired.
Education and persuasion				Impact generally evaluated in terms of knowledge and attitudes; effect on onset of drinking and drinking problems is equivocal or minimal. Target population is young drinkers unless otherwise noted.

Classroom education	0	+++	++	May increase knowledge and change attitudes but has no long-term effect on drinking.
College student normative education and multicomponent programmes	+	+++	0	Individualized multi-component approaches that include feedback on norms, expectancies, motives, or decisional balance have short-term effects on consumption and problems. Programmes usually targeted heavy drinkers and thus may overlap with brief interventions targeted at high risk drinkers. Purely informational approaches may increase knowledge and change attitudes, but have no effect on drinking.
Brief interventions with high-risk students	+	+	0	Brief motivational interventions can impact drinking behaviour.
Mass media campaigns, including drink-driving campaigns	0	+++	++	No evidence of impact of messages to the drinker about limiting drinking; some evidence of increased effectiveness of random breath testing when media publicize it.
Warning labels and signs	0	+	0	Raise public awareness, but do not change drinking behaviour.
Social marketing	0	++	0	Raises public awareness but alcohol-specific campaigns do not change behaviour.
Treatment and early intervention				Usually evaluated in terms of days or months of abstinence, reduced intensity and volume of drinking, and improvements in health and life functioning. Target population is harmful and dependent drinkers, unless otherwise noted.
Brief intervention with at-risk drinkers	+++	+++	+++	Can be effective but most primary care practitioners lack training and time to conduct screening and brief interventions.
Mutual help/self-help attendance	++	++	++	A feasible, cost-effective complement or alternative to formal treatment in many countries.
Mandatory treatment of drink-driving repeat offenders	+	++	0	Punitive and coercive approaches have time-limited effects, and sometimes distract attention from more effective interventions.

(continued)

Table 16.1 (Continued) Ratings of policy-relevant strategies and interventions

Strategy or intervention	Effectiveness	Breadth of research support	Cross-national testing	Comments
Medical and social detoxification	+++	++	++	Safe and effective for treating withdrawal symptoms. Reduces alcohol-related harms through prevention of mortality. Little effect on long-term alcohol consumption unless combined with other therapies.
Talk therapies	++	+++	++	A variety of theoretically based therapies to treat persons with alcohol dependence in outpatient and residential settings. Population reach is low because most countries have limited treatment facilities.
Pharmaceutical therapies	+	++	++	Consistent evidence for a modest improvement over talk therapies and clinical management only for naltrexone.

BAC, blood alcohol concentration.

Possible strategies include enforcement of bans against illicit production and use of tax stamps to verify that appropriate duties have been paid. Nevertheless, given the broad reach of pricing and taxation strategies, and the relatively low expense of implementing them, the expected impact of these measures on public health is relatively high.

In addition to alcohol taxes, the evidence is strong for the regulation of physical availability designed to prevent easy access to alcohol. Availability theory suggests that alcohol consumption and related problems increase when alcohol becomes more accessible and convenient to use (see Chapter 9). By restricting hours, days, and locations of sale, as well as the density or concentration of on-premises and retail drinking establishments, policymakers can reduce overall exposure to alcohol's intoxicating and toxic effects, and thereby reduce alcohol-related problems. Total bans on all alcoholic beverages have been attempted in various countries at different times with varying degrees of effectiveness, and they are still used in countries with large Muslim populations and in communities with large indigenous populations. However, partial bans on the sale or use of alcohol in particular circumstances (e.g. operating machinery), locations (e.g. parks), or population groups (e.g. young persons below a certain age) are more typical of the availability restrictions employed in most countries. Government monopolies on alcohol production and sales provide an effective way to control availability if public health objectives rather than revenue maximization are the primary rationale for the system. In the absence of a monopoly, licensing systems have been used to control availability through regulation and sanctions (e.g. license revocation). A strategy employed in almost all nations to control access to alcohol by adolescents is the enforcement of age restrictions for the purchase of alcohol. Where age restrictions can be enforced consistently, and the legal purchase age is set later in the period of greatest exposure risk (e.g. age 21 years), research in the USA has demonstrated significant reductions in drink-driving casualties and other alcohol-related harms. Availability theory suggests that the greater the restriction on youth access to alcohol, the less harm will be likely to occur.

Many countries have inadvertently influenced the availability of alcohol in their populations through economic policies such as those encouraging development of the late-night economy in urban areas. The research shows that the density of drinking outlets is correlated with the prevalence of alcohol-related problems, and therefore restrictions on density may be an effective antidote to intoxication, injuries and violence because they reduce the attractiveness and convenience of heavy drinking.

Beyond alcohol taxes and availability restrictions, Table 16.1 shows that most drink-driving countermeasures also received high ratings on effectiveness. Not only is there good research support for these programmes but they also seem to be applicable in most countries and are relatively inexpensive to implement and sustain. As a general principle, drink-driving countermeasures that increase the certainty and visibility of enforcement (e.g. random breath testing) as well as the rapidity of sanctions (e.g. administrative licence suspension), are effective ways to prevent alcohol-related automobile casualties.

16.3.2 Alcohol marketing restrictions

Although prior research using econometric methods provided only limited support for restrictions on youth exposure to alcohol marketing, more recent studies, reviewed in Chapter 12, have demonstrated that exposure to marketing practices can affect early initiation of alcohol use as well as riskier drinking patterns. There is less evidence to show that the imposition of a ban will reduce consumption or prevent the onset of hazardous drinking in young persons; however, such bans are rarely imposed, enforced, or studied systematically. Nevertheless, the weight of evidence suggests that a total ban on the full range of marketing practices could have a modest effect on drinking by young people. On the other hand, there is no evidence that voluntary self-regulation codes, the alcohol industry's favoured alternative to alcohol marketing bans, have been successful in protecting vulnerable populations from exposure to alcohol advertising and other youth-oriented marketing practices.

16.3.3 Treatment and early intervention services

Treatment and early intervention services have been, in many countries, the first line of response to alcohol-related problems, under the assumption that if those who develop alcohol dependence could be helped to stop drinking, there would be a significant reduction in alcohol-related problems in society. From the literature reviewed in Chapter 14, it was shown that alcohol treatment services have good evidence of effectiveness, but most treatment options are expensive to implement and maintain, with the exception of mutual help organizations. At the population level, their impact is limited relative to other policy options, since full treatment for alcohol problems can only benefit the small fraction of the population who come to treatment. Even brief interventions, which have good evidence for effectiveness, are restricted to those who use the services within which brief interventions are offered. Whereas providing treatment is an obligation of a humane society, its effect on the actual drinking problem rates of the population at large is necessarily limited.

16.3.4 Altering the drinking context

The amount of evidence on the effects of altering the drinking context has been growing, leading to the conclusion that strategies in this area have modest effects. The fact that these strategies are primarily applicable to on-premises drinking in bars and restaurants somewhat limits their public health significance. Although drinking in licensed premises is associated with high risk of problems, only a minority of drinking is done on licensed premises in most developed countries. One recurring theme in this literature is the importance of enforcement to the success of strategies that alter the context of drinking. This theme also applies to strategies regulating physical availability. Passing a minimum purchasing age law, for instance, will have less effect than if it is reinforced with a credible threat to suspend or cancel the licenses of outlets that repeatedly sell to minors. Likewise, training in responsible beverage service is unlikely to have an effect unless it is backed by a threat to suspend the licenses of those establishments that continue to serve already intoxicated patrons.

Monitoring and enforcement as a condition of licensing have some costs, of course, but the governmental costs are frequently defrayed by such means as license fees on bars and restaurants.

16.3.5 Less effective measures: education and public service messages

The expected impact is low for education and for public service messages about drinking. Despite a growing amount of research using randomized controlled research designs (see Chapter 13), there is only weak evidence for the effectiveness of programmes that combine alcohol education with more intensive family and community involvement. Education strategies also have a moderate to high cost due to the expense of training and implementation for a full education programme. From the viewpoint of a state or local government, the costs may be lower than this because the teaching costs are part of the education budget, or may be paid by a different level of government, or because the education programme is viewed as a low-cost add-on to existing commitments. But in terms of impact or value-for-money, the cost hardly matters: education strategies have shown little or no effect, regardless of the investment. Although the reach of school-based educational programmes is thought to be excellent (because of the availability of captive audiences in schools), the population impact of these programmes in reducing harm is poor. Similarly, while feasibility is good, cost-effectiveness and cost-benefit are poor.

16.4 Enhancing the likelihood of effectiveness

Alcohol policies rarely operate independently or in isolation from other measures, as might be implied by the listing of individual strategies in Table 16.1. Policy options are often moulded to existing conditions and are typically implemented over time in a way that is fragmented, piecemeal, and not co-ordinated, in part because of the range of policy areas covered. As noted in Chapter 15, different ministries, departments, and administrative agencies each have some aspect of alcohol policy under their purview. As a result, most countries do not have a single comprehensive policy toward alcohol but rather dozens of policies that sometimes involve profoundly different assumptions about the role of alcohol in society and the nature of alcohol-related problems. To enhance the likelihood of effectiveness, alcohol policies would benefit from greater integration and co-ordination.

Research on local prevention efforts suggests that alcohol problems are best considered in terms of the community systems that produce them. Local strategies have great potential to be effective when prior scientific evidence is used and multiple policies are implemented in a systematic way. Thus, a complementary system of strategies that seek to restructure the total drinking environment is more likely to be effective than single strategies. Finally, prevention strategies with a natural capacity for long-term institutionalization should be favoured over those that are only in place for the life of a project. This line of reasoning suggests that full-spectrum interventions are needed to achieve the greatest population impact.

16.5 Cost and cost-effectiveness of alcohol policies

Harmful alcohol use has enormous social as well as medical costs in many countries, as described in Chapters 3 and 4. Based on an earlier analysis prepared for the World Health Organization (WHO), Anderson *et al.* (2009) used economic modelling procedures to estimate the cost and cost-effectiveness of seven of the interventions reviewed in Chapters 8–14: school-based education, brief interventions for heavy drinkers, mass media campaigns, enforcement of random breath testing, reduced access to retail outlets, a comprehensive advertising ban, and four levels of tax pricing policies. Population-level costs to implement the interventions included legislation, enforcement, administration, training, and service provision (in the case of treatment). The health benefits of the interventions were expressed in **disability-adjusted life-years** (DALYs) saved, relative to a hypothetical situation of no alcohol control measures in the population. In addition, non-health effects of the measures, such as reduced property damage and increased work productivity, were added to the model. The findings, presented in Table 16.2, are provided for three regions defined by the World Health Organization (WHO): the Americas (e.g. Brazil and Mexico), Eastern Europe (e.g. Russia, Ukraine), and the Western Pacific (e.g. China and Vietnam). The following points summarize the findings:

1) Two strategies (school-based education and mass-media awareness campaigns) were found not to be cost-effective because they do not affect alcohol consumption or health outcomes.

2) Population-level alcohol policies (e.g. pricing and availability policies) are more cost-effective than individual-level policies, such as brief interventions for hazardous alcohol use.

3) Tax increases represent a highly cost-effective response in regions with a high prevalence of heavy drinking, such as Latin America and Eastern Europe.

4) In countries with high levels of unrecorded production and consumption, increasing the proportion of consumption that is taxed could be more effective than a simple increase in excise taxes.

5) The impact of reducing access to retail outlets for specified periods of the week and implementing a comprehensive advertising ban have the potential to be cost-effective countermeasures, but only if they are fully enforced.

16.6 Policy independent of commercial interests

Chapter 5 described the growth of the alcohol industry in terms of its economic concentration among the large producers, its global reach across the world's major economies, and its use of new product designs and sophisticated marketing techniques to recruit new drinkers. As noted in Chapter 15, the industry and its front organizations also play an increasingly influential role in the policymaking process, promoting an approach that includes 'partnerships' with public health professionals, government agencies, and the scientific community. Two major industry objectives

Table 16.2 Cost and cost-effectiveness of interventions relating to different target areas for alcohol public health policy

	Coverage	Americas (e.g. Brazil, Mexico)		Europe (e.g. Russia, Ukraine)		Western Pacific (e.g. China, Vietnam)	
		Yearly cost per head (I$)[a]	Cost per DALY saved (I$)[b]	Yearly cost per head (I$)[a]	Cost per DALY saved (I$)[b]	Yearly cost per head (I$)[a]	Cost per DALY saved (I$)[b]
School-based education	80%	0.29	NA[c]	0.34	NA[c]	0.53	NA[c]
Brief interventions for heavy drinkers	30%	1.04	3870	1.78	2671	0.42	2016
Mass media coverage	80%	0.31	NA[c]	0.79	NA[c]	0.19	NA[c]
Drink-driving legislation and enforcement (via random breath-testing campaigns)	80%	0.44	924	0.72	781	0.24	1262
Reduced access to retail outlets	80%	0.24	515	0.47	567	0.16	1307
Comprehensive advertising ban	95%	0.24	931	0.47	961	0.16	955
Increased excise taxation (by 20%)	95%	0.34	277	0.67	380	0.20	1358
Increased excise taxation (by 50%)	95%	0.34	241	0.67	335	0.20	1150
Tax enforcement (20% less unrecorded)	95%	0.56	468	0.87	498	0.37	2603
Tax enforcement (50% less unrecorded)	95%	0.63	476	0.93	480	0.43	2733

[a] Implementation cost in 2005 international dollars (I$).

[b] Cost-effectiveness ratio, expressed in international dollars per disability-adjusted life-year (DALY) saved for the year 2005.

[c] Not applicable (NA) because effect size not significantly different from zero (cost-effectiveness ratio would therefore approach infinity).

Source: Anderson et al. (2009), with permission.

are to keep alcohol taxation as low as possible and to avoid government regulation of marketing and other activities.

There are opportunities for the industry to demonstrate an ethical responsibility to minimize the harm caused by its products at all stages of the production chain, including product design and marketing (Stenius and Babor 2009). However, there is often a conflict between this aim and the need to generate profit for the industry's stockholders. For these reasons, a WHO Expert Committee has spelled out an appropriate role for the alcohol industry that applies to governments as well as the WHO. The WHO Expert Committee on Problems Related to Alcohol Consumption (2007, p. 48) recommended

> . . . that WHO continue its practice of no collaboration with the various sectors of the alcohol industry. Any interaction should be confined to discussion of the contribution the alcohol industry can make to the reduction of alcohol-related harm only in the context of their roles as producers, distributors and marketers of alcohol, and not in terms of alcohol policy development or health promotion.

This implies that the most appropriate role of the industry would be to support evidence-based policies that minimize alcohol-related problems, regardless of their impact on alcohol consumption and alcohol sales, and that governments and the WHO engage in policymaking activities in ways that maintain their independence from the alcohol industry.

16.7 The need to make science more accessible to policymakers

Because alcohol availability and control occur in a complex cultural, social, and political environment, policy changes should be made with caution and with a sense of experimentation to determine whether they have their intended effects. The knowledge needed to address health and social problems is unlikely to reside in a single discipline or research methodology. Interdisciplinary research is capable of playing a critical role in the progress of public health by applying the methodologies of the medical, behavioural, social, and population sciences to an understanding of alcohol-related problems and their prevention.

Policymakers have neither the time nor the training to read, digest, and base their decisions upon the research findings reported in the scientific literature. Responsibility for translating scientific research into effective policy is distributed across a wide variety of government agencies and public interest groups. As described in Chapter 15, this process rarely follows a rational plan of action. In one analysis of alcohol policy implementation in North and South America (Babor and Caetano 2005), there were large variations among the 27 nations studied in the extent to which evidence-based alcohol policies are implemented and enforced. If the public's health is to be served, it will be necessary to strengthen the links between science and policy through an innovative strategy in which promising research findings are identified, synthesized, and communicated effectively to both the policymakers and the public. In this book we have tried to illustrate such an approach by identifying the critical health needs in the alcohol field, describing the principal factors responsible for alcohol problems, integrating the disparate findings that point to causal mechanisms, identifying what is known (and unknown) about the prevention and management of alcohol-related problems, and describing critical barriers to effective public health policy. We do not claim this text to be the final and exemplary model of its kind, but we do believe that it shows how science can be made more useful in this arena.

Alcohol policies will, of course, always be based on more than pure science. They are likely to arise from a combination of political expediency, commercial interests, common sense, and concerns for public safety, public order, and public health. But that realization should not discourage governments from giving much closer attention to ways in which the scientific asset can be intelligently used.

16.8 The 'precautionary principle'

The 'precautionary principle' is a general public health concept that we believe should be put to use in the alcohol policy arena (Kriebel and Tickner 2001). The main tenets of this principle are to take preventive action even in the face of uncertainty, to shift the burden of proof to the proponents of a potentially harmful activity, to offer alternatives to harmful actions, and to increase public involvement in decision-making.

When applied to alcohol policy, the precautionary principle implies that decision-making in areas such as international trade agreements, the introduction of new alcohol products, the removal of restrictions on hours of sale, and the promotion of alcohol through advertising, should be guided by the likelihood of risk, rather than the potential for profit. The application of the precautionary principle to alcohol policy will help to increase both public participation in the policymaking process and the transparency of decision-making, currently guided too often by the economic considerations of the few rather than the public health concerns of the many.

16.9 Alcohol policy and alcohol science in low- and middle-income countries

This book is largely based on research conducted in the mature alcohol markets of high-income countries. Although the burden of illness attributable to alcohol is smaller in most regions with emerging markets for alcohol, it nonetheless accounts for a considerable amount of premature death and disability, especially in Latin America (see Chapter 4 and Room *et al.* 2002). Relatively low levels of aggregate consumption reflect higher levels of abstention and, among drinkers, a pattern of heavy occasion consumption in many developing nations is associated with injuries and other acute alcohol problems. This places a heavy burden on the limited resources available to protect health, welfare, and public safety. The findings suggest that as economic development occurs, alcohol consumption is likely to increase with rising incomes, increased availability, and alcohol marketing. This process confronts these nations with greater levels of alcohol-related problems and new challenges to fashion effective alcohol policies. Global and regional trade agreements are also likely to have an adverse influence on developing nations. With the growing emphasis on free trade and market access, international institutions such as the World Trade Organization have pushed to dismantle effective alcohol control measures, including state alcohol monopolies and other restrictions on the supply of alcoholic beverages. Despite the relative weaknesses in the alcohol policy research base in many such countries, the strategies recommended by the analysis offered in this book are applicable with due modification (Room *et al.* 2002).

Countries with growing economies, especially those providing expanding markets for alcohol, need individual assessments of their own alcohol policy experiences and their own alcohol science. The scarcity of indigenous health science is a general handicap affecting policy formulation in low-income countries, and it goes beyond the alcohol arena. The world research community, in partnership with international agencies, has a special responsibility to rectify this situation.

16.10 **Extraordinary opportunities**

On the basis of the evidence arrayed in this book, extraordinary opportunities exist to strengthen the policy response to alcohol-related problems. The following considerations support this conclusion:

◆ *Multiple opportunities.* The policy options listed in the left-hand column of Table 16.1 speak to the wide range of available strategies from which policymakers can choose. Each of those entries deserves separate scrutiny as we have argued above, but the extensiveness of the list carries its own message.

◆ *Opportunity to make choices rationally.* The compendium of intervention strategies should not be read as an invitation to apply the listed approaches randomly and at whim. On the contrary, the research enables an informed and discriminating choice based on multiple lines of evidence.

◆ *Opportunity to combine rationally selected strategies into an integrated overall policy.* Tables 16.1 and 16.2 provide a basis for the selection of a set of integrated and mutually supportive strategies that are also cost-effective. Alcohol policy is likely to be most effective when it uses a variety of complementary strategies such as the combination of lower BAC limits, random breath testing of drivers, and minimum legal purchasing age restrictions in order to prevent alcohol-related road casualties. We strongly recommend the creation of such broadly based alcohol policies.

◆ *The research base is strong.* Research technologies are now available to monitor policy effectiveness. Rather than viewing alcohol interventions as certain solutions or hopeful 'shots in the dark', it is now possible and highly desirable that outcomes be measured and policies be self-correcting. There are numerous and evolving opportunities for further application of prevention science to policy questions.

◆ *Opportunities to implement policies at multiple levels.* Alcohol policies can be effective at both the community level and the national level. Within each of these levels, policies will affect the general population, high-risk drinkers, and people already experiencing alcohol-related problems. Synergistic types of activity are likely to obtain the best results. International policies provide the third level. When responding to alcohol problems, there is thus always somewhere to start, always a layer to be strengthened.

♦ *Opportunities to strengthen public awareness and support.* The consumers of the research reported in this book should be, in part, the general public. Significant, but so far largely neglected, opportunities exist to translate the scientific evidence into plain language for the media, opinion leaders, community groups, and the man and woman in the street. An informed public climate can help build support for public policies on alcohol.

♦ *Enhancing international collaboration in the response to alcohol.* This book has taken an international perspective throughout. The research we have presented and the policy experience we have described come from many different countries. International trade agreements and the global activities of the alcohol industry make an international view of alcohol-related problems mandatory. There are considerable opportunities to strengthen international collaboration and the sharing of experiences in this arena. The role of the WHO is paramount. In our view, the findings assembled in this book make a strong case for strengthened WHO initiatives on alcohol and public health.

In sum, opportunities for evidence-based alcohol policies that better serve the public good are more widely available than ever before, as a result of accumulating knowledge on those strategies that work and on how to make them work. This conclusion provides ample cause for optimism. However, this book must also be seen as carrying another well-evidenced and not so cheerful message. It provides the world community with new documentation that alcohol problems are inflicting, on a global scale, vast damage to the public health. It also shows that the policies to address these problems are too seldom informed by science, and there are still too many instances of policy vacuums filled by unevaluated or ineffective strategies and interventions.

Optimism or pessimism: which is it to be? The answer to that question may depend significantly on whether the future brings increased use of evidence-based alcohol policies. That is what the citizens of alcohol-using countries have a right to expect.

References

Aarens M., Cameron T., Roizen J., Roizen R., Room R., Schneberk D., and Wingard D. (1977) *Alcohol, casualties and crime.* Report C18. Berkeley, CA: Social Research Group.

Abbey A., Scott R.O., and Smith M. J. (1993) Physical, subjective, and social availability: Their relationship to alcohol consumption in rural and urban areas. *Addiction* **88**, 489–99.

Adlaf E.M. and Ialomiteanu A. (2007) *CAMH monitor e-*report*: Addiction and mental health indicators among Ontario adults in 2001, and changes since 1977.* CAMH Research Document Series No. 12. Toronto, Canada: Centre for Addiction and Mental Health.

Adrian M., Ferguson B.S., and Her M. (1996) Does allowing the sale of wine in Quebec grocery stores increase consumption? *Journal of Studies on Alcohol* **57**, 434–48.

Adrian M., Ferguson B.S., and Her M. (2001) Can alcohol price policies be used to reduce drunk driving?: Evidence from Canada. *Substance Use and Misuse* **36**, 1923–57.

Advocacy Institute (1992) *Taking initiative: The 1990 citizen's movement to raise California alcohol excise taxes to save lives.* Washington, DC: Advocacy Institute.

Agostinelli G. and Grube J. (2002) Alcohol counter-advertising and the media: A review of recent research. *Alcohol Research and Health* **26**, 15–21.

Agostinelli G., Brown J.M., and Miller W.R. (1995) Effects of normative feedback on consumption among heavy drinking college students. *Journal of Drug Education* **25**, 31–40.

Ahtola J., Ekholm A., and Somervuori A. (1986) Bayes estimates for the price and income elasticities of alcoholic beverages in Finland from 1955 to 1980. *Journal of Business and Economic Statistics* **4**, 199–208.

Alaniz M.L. (1998) Alcohol availability and targeted advertising in racial/ethnic minority communities. *Alcohol Health and Research World* **22**, 286–9.

Alavaikko M. and Österberg E. (2000) The influence of economic interests on alcohol control policy: A case study from Finland. *Addiction* **95** (Suppl. 4), 565–79.

Albalate D. (2006) *Lowering blood alcohol content levels to save lives: The European experience.* IREA Working Paper No 200603. Barcelona, Spain: University of Barcelona, Research Institute of Applied Economics. Available at: http://www.ub.edu/irea/working_papers/2006/200603.pdf (accessed 13 July 2009).

Alcohol Concern (1996) Toughen rules on toughened glasses, in light of 5000 serious bar injuries. Press release (July 5). Available at: http://www.alcoholconcern.org.uk/information/pressrel/1996/05-07-96.htm.

American Psychiatric Association (1994) *Diagnostic and statistical manual of mental disorders,* 4th edn (DSM-IV). Washington, DC: American Psychiatric Association.

Ames G.M. and Janes C. (1992) Cultural approach to conceptualizing alcohol and the workplace. *Alcohol Health and Research World* **16**, 112–19.

Andenaes J. (1988) The Scandinavian experience. In: Laurence M.D., Snortum J.R., and Zimring F.E. (eds), *Social Control of the Drinking Driver,* pp. 43–63. Chicago, IL: University of Chicago Press.

Anderson P. (2002) The beverage alcohol industry's social aspects organisations: A public health warning. St. Ives, UK: Eurocare.

Anderson P. (2004) The beverage alcohol industry's social aspects organizations: A public health warning. (Commentary.) *Addiction* **99**, 1376–7.

Anderson P. (2007) A safe, sensible and social AHRSE: New Labour and alcohol policy. *Addiction* **102**, 1515–21.

Anderson P. (2008) Consulting with the alcohol industry. *Drug and Alcohol Review* **27**, 463–5.

Anderson P. and Baumberg B. (2006a) *Alcohol in Europe: A public health perspective.* London, UK: Institute of Alcohol Studies. Available at: http://dse.univr.it/addiction/documents/External/alcoholineu.pdf (accessed 6 July 2009).

Anderson P. and Baumberg B. (2006b) Stakeholders' views of alcohol policy. *Nordic Studies on Alcohol and Drugs* **23**, 393–414.

Anderson P., Chisholm D., and Fuhr D.C. (2009a) Alcohol and global health 2: Effectiveness and cost-effectiveness of policies and programmes to reduce the harm caused by alcohol. *Lancet* **373**, 2234–46.

Anderson P., de Bruijn A., Angus K., Gordon R., and Hastings G. (2009b) Impact of alcohol advertising and media exposure on adolescent alcohol use: A systematic review of longitudinal studies. *Alcohol and Alcoholism* **44**, 229–43.

Anderson P., Drummond C., Mellman M. and Rosenqvist P. (2009c) Introduction to the issue: The alcohol industry and alcohol policy. *Addiction* **104**, S1–2.

Andréasson S., Allebeck P., and Romelsjö A. (1988) Alcohol and mortality among young men: Longitudinal study of Swedish conscripts. *British Medical Journal* **296**, 1021–5.

Andrews J.C. (1995) Effectiveness of alcohol warning labels: A review and extension. *American Behavioral Scientist* **38**, 622–32.

Andriamananjara S. (2001) International trade developments: Preferential trade agreements and the multilateral trading system. In: *International Economic Review*, pp. 1–4. Washington, DC: United States International Trade Commission, Publication 3402.

Andrienko Y. and Nemtsov A. (2005) *Estimation of individual demand for alcohol.* Working paper series. Moscow, Russia: Economics Education and Research Consortium. Available at: http://www.eerc.ru/details/EERCWorkingPaper.aspx?id=421 (accessed 8 July 2009).

Anton R.F., O'Malley S.S., Ciraulo D.A., Cisler R.A., Couper D., Donovan D.M., Gastfriend D.R., Hosking J.D., Johnson B.A., LoCastro J.S., Longabaugh R., Mason B.J., Mattson M.E., Miller W.R., Pettinati H.M., Randall C.L., Swift R., Weiss R.D., Williams L.D., and Zweben A., for the COMBINE Study Research Group (2006) Combined pharmacotherapies and behavioral interventions for alcohol dependence: The COMBINE Study: A randomized controlled trial. *Journal of the American Medical Association* **295**, 2003–17.

Argo J.J. and Main K.J. (2004) Meta-analyses of the effectiveness of warning labels. *Journal of Public Policy and Marketing* **23**, 193–208.

Arranz J.M. and Gil A.I. (2008) Traffic accidents, deaths and alcohol consumption. Applied Economics (online early access). DOI: 10.1080/00036840701222652.

Asbridge M., Mann R.E., Stoduto G. and Flam-Zalcman R. (2004) The criminalization of impaired driving in Canada: Assessing the deterrent impact of Canada's first *per se* law. *Journal of Studies on Alcohol* **65**, 450–9.

Asbridge M., Mann R.E., Smart R.G., Stoduto G., Vingilis E., Beirness D., and Lamble R. (2009) The effects of Ontario's administrative driver's licence suspension law on total driver fatalities: A multiple time series evaluation of Ontario and two control provinces. *Drugs: Education, Prevention and Policy* **16**, 140–51.

Ashe M., Jernigan D., Kline R., and Galaz R. (2003) Land use planning and the control of alcohol, tobacco, firearms, and fast food restaurants. *American Journal of Public Health* **93**, 1404–8.

Ashley M.J., Rehm J., Bondy S., Single E., and Rankin J. (2000) Beyond ischemic heart disease: Are there other health benefits from drinking alcohol? *Contemporary Drug Problems* **27**, 735–77.

Ashton T., Casswell S., and Gilmore L. (1989) Alcohol taxes: Do the poor pay more than the rich? *Addiction* **84**, 759–66.

Asplund M., Friberg R., and Wilander F. (2007) Demand and distance: Evidence on cross-border shopping. *Journal of Public Economics* **91**, 141–57.

Astley S.J. and Clarren S.K. (2000) Diagnosing the full spectrum of fetal alcohol-exposed individuals: Introducing the 4-Digit Diagnostic Code. *Alcohol and Alcoholism* **35**, 400–10.

Audience Research & Analysis (2004) The $9 billion economic impact of the nightlife industry in New York City: A study of spending by bar/lounges and clubs/music venues and their attendees. Available at: http://www.audienceresearch.com/News/ NightLifeEconomicImpact2003.pdf.

Austin E. and Hurst S. (2005) Targeting adolescents?: The content and frequency of alcoholic and nonalcoholic beverage ads in magazine and video formats, November 1999–April 2000. *Journal of Health Communication* **10**, 1–18.

Austin E. and Johnson K.K. (1997) Immediate and delayed effects of media literacy training on third graders' decision making for alcohol. *Health Communication* **9**, 323–49.

Austin E. and Knaus C. (2000) Predicting the potential for risky behavior among those 'too young' to drink as the result of appealing advertising. *Journal of Health Communications* **5**, 13–27.

Austin E., Chen M.-J., and Grube J. (2006) How does alcohol advertising influence underage drinking?: The role of desirability, identification and skepticism. *Journal of Adolescent Health* **38**, 376–84.

Australian Tax Office (2006) *The alcohol industry—excise technical guidelines.* Canberra, Australia: Australian Tax Office.

Ayer S., FranHois Y., and Rehm J. (1994) *Opération Nez Rouge, hiver 1993–1994: Evaluation auprés des usagers.* Lausanne, Switzerland: Insitut suisse de prévention de l'alcoolisme et autres toxicomainies.

Ayres I. and Braithwaite J. (1992) *Responsive regulation: Transcending the deregulation debate.* Oxford: Oxford University Press.

Baan R., Straif K., Grosse Y., Secretan B., El Ghissassi F., Bouvard V., Altieri A., and Cogliano V., on behalf of the WHO International Agency for Research on Cancer Monograph Working Group (2007) Carcinogenicity of alcoholic beverages. *Lancet Oncology* **8**, 292–3.

Babb P. (2007) *Violent crime, disorder and criminal damage since the introduction of the Licensing Act 2003*, 2nd edition. Home Office On-line Report 16/07. London, UK: Home Office. Available at: http://www.homeoffice.gov.uk/rds/pdfs07/rdsolr1607.pdf (accessed 6 July 2009).

Babor T.F. (1993) Megatrends and dead ends: Alcohol research in global perspective. *Alcohol Health and Research World* **17**, 177–86.

Babor T.F. (2004) Admirable ends, ineffective means: Comments on the alcohol harm reduction strategy for England. *Drugs: education, prevention and policy* **11**, 361–5.

Babor T.F. (2006) Diageo, University College Dublin and the integrity of alcohol science: It's time to draw the line between public health and public relations. *Addiction* **101**, 1375–7.

Babor T.F. (2008a) Tackling alcohol misuse in the UK. *BMJ* **336**, 455. Doi: 10.1136/bmj.39496.556435.80.

Babor T.F. (2008b) Treatment for persons with substance use disorders: Mediators, moderators and the need for a new research approach. *International Journal of Methods in Psychiatric Research* **17** (Suppl. 1), S45–9.

Babor T.F. (2009) Alcohol research and the alcoholic beverage industry: Issues, concerns and conflicts of interest. *Addiction* **104**, 34–47.

Babor T.F. and Caetano R. (2005) Evidence-based alcohol policy in the Americas: Strengths, weaknesses and future challenges. *Revista Panamericana de Salud Pública/Pan American Journal of Public Health* **18**, 327–37.

Babor T.F. and Del Boca, F.K. (eds) (2003) *Treatment matching in alcoholism*. Cambridge: Cambridge University Press.

Babor T.F. and Rosenkrantz B.G. (1991) Public health, public morals and public order: Social science and liquor control in Massachusetts: 1880–1916. In: Barrows S. and Room R. (eds), *Drinking behavior and belief in modern history*, pp. 265–86. Berkeley, CA: University of California Press.

Babor T.F., Mendelson J.H., Greenberg I., and Kuehnle J. (1978) Experimental analysis of the 'happy hour': Effects of purchase price on alcohol consumption. *Psychopharmacology* **58**, 35–41.

Babor T.F., Mendelson J.H., Uhly B., and Souza E. (1980) Drinking patterns in experimental and barroom settings. *Journal of Studies on Alcohol* **41**, 635–51.

Babor T.F., Campbell R., Room R., and Saunders J. (1994) *Lexicon of alcohol and drug terms*. Geneva, Switzerland: World Health Organization.

Babor T.F., Edwards G., and Stockwell T. (1996) Science and the drinks industry: Cause for concern. (Editorial.) *Addiction* **91**, 5–9.

Babor T., Caetano R., Casswell S., Edwards G., Giesbrecht N., Graham K., Grube J., Gruenewald P.J., Hill L., Holder H., Homel R., Österberg E., Rehm J., Room R., and Rossow I. (2003) *Alcohol: no ordinary commodity—Research and public policy*, 1st edn. Oxford: Oxford University Press.

Babor T.F., McRee B., Kassebaum P., Grimaldi P., Ahmed K., and Bray J. (2007) Screening, brief intervention, and referral to treatment (SBIRT): Toward a public health approach to the management of substance abuse. *Substance Abuse* **28**, 7–30.

Babor T.F., Hernandez-Avlia C.A., and Ungemack J.A. (2008a) Substance abuse: Alcohol use disorders: Alcohol dependence, alcohol abuse. In: Tasman A., Kay J., and Lieberman J.A. (eds), *Psychiatry*, 3rd edn, Vol. 1, pp. 971–1004. Chichester, UK: Wiley.

Babor T.F., Morisano D., Stenius K., Winstanley E.L., and O'Reilly J. (2008b) How to choose a journal: Scientific and practical considerations. In: Babor T.F., Stenius K., Savva S., and O'Reilly J. (eds), *Publishing addiction science: A guide for the perplexed*, 2nd edn, pp. 12–35. London: Multi-Science.

Babor T.F., Stenius K., and Romelsjö A. (2008c) Alcohol and drug treatment systems in public health perspective: Mediators and moderators of population effects. *International Journal of Methods in Psychiatric Research* **17** (Suppl. 1), S50–9.

Babor T.F., Xuan Z., and Proctor D. (2008d) Reliability of a rating procedure to monitor industry self-regulation codes governing alcohol advertising content. *Journal of Studies on Alcohol and Drugs* **69**, 235–42.

Babor T.F., Xuan Z., and Damon D. (in press) Changes in the self-regulation guidelines of the US Beer Code reduce the number of content violations reported in TV advertisements. *Journal of Public Policy*.

Baer J.S., Kivlahan D.R., Blume A.W., McNight P., and Marlatt G.A. (2001) Brief intervention for heavy-drinking college students: Four-year follow-up and natural history. *American Journal of Public Health* **91**, 1310–16.

Baggott R. (1986) By voluntary agreement: The politics of instrument selection. *Public Administration* **64**, 51–67.

Baggott R. (1989) Regulatory reform in Britain: The changing face of self-regulation. *Public Administration* **67**, 435–54.

Baggott R. (1990) *Alcohol, politics and social policy*. Aldershot, UK: Avebury.

Bagnardi V, Zatonski W, Scotti L, La Vecchia C, and Corrao G. (2008) Does drinking pattern modify the effect of alcohol on the risk of coronary heart disease?: Evidence from a meta-analysis. *Journal of Epidemiology and Community Health* **62**, 615–9.

Baker T.K., Johnson M.B., Voas R.B., and Lange J.E. (2000) Reduce youthful binge drinking: Call an election in Mexico. *Journal of Safety Research* **31**, 61–9.

Bakke Ø., and Endal D. (in press) Alcohol policies out of context: Drinks industry supplanting government role in alcohol policies in sub-Saharan Africa. *Addiction*.

Bandera E.V., Freudenheim J.L., and Vena J.E. (2001) Alcohol and lung cancer: A review of the epidemiologic evidence. *Cancer Epidemiology, Biomarkers and Prevention* **10**, 813–21.

Barber J.G. and Gilbertson R. (1999) Drinker's children. *Substance Use and Misuse* **34**, 383–402.

Barlow T. and Wogalter M.S. (1993) Alcoholic beverage warnings in magazine and television advertisements. *Journal of Consumer Research* **20**, 147–56.

Baumberg B. and Anderson P. (2008) Health, alcohol and EU law: Understanding the impact of European single market law on alcohol policies. *European Journal of Public Health* **18**, 392–8.

Beccaria F. (1999) 'Bait' or 'prey': Women in Italian alcohol advertising at the end of millennium. *Alcologia* **11**, 101–6.

Beck K. (2009) Lessons learned from evaluating Maryland's anti-drunk driving campaign: Assessing the evidence for cognitive, behavioral, and public health impact. *Health Promotion Practice* **10**, 370–7.

Beck K. and Moser M. (2006) Does the type of exposure to a roadside sobriety checkpoint influence driver perceptions regarding drunk driving? *American Journal of Health Behavior* **30**, 268–77.

Bellis M.A., Hughes K., Morleo M., Tocque K., Hughes S., Allen T., Harrison D., and Fe-Rodriguez E. (2007) Predictors of risky alcohol consumption in schoolchildren and their implications for preventing alcohol-related harm. *Substance Abuse Treatment, Prevention, and Policy* **2** (doi:10.1186/1747-597X-2-15).

Bello W. (2006) The capitalist conjuncture: Overaccumulation, financial crises, and the retreat from globalization. *Third World Quarterly* **27**, 1345–67.

Benegal V. (2005) India: Alcohol and public health. *Addiction* **100**, 1051–6.

Benegal V., Nayak M., Murthy P., Chandra P. and Gururaj G. (2005) Women and alcohol use in India. In: Obot I.S. and Room R. (eds), *Alcohol, gender and drinking problems:*

Perspectives from low and middle income countries, pp. 89–123. Geneva: World Health Organization.

Benson B.L., Rasmussen D.W., and Mast B.D. (1999) Deterring drunk driving fatalities: An economics of crime perspective. *International Review of Law Economics* **19**, 205–25.

Berkowitz A.D. (1997) From reactive to proactive prevention: Promoting an ecology of health on campus. In: Rivers P.C. and Shore E.R. (eds), *Substance abuse on campus: A handbook for college and university personnel*, pp. 119–39. Westport, CT: Greenwood Press.

Bernat D., Dunsmuir W., and Wagenaar A.C. (2004) Effects of lowering the legal BAC to 0.08 on single-vehicle-nighttime fatal traffic crashes in 19 jurisdictions. *Accident Analysis and Prevention* **36**, 1089–97.

Bjerre B. (2005) Primary and secondary prevention of drinking and driving by the use of alcolock device and program: Swedish experiences. *Accident Analysis and Prevention* **37**, 1145–52.

Bjerre B. and Kostela J. (2008) Primary prevention of drink driving by the large-scale use of alcolocks in commercial vehicles. *Accident Analysis and Prevention* **40**, 1294–9.

Bjerre B. and Thorsson U. (2008) Is an alcohol ignition interlock programme a useful tool for changing the alcohol and driving habits of drink-drivers? *Accident Analysis and Prevention* **40**, 267–73.

Blake D. and Nied A. (1997) The demand for alcohol in the UK. *Applied Economics* **29**, 1655–72.

Blecher E. (2008) The impact of tobacco advertising bans on consumption in developing countries. *Journal of Health Economics* **27**, 930–42.

Blomberg R.D., Peck R.C., Moskowitz H., Burns M., and Fiorentino D. (2005) *Crash risk of alcohol involved driving: A case–control study*. Stamford, CT: Dunlap & Associates.

Bloomfield K. (1998) West German drinking patterns in 1984 and 1990. *European Addiction Research* **4**, 163–71.

Bloomfield K., Gmel G., Neve R., and Mustonen H. (2001) Investigating gender convergence in alcohol consumption in Finland, Germany, The Netherlands, and Switzerland: A repeated survey analysis. *Substance Abuse* **22**, 39–54.

Blose J.O. and Holder H.D. (1987) Liquor-by-the-drink and alcohol-related traffic crashes: A natural experiment using time-series analysis. *Journal of Studies on Alcohol and Drugs* **48**, 52–60.

Bofetta P. and Hashibe M. (2006) Alcohol and cancer. *Lancet Oncology* **7**, 149–56.

Bondy S.J. and Lange P. (2000) Measuring alcohol-related harm: Test–retest reliability of a popular measure. *Substance Use and Misuse* **35**, 1263–75.

Bondy S.J., Rehm J., Ashley M.J., Walsh G., Single E., and Room R. (1999) Low-risk drinking guidelines: Scientific evidence. *Canadian Journal of Public Health* **90**, 264–70.

Booth A., Meier P., Stockwell T., Sutton A., Wilkinson A., and Wong R. (2008) Independent review of the effects of alcohol pricing and promotion. part a: Systematic reviews. Sheffield, UK: School of Health and Related Research, University of Sheffield. Available at: http://www.dh.gov.uk/en/Publichealth/Healthimprovement/Alcoholmisuse/DH_4001740 (accessed 30 January 2009).

Bormann C.A. and Stone M.H. (2001) The effects of eliminating alcohol in a college stadium: the Folsom Field beer ban. *Journal of American College Health* **50**, 81–8.

Borsari B. and Carey K.B. (2000) Effects of a brief motivational intervention with college student drinkers. *Journal of Consulting and Clinical Psychology* **68**, 728–33.

Botvin G. J. and Botvin E. M. (1992) Adolescent tobacco, alcohol, and drug abuse: Prevention strategies, empirical findings, and assessment issues. *Developmental and Behavioral Pediatrics* **13**, 290–301.

Botvin G.J. and Griffin K.W. (2007) School-based programmes to prevent alcohol, tobacco and other drug use. *International Review of Psychiatry* **19**, 607–15.

Botvin G.J., Baker E., Dusenbury L., Botvin E.M., and Diaz T. (1995) Long-term follow-up results of a randomized drug abuse prevention trial in a white middle-class population. *Journal of the American Medical Association* **273**, 1106–12.

Bourgeois J. and Barnes J. (1979) Does advertising increase alcohol consumption? *Journal of Advertising Research* **19**, 19–29.

Brady M. (2000) Alcohol policy issues for indigenous people in the United States, Canada, Australia and New Zealand. *Contemporary Drug Problems* **27**, 435–509.

Brain K. (2000) Youth, alcohol and the emergence of the post-modern alcohol order. Occasional Paper No. 1. London, UK: Institute of Alcohol Studies.

Braithwaite J. (2002) *Restorative justice and responsive regulation.* Oxford, UK: Oxford University Press.

Bramley D., Broad J., Harris R., Reid P., and Jackson R. (2003) Differences in patterns of alcohol consumption between Maori and non-Maori in Aotearoa (New Zealand). *New Zealand Medical Journal* **116**, U645.

Braun K. and Graham K., with Bois C., Tessier C., Hughes S., Prentice L. (2000) *Safer bars trainer's guide.* Toronto: Centre for Addiction and Mental Health.

Breen R. (2008) Code of practice on alcohol marketing, communications and sponsorship in Ireland. Presentation delivered at the Conference on Alcohol advertising—impact and self-regulation (Berlin, 25 September). Available at: http://www.eurocare.org/press/newsletter/september_november_2008/news_from_the_member_states/germany_conference_on_alcohol_advertising_impact_and_self_regulation_berlin (accessed 14 July 2009).

Brewers Association of Canada (1997) *Alcoholic beverage taxation and control policies. international survey,* 9th edn. Ottawa: Brewers Association of Canada.

Brody G.H., Murry V.M., Kogan S.M., Gerrard M., Gibbons F.X., Molgaard V., Brown A.C., Anderson T., Chen Y.-F., Luo Z., and Wills T.A. (2006) The Strong African American Families Program: A cluster-randomized prevention trial of long-term effects and a mediational model. *Journal of Consulting and Clinical Psychology* **74**, 356–66.

Brook R.H. and McGlynn E.A. (1991) Maintaining quality of care. In: Ginzberg E. (ed.), *Health services research: Key to health policy,* pp. 784–817. Cambridge, MA: Harvard University Press.

Broughton E.A. (1997) Impact of informational methods among drinking college students applying the Health Belief Model. *Dissertation Abstracts International* **57**, 3839–40A.

Brown J.H. and Kreft I.G.G. (1998) Zero effects of drug prevention programs: Issues and solutions. *Evaluation Review* **22**, 3–14.

Brunet A.R. (2007) Violence amongst juveniles in leisure areas: A comparative approach. In: Recasens A. (ed.), *Violence between young people in night-time leisure zones: A European comparative study,* pp. 9–30. Brussels: VUB Press.

Bruun K. (1973) Social research, social policy and action. In: *The epidemiology of drug dependence: report on a conference,* London 25–29 September 1972, pp. 115–19. Copenhagen Denmark: WHO, Regional Office for Europe, EURO 5436 IV.

Bruun K., Edwards G., Lumio M., Mäkelä K., Pan L., Popham R.E., Room R., Schmidt W., Skog O.-J., Sulkunen P., and Österberg E. (1975a) *Alcohol control policies in public health perspective*. Helsinki: Finnish Foundation for Alcohol Studies.

Bruun K., Pan L., and Rexed I. (1975b) *The gentlemen's club: International control of drugs and alcohol*. Chicago: University of Chicago Press.

Bryding G. and Rosén U. (1969) *Konsumtionen av alkoholhaltiga drycker 1920–1951, en efterfrågeananalytisk studie* (Consumption of alcohol beverages in Sweden 1920–1951, an econometric study). Uppsala: Universitetets Statistiska Institution (stencil).

Buchanan D. and Lev J. (1989) *Beer and fast cars: How brewers targets blue-collar youth through motor sports sponsorship*. Washington, DC: AAA Foundation for Traffic Safety.

Buka S.L. and Birdthistle I.J. (1999) Long-term effects of a community-wide alcohol server training intervention. *Journal of Studies on Alcohol* **60**, 27–36.

Bucuvalas M. and Weiss C. (1980) Truth tests and utility tests: Decision makers' frames of reference for social science research. *American Sociological Review* **45**, 302–13.

Burns L., Flaherty B., Ireland S., and Frances M. (1995) Policing pubs: What happens to crime? *Drug and Alcohol Review* **14**, 369–75.

Bushman B.J. (1997) Effects of alcohol on human aggression: Validity of proposed mechanisms. In: Galanter M. (ed.) *Recent Developments in Alcoholism*, Vol. 13, *Alcohol and violence*, pp. 227–44. New York: Plenum Press.

Bushman B.J. and Cooper H.M. (1990) Effects of alcohol on human aggression: An integrative research review. *Psychological Bulletin* **107**, 341–54.

Caetano R. (1997) Prevalence, incidence and stability of drinking problems among whites, blacks and Hispanics: 1984–1992. *Journal of Studies on Alcohol* **58**, 565–72.

Caetano R. and Laranjeira R. (2005) A 'perfect storm' in developing countries: Economic growth and the alcohol industry. *Addiction* **101**, 149–52.

Caetano R., Tam T., Greenfield T., Cherpitel C., and Midanik L. (1997) DSM-IV alcohol dependence and drinking in the US population: A risk analysis. *Annals of Epidemiology* **7**, 542–9.

Cahalan D. and Room R. (1974) *Problem drinking among American men*. New Brunswick, NJ: Rutgers Center of Alcohol Studies.

Cameron J., Whitehead P.C., and Hayes M.J. (1993) Evaluation of a program to modify alcohol-related knowledge, attitudes, intentions and behaviors among first-year university students. In: Greenfield T.K. and Zimmerman R. (eds), *Second International Research Symposium on Experiences with Community Action Projects for the Prevention of Alcohol and Other Drug Problems*, pp. 167–73. Washington, DC: US Department of Health and Human Services.

Campos V.R., Salgado R., Rocha M.C., Duailibi S., and Laranjeira R. (2008) Prevalência do beber e dirigir em Belo Horizonte, Minas Gerais, Brasil [Drinking-and-driving prevalence in Belo Horizonte, Minas Gerais State, Brazil]. *Cadernos de Saúde Pública* **24**, 829–34.

Canzer B. (1996) Social marketing approach to media intervention design in health and lifestyle education. *Dissertation Abstracts International* **57**, 647A.

Carey K.B, Carey, M. P., Maisto S.A., and Henson J.M. (2006) Brief motivational interventions for heavy college drinkers: A randomized controlled trial. *Journal of Consulting and Clinical Psychology* **74**, 943–54.

Carey K.B., Scott-Sheldon L.A.J., Carey M.P., and DeMartini K.S. (2007) Individual-level interventions to reduce college student drinking: A meta-analytic review. *Addictive Behaviors* **32**, 2469–94.

Carlsberg (2006) *Annual Report 2005*. Copenhagen, Denmark: Carlsberg A/S. Available at: http://www.carlsberggroup.com/Investor/DownloadCentre/Pages/Annualreports.aspx (accessed 14 July 2009).

Carpenter C.S. and Dobkin C. (2007) *The effect of alcohol consumption on mortality: Regression discontinuity evidence from the minimum drinking age.* NBER Working Paper 13374. Cambridge, MA: National Bureau of Economic Research.

Carpenter C.S., Kloska D.D., O'Malley P., and Johnston L. (2007) Alcohol control policies and youth alcohol consumption: Evidence from 28 years of Monitoring the Future. *The BE Journal of Economic Analysis and Policy* 7, 1–21.

Carvolth R. (1995) *The contribution of risk assessment to harm reduction through the Queensland safety action approach.* Proceedings of the 'Window of Opportunity Congress', Brisbane, Australia.

Cases F.M., Harford T.C., Williams G.D., and Hanna E.Z. (1999) Alcohol consumption and divorce rates in the United States. *Journal of Studies on Alcohol* 60, 647–52.

Casswell S. (1993) Public discourse on the benefits of moderation: Implications for alcohol policy development. *Addiction* 88, 459–65.

Casswell S. (1995) Public discourse on alcohol: Implications for public policy. In: Holder H.D. and Edwards G. (eds), *Alcohol and Public Policy: Evidence and Issues*, pp. 190–214. Oxford: Oxford University Press.

Casswell S. (1997) Public discourse on alcohol. *Health Promotion International* 12, 251–7.

Casswell S. (2004) Alcohol brands in young people's everyday lives: New developments in marketing. *Alcohol and Alcoholism* 39, 471–6.

Casswell S. (2009) Alcohol industry and alcohol policy: The challenge ahead. *Addiction* 104 (Suppl. 1), 3–5.

Casswell S. and Gilmore L. (1989) An evaluated community action project on alcohol. *Journal of Studies on Alcohol* 50, 339–46.

Casswell S. and Stewart L. (1989) A Community Action Project on alcohol: Community organisation and its evaluation. *Community Health Studies* 13, 39–48.

Casswell S. and Thamarangsi T. (2009) Reducing harm from alcohol: Call to action. *The Lancet* 373, 2247–57.

Casswell S. and Zhang J. (1998) Impact of liking for advertising and brand allegiance on drinking and alcohol-related aggression: A longitudinal study. *Addiction* 93, 1209–17.

Casswell S., Gilmore L., Maguire V., and Ransom R. (1989) Changes in public support for alcohol policies following a community based campaign. *British Journal of Addiction* 84, 515–22.

Casswell S., Stewart L., and Duignan P. (1993) The negotiation of New Zealand alcohol policy in a decade of stabilized consumption and political change: The role of research. *Addiction* 88 (Suppl.), 9–17S.

CATALYST (2001) Alcohol misuse in Scotland: Trends and costs: Final report. Northwood, UK: Catalyst Health Economics Consultants. Available at: http://www.alcoholinformation.isdscotland.org/alcohol_misuse/files/Catalyst_Full.pdf (accessed 11 July 2009).

Caudill B.D., Harding W.M., and Moore B.A. (2000a) DWI prevention: Profiles of drinkers who serve as designated drivers. *Psychology of Addictive Behaviors* 14, 143–50.

Caudill B.D., Harding W.M., and Moore B.A. (2000b) At-risk drinkers use safe ride services to avoid drinking and driving. *Journal of Substance Use* 11, 149–59.

Cauzard J.-P. (ed.) (2004) *European drivers and road risk SARTRE 3 reports Part 1: Report on principal analyses.* Arcueil, France: Institut National de Recherche sur les Transports et leur Sécurité. Available at: http://sartre.inrets.fr/documents-pdf/repS3V1E.pdf (accessed 13 July 2009).

Cavan S. (1966) Bar sociability. In: Cavan S. (ed.), *Liquor license: An ethnography of a bar,* pp. 49–87. Chicago, IL: Aldine.

C'de Baca J., Lapham S.C., Liang H.C., and Skipper B.J. (2001) Victim impact panels: Do they impact drunk drivers? A follow-up of female and male, first-time and repeat offenders. *Journal of Studies on Alcohol* **62**, 615–20.

Center for Disease Control and Prevention (2003) Point-of-purchase alcohol marketing and promotion by store type, United States, 2000–2001. *Morbidity and Mortality Weekly Reports* **54**, 310–13.

Center on Alcohol Marketing and Youth (2003) *Drops in the bucket: Alcohol industry "responsibility" advertising on television in 2001.* Washington, DC: CAMY. Available at: http://camy.org/research/files/drops0203.pdf (accessed 14 July 2009).

Center on Alcohol Marketing and Youth (2006) *Exposure of African-American youth to alcohol advertising, 2003 to 2004* Washington, DC: CAMY. Available at: http://camy.org/research/afam0606/ (accessed 14 July 2009).

Center on Alcohol Marketing and Youth (2008) *Youth exposure to alcohol advertising on television, 2001 to 2007.* Washington, DC: CAMY. Available at: http://camy.org/research/tv0608/ (accessed 14 July 2009).

Chadwick D.J. and Goode J.A. (1998) *Alcohol and cardiovascular disease.* Novartis Foundation Symposium No. 216, London, 7–9 October 1997. Chichester, UK: John Wiley & Sons.

Chaloupka F.J. and Wechsler H. (1996) Binge drinking in college: The impact of price, availability, and alcohol control policies. *Contemporary Economic Policy* **14**, 112–24.

Chaloupka F.J., Saffer H., and Grossman M. (1993) Alcohol-control policies and motor-vehicle fatalities. *Journal of Legal Studies* **22**, 161–86.

Chaloupka F.J., Grossman M., and Saffer H. (2002) The effects of price on alcohol consumption and alcohol-related problems. *Alcohol Research and Health* **26**, 22–34.

Chamberlain E. and Solomon R. (2008) Zero blood alcohol concentration limits for drivers under 21: Lessons from Canada. *Injury Prevention* **14**, 123–8.

Chang H.-L. and Yeh C.-C. (2004) The life cycle of policy for preventing road accidents: An empirical example of the policy for reducing drunk driving crashes in Taipei. *Accident Analysis and Prevention* **36**, 809–18.

Chapman S. and Lupton D. (1994) *The fight for public health: Principles and practice of media advocacy.* London, UK: BMJ.

Chatterton P. and Hollands R. (2002) Theorising urban playscapes: Producing, regulating and consuming youthful nightlife city spaces. *Urban Studies* **39**, 95–116.

Chen M.-J., Grube J., Bersamin M., Waiters E., and Keefe D. (2005) Alcohol advertising: What makes it attractive to youth? *Journal of Health Communication* **10**, 553–65.

Cherpitel C.J. (1996) Drinking patterns and problems and drinking in the event: An analysis of injury by cause among casualty patients. *Alcoholism: Clinical and Experimental Research* **20**, 1130–7.

Chesson H., Harrison P., and Kassler W.J. (2000) Sex under the influence: The effect of alcohol policy on sexually transmitted disease rates in the United States. *Journal of Law and Economics* **43**, 215–38.

Chikritzhs T. (2009) Australia. In: Hadfield P. (ed.), *Nightlife and crime: Social order and governance in international perspective.* Oxford: Oxford University Press.

Chikritzhs T. and Stockwell T. (2002) The impact of later trading hours for Australian public houses (hotels) on levels of violence. *Journal of Studies on Alcohol* **63**, 591–9.

Chikritzhs T. and Stockwell T. (2006) The impact of later trading hours for hotels on levels of impaired driver road crashes and driver breath alcohol levels. *Addiction* **101**, 1254–64.

Chikritzhs T. and Stockwell T. (2007) The impact of later trading hours for hotels (public houses) on breath alcohol levels of apprehended impaired drivers. *Addiction* **102**, 1609–17.

Chikritzhs T.N., Stockwell T., and Pascal R. (2005) The impact of the Northern Territory's Living With Alcohol program, 1992–2002: Revisiting the evaluation. *Addiction* **100**, 1625–36.

Chikritzhs T., Gray D, Lyons Z., and Saggers S. (2007) *Restrictions on the sale and supply of alcohol: Evidence and outcomes.* Perth, Australia: National Drug Research Institute, Curtin University of Technology.

Chikritzhs T.N., Dietze P.M., Allsop S.J., Daube M.M., Hall W.D. and Kypri K. (2009) The "alcopops" tax: Heading in the right direction. *Medical Journal of Australia* **190**, 294–5.

Chisholm D., Rehm J., Van Ommeren M., and Monteiro M. (2004) Reducing the global burden of hazardous alcohol use: A comparative cost-effectiveness analysis. *Journal of Studies on Alcohol* **65**, 782–93.

Chisholm D., Doran C., Shibuya K., and Rehm J. (2006) Comparative cost-effectiveness of policy instruments for reducing the global burden of alcohol, tobacco and illicit drug use. *Drug and Alcohol Review* **25**, 553–65.

Chiu A.Y., Perez P.E., and Parker R.N. (1997) Impact of banning alcohol on outpatient visits in Barrow, Alaska. *Journal of the American Medical Association* **278**, 1775–7.

Choice (2008) Alcopops. *Trusted information for Australian consumers.* February. Available at: http://www.iterasi.net/openviewer.aspx?sqrlitid=kaf6rrv0kei5jpmxgrepwa (accessed 3 July 2009).

Christie N. and Bruun K. (1969) Alcohol problems: The conceptual framework. In: Keller M. and Coffey T. (eds), *Proceedings of the 28th International Congress on Alcohol and Alcoholism*, Vol. 2, pp. 65–73. Highland Park, NJ: Hillhouse Press.

Cimini M.D., Page J.C., and Trujillo D.A. (2002) Using peer theater to deliver social norms information: The middle earth players program. *Report on Social Norms* **2**, 1 (Working Paper No. 8).

Cisneros Örnberg J. and Ólafsdóttir H. (2008) How to sell alcohol? Nordic alcohol monopolies in a changing epoch. *Nordisk alkohol- och narkotikatidskrift* **25**, 129–53 (in English).

Clarke R.V. (ed.) (1997) *Situational crime prevention: Successful case studies*, 2nd edn. Guilderland, NY: Harrow & Heston.

Clarke R.V. and Homel R. (1997) A revised classification of techniques of situational crime prevention. In: Lab S.P. (ed.), *Crime prevention at a crossroads*, pp. 21–35. Cincinnati, OH: Anderson.

Clarren S.K. and Smith D.W. (1978) The fetal alcohol syndrome. *New England Journal of Medicine* **298**, 1063–7.

Clausen T., Rossow I., Naidoo N. and Kowal P. (2009) Diverse alcohol drinking patterns in 20 African countries. *Addiction* **104**, 1147–54.

Coate D. and Grossman M. (1988) Effects of alcoholic beverage prices and legal drinking ages on youth alcohol use. *Journal of Law and Economics* **31**, 145–71.

Coffield A., Maciosek M.V., McGinnis J.M., Harris J.R., Caldwell M.B., Teutsch S.M., Atkins D., Richland J.H., and Haddix A. (2001) Priorities among recommended clinical preventive services. *American Journal of Preventive Medicine* **21**, 1–9.

Cohen D.A., Ghosh-Dastidar B., Scribner R.A., Miu A., Scott M., Robinson P., Farley T.A., Blumenthal R.N., and Brown-Taylor D. (2006) Alcohol outlets, gonorrhea, and the Los Angeles civil unrest: A longitudinal analysis. *Social Science and Medicine* **62**, 3062–71.

Cohen L.E. and Felson M. (1979) Social change and crime rate trends: A routine activity approach. *American Sociological Review* **44**, 588–608.

Collins D.J. and Lapsley H.M. (2008) *The avoidable costs of alcohol abuse in Australia and the potential benefits of effective policies to reduce the social costs of alcohol.* National Drug Strategy Monograph No. 70. Canberra, Australia: Department of Health & Ageing. Available at: http://www.nationaldrugstrategy.gov.au/internet/drugstrategy/publishing.nsf/Content/0A14D387E42AA201CA2574B3000028A8/$File/mono70.pdf (accessed 8 July 2009).

Collins R., Schell T., Ellickson P., and McCaffrey D. (2003) Predictors of beer advertising awareness among eighth graders. *Addiction* **98**, 1297–1306.

Collins S.E., Carey K.B., and Sliwinski M.J. (2002) Mailed personalized normative feedback as a brief intervention for at-risk college drinkers. *Journal of Studies on Alcohol* **63**, 559–67.

Connolly G.M., Casswell S., Zhang J.F., and Silva P.A. (1994) Alcohol in the mass media and drinking by adolescents: A longitudinal study. *Addiction* **89**, 1255–63.

Conway K. (2002) Booze and beach bans: Turning the tide through community action in New Zealand. *Health Promotion International* **17**, 171–7.

Cook P.J. (1981) The effect of liquor taxes on drinking, cirrhosis and auto accidents. In: Moore M.H. and Gerstein D.R. (eds), *Alcohol and public policy: Beyond the shadow of prohibition*, pp. 255–85. Washington, DC: National Academy Press.

Cook P.J. (2007) *Paying the tab: The costs and benefits of alcohol control.* Princeton, NJ: Princeton University Press.

Cook P.J. and Moore, M.J. (1993) Taxation of alcoholic beverages. In: Hilton M.E. and Bloss G. (eds), *Economics and the prevention of alcohol-related problems: Proceedings of a workshop on economic and socioeconomic issues in the prevention of alcohol-related problems*, October 10–11, 1991, Bethesda, MD. NIAAA Research Monograph No. 25. Rockville, MD: National Institute on Alcohol Abuse and Alcoholism.

Cook P.J. and Tauchen G. (1982) The effect of liquor taxes on heavy drinking. *Bell Journal of Economics* **13**, 379–90.

Cooney N.L., Babor T.F., DiClemente C.C., and Del Boca F.K. (2003) Clinical and scientific implications of Project MATCH. In: Babor T.F. and Del Boca F.K. (eds), *Treatment Matching in Alcoholism*, pp. 222–37. Cambridge: Cambridge University Press.

Copeland J., Stevenson R.J., Gates P., and Dillon P. (2007) Young Australians and alcohol: The acceptability of ready-to-drink (RTD) alcoholic beverages among 12–30 year-olds. *Addiction* **102**, 1740–6.

Cornish D.B. and Clarke R.V. (2003) Opportunities, precipitators and criminal decisions: A reply to Wortley's critique of situational crime prevention. In: Smith M.J. and Cornish D.B. (eds), *Theory for practice in situational crime prevention*, vol. 16, pp. 41–96. Monsey, NY: Criminal Justice Press.

Corrao G., Bagnardi V., Zambon A., and Arico S. (1999) Exploring the dose–response relationship between alcohol consumption and the risk of several alcohol-related conditions: A meta-analysis. *Addiction* **94**, 1551–73.

Corrao G., Rubbiati L., Bagnardi V., Zambon A., and Poikolainen K. (2000) Alcohol and coronary heart disease: A meta-analysis. *Addiction* **95**, 1505–23.

Cosper R.L., Okraku I.O., and Neumann B. (1987) Tavern going in Canada: A national survey of regulars at public drinking establishments. *Journal of Studies on Alcohol* **48**, 252–9.

Craplet M. (1997) Alcohol advertising: The need for European regulation. *Commercial Communications: The Journal of Advertising and Marketing Policy and Practice in the European Community* **9**, 1–3.

Creyer E.H., Kozup J.C., and Burton S. (2002) An experimental assessment of the effects of two alcoholic beverage health warnings across countries and binge-drinking status. *Journal of Consumer Affairs* **36**, 171–202.

Criqui M.H. (1994) Alcohol and the heart: Implications of present epidemiologic knowledge. *Contemporary Drug Problems* **21**, 125–42.

Criqui M.H. (1996) Alcohol and coronary heart disease: Consistent relationship and public health implications. *Clinica Chimica Acta* **246**, 51–7.

Cuijpers P. (2003) Three decades of drug prevention research. *Drugs: Education, Prevention and Policy* **10**, 7–20.

Cummings S. (1997) Empowerment model for collegiate substance abuse prevention and education programs. *Journal of Alcohol and Drug Education* **43**, 46–62.

d'Abbs P. and Togni S. (2000) Liquor licensing and community action in regional and remote Australia: A review of recent initiatives. *Australian and New Zealand Journal of Public Health* **24**, 45–53.

D'Amico E.J. and Fromme K. (2002) Brief prevention for adolescent risk-taking behaviour. *Addiction* **97**, 563–74.

Dal Cin S., Worth K.A., Dalton M.A., and Sargent J.D. (2008) Youth exposure to alcohol use and brand appearances in popular contemporary movies. *Addiction* **103**, 1925–32.

Daly J.B., Campbell E.M., Wiggers J.H., and Considine R.J. (2002) Prevalence of responsible hospitality policies in licensed premises that are associated with alcohol-related harm. *Drug and Alcohol Review* **21**, 113–20.

Dang J.N. (2008) *Statistical analysis of alcohol-related driving trends, 1982–2005*. Publication No. DOT HS 810 942. Washington, DC: National Highway Traffic safety Administration.

Darkes J. and Goldman M.S. (1993) Expectancy challenge and drinking reduction: Experimental evidence for a mediational process. *Journal of Consulting and Clinical Psychology* **61**, 344–53.

Datamonitor (2007). Available at http://www.datamonitor.com/ (accessed 25 September 2007).

Davies P. and Mummery H. (2006) Nightvision. Town centres for all. London, UK: Civic Trust. Available at: http://www.bcsc.org.uk/publication.asp?pub_id=212 (accessed 3 July 2009).

Davies P. and Walsh D. (1983) *Alcohol problems and alcohol control in Europe*. New York: Gardner.

Davis A., Quimby A., Odero W., Gururaj G., and Hijar M. (2003) *Improving road safety by reducing impaired driving in developing countries: A scoping study*. Project report pr/int/724/03. Crowthorne, UK: Transportation Research Laboratory Available at: http://www.grsproadsafety.org/themes/default/pdfs/Impaired%20driving%20final.pdf (accessed 13 July 2009).

Dawson D.A. (1997) Alcohol, drugs, fighting and suicide attempt/ideation. *Addiction Research* **5**, 451–72.

Dawson D.A. (1998) Beyond black, white and Hispanic: Race, ethnic origin and drinking patterns in the United States. *Journal of Substance Abuse* **10**, 321–39.

Dawson D.A. (2000) Drinking patterns among individuals with and without DSM-IV alcohol use disorders. *Journal of Studies on Alcohol* **61**, 111–20.

Dawson D.A. and Archer L.D. (1993) Relative frequency of heavy drinking and the risk of alcohol dependence. *Addiction* **88**, 1509–18.

Dawson D.A., Grant B.F., Stinson F.S., and Chou P.S. (2004) Toward the attainment of low-risk drinking goals: A 10-year progress report. *Alcoholism: Clinical and Experimental Research* **28**, 1371–8.

Decoster A. (2005) How progressive are indirect taxes in Russia? *Economics of Transition* **13**, 705–29.

De Crespigny C., Vincent N., and Ask A. (1998) *Young women and drinking*, Vol. 1. Adelaide, Australia: The Flinders University of South Australia School of Nursing.

Dee T.S. (1999) State alcohol policies, teen drinking and traffic fatalities. *Journal of Public Economics* **72**, 289–315.

Dee T.S. (2001) Alcohol abuse and economic conditions: Evidence from repeated cross-sections of individual-level data. *Health Economics* **10**, 257–70.

DeJong W. and Langford L.M. (2002) A typology for campus-based alcohol prevention: Moving toward environmental management strategies. *Journal of Studies on Alcohol* Suppl. 14, 140–7.

DeJong W. and Russell A. (1995) MADD's position on alcohol advertising: A response to Marshall and Oleson. *Journal of Public Health Policy* **16**, 231–8.

Delaney H., Kunitz S., Zhao H., Woodall W., Westerberg V., Rogers E., and Wheeler D.R. (2005) Variations in jail sentences and the probability of re-arrest for driving while intoxicated. *Traffic Injury Prevention* **6**, 105–9.

Demers A. (1997) When at risk?: Drinking contexts and heavy drinking in the Montreal adult population. *Contemporary Drug Problems* **24**, 449–71.

Demers A., Kairouz S., Adlaf E.M., Gliksman L., Newton-Taylor B., and Marchand A. (2002) Multilevel analysis of situational drinking among Canadian undergraduates. *Social Science and Medicine* **55**, 415–24.

Demers A., Room R., and Bourgault C. (eds) (2001) *Surveys of drinking patterns and problems in seven developing countries*. WHO/MSD/MSB/01.2. Geneva: WHO Department of Mental Health and Substance Dependence.

Dent C.W., Grube J.W., and Biglan A. (2005) Community level alcohol availability and enforcement of possession laws as predictors of youth drinking. *Preventive Medicine* **40**, 355–62.

Derks J.T.M., Marten J., Hoekstra J., and Kaplan C.D. (1998) Integrating care, cure and control: The drug treatment system in The Netherlands. In: Klingemann H. and Hunt G. (eds), *Drug treatment systems in an international perspective: Drugs, demons and delinquents*, pp. 81–93. London: SAGE Publications.

Derweduwen P., Brichet M., and Wagner H.B. (2003) *Designated driver campaigns against drink-driving in Europe 2003*. Belgian Road Safety Institute. Available at: http://www.efrd.org/communication/docs/Drink-Driving_Campaigns.pdf (accessed 13 July 2009).

Desapriya E.B.R., Iwase N., Brussoni M., Shimizu S., and Belayneh T.N. (2003) International policies on alcohol impaired driving: Are legal blood alcohol concentration (BAC) limits in motorized countries compatible with the scientific evidence? *Nihon Arukoru Yakubutsu Igakkai* (Japanese Journal of Alcohol Studies and Drug Dependence) **38**, 83–102.

Desapriya E.B.R., Shimizu S., Pike I., Subzwari S., and Scime G. (2007) Impact of lowering the legal blood alcohol concentration limit to 0.03 on male, female and teenage drivers involved alcohol-related crashes in Japan. *International Journal of Injury Control and Safety Promotion* **14**, 181–7.

Deutsche Bundesregierung (2005) Bericht der bundesregierung uber die auswirkungen des alkopopsteuergesetzes auf den alkoholkonsum von jugendlichen unter 18 jahren sowie die marktentwicklung von alkopops und vergleichbaren getranken (Report of the federal government on the effects of alcopop taxes on alcohol consumption of young people under 18 years as well as the market development of alcopops and comparable beverages). Koln: Bundeszentrale fur gesundheitliche Aufklarung Available from: http://www.bzga.de/pdf. php?id=7af8a23ce8cb7787afc0b9165edd69fd (accessed 9 July 2009).

DeYoung D.J. (1997) An evaluation of the effectiveness of alcohol treatment, driver license actions and jail terms in reducing drunk driving recidivism in California. *Addiction* **92**, 989–97.

DeYoung D.J. (2002) An evaluation of the implementation of ignition interlock in California. *Journal of Safety Research* **33**, 473–82.

DeYoung D.J., Tashima H.N., and Maston S.V. (2005) An evaluation of the effectiveness of ignition interlock in California. In: Marques P.R. (ed.), *Alcohol ignition interlock devices. Volume II: Research, policy, and program status 2005*, pp. 42–52. Oosterhout, The Netherlands: International Council on Alcohol, Drugs and Traffic Safety.

Di Castelnuovo A., Costanzo S., Bagnardi V., Donati M.B., Iacoviello L., and de Gaetano G. (2006) Alcohol dosing and total mortality in men and women: An updated meta-analysis of 34 prospective studies. *Archives of Internal Medicine* **166**, 2437–45.

Dielman T.E. (1995) School-based research on the prevention of adolescent alcohol use and misuse: Methodological issues and advances. In: Boyd G.M., Howard J., and Zucker R.A. (eds) *Alcohol problems among adolescents: Current directions in prevention research*, pp. 125–46. Hillsdale, NJ: Erlbaum.

Dill P. and Wells-Parker E. (2006) Court-mandated treatment for convicted drinking drivers. *Alcohol Research and Health* **29**, 41–8.

Dinh-Zarr T., Goss C., Heitman E., Roberts I., and DiGuiseppi C. (2004) Interventions for preventing injuries in problem drinkers. *Cochrane Database Systematic Reviews*, Issue 2. Art. No. CD001857. doi: 10.1002/14651858.CD001857.pub2 CD001857.

Distilled Spirits Council of the United States (2007) Economic contributions of the distilled spirits industry. Available at: http://www.discus.org/ economics/ (accessed 23 June 2009).

Ditter S.M., Elder R.W., Shults R.A., Sleet D.A., Compton R., Nichols J.L., and the Task Force on Community Preventive Services. (2005) Effectiveness of designated driver programs for reducing alcohol-impaired driving: A systematic review. *American Journal of Preventive Medicine* **28**(Suppl. 5), 280–7.

Donaldson S.I., Graham J.W., Piccinin A.M., and Hansen W.B. (1997) Resistance-skills training and onset of alcohol use: Evidence for beneficial and potentially harmful effects in public schools and private Catholic schools. In: Marlatt G.A and VandenBos G.R. (eds), *Addictive behaviors: Readings on etiology, prevention, and treatment*, pp. 215–38. Washington, DC: American Psychological Association.

Donnar R. and Jakee K. (2004) Australian beer wars and pub demand: How vertical restraints improved the drinking experience. *Applied Economics* **36**, 1613–22.

Donohue B., Allen D.N, Maurer A., Ozols J., and DeStefano G. (2004) A controlled evaluation of two prevention programs in reducing alcohol use among college students at low and high risk for alcohol related problems. *Journal of Alcohol and Drug Education* **48**, 13–33.

Dresser J. and Gliksman L. (1998) Comparing statewide alcohol server training systems. *Pharmacology, Biochemistry, and Behavior* **61**, 150.

Dring C. and Hope A. (2001) *The impact of alcohol advertising on teenagers in Ireland.* Dublin, Ireland: Health Promotion Unit, Department of Health and Children.

Drummond D.C. (2000) UK Government announces first major relaxation in the alcohol licensing laws for nearly a century: Drinking in the UK goes 24–7. *Addiction* **95**, 997–8.

Drummond M.F., O'Brien B., Stoddart G.L., and Torrance G.W. (1997) *Methods for the economic evaluation of health care programmes*, 2nd ed. Oxford: Oxford University Press.

Duailibi S., Pinsky I., and Laranjeira R. (2007a) Prevalence of drinking and driving in a city of Southeastern Brazil. *Revista de Saúde Públic* **41**, 1058–61.

Duailibi S., Ponicki W., Grube J., Pinsky I., Laranjeira R., and Raw M. (2007b) The effect of restricting opening hours on alcohol-related violence. *American Journal of Public Health* **97**, 2276–80.

Dubois G., Got C., Gremy F., Hirsch A., and Tubiana M. (1989) Non au ministere de la maladie! (No to a ministry office for disease!) Le Monde 15 November.

Duff C. (2003) Alcohol marketing and the media: What are alcohol advertisements telling us? *Media International Australia* **108**, 13–21.

Duffy J.C. and Pinot De Moira A.C. (1996) Changes in licensing law in England and Wales and indicators of alcohol-related problems. *Addiction Research and Theory* **4**, 245–71.

Duffy J.C. and Plant M.A. (1986) Scotland's liquor licensing changes: an assessment. *British Medical Journal (Clinical Research Edition)* **292**, 36–9.

Duffy M. (2001) Advertising in consumer allocation models: Choice of functional form. *Applied Economics* **33**, 437–56.

Duignan P., Casswell S., and Stewart L. (1993) Evaluating community projects: Conceptual and methodological issues illustrated from the Community Action Project and the Liquor Licensing Project in New Zealand. In: Greenfield T. and Zimmerman R. (eds), *Experiences with community action projects: New research in the prevention of alcohol and other drug problems*, pp. 20–30. CSAP Prevention Monograph 14. Rockville, MD: US Department of Health and Human Services.

Eck J.E. and Weisburd D. (1995) Crime places in crime theory. In: Eck J.E. and Weisburd D. (eds), *Crime and place: Crime prevention studies*, Vol. 4, pp. 1–34. Monsey, NY: Criminal Justice Press.

Eckardt M.J., File S.E., Gessa G.L., Grant K.A., Guerri C., Hoffman P.L., Kalant H., Koob G.F., Li T.-K., and Tabakoff B. (1998) Effects of moderate alcohol consumption on the central nervous system. *Alcoholism: Clinical and Experimental Research* **22**, 998–1040.

Econtech (2004) *Modelling health-related reforms to taxation of alcoholic beverages.* Canberra: Econtech.

Edwards G. (1998) Should the drinks industry sponsor research?: If the drinks industry does not clean up its act, pariah status is inevitable. *British Medical Journal* **317**, 336.

Edwards G. (2000) *Alcohol: The ambiguous molecule.* Harmondsworth, UK: Penguin.

Edwards G. and Gross M.M. (1976) Alcohol dependence: Provisional description of a clinical syndrome. *British Medical Journal* **1**, 1058–61.

Edwards G. and Holder H.D. (2000) The alcohol supply: Its importance to public health and safety, and essential research questions. *Addiction* **95**, S621–7.

Edwards G., Anderson P., Babor T.F., Casswell S., Ferrence R., Giesbrecht N., Godfrey C., Holder H.D., Lemmens P., Mäkelä K., Midanik L.T., Norström T., Österberg E., Romelsjö A.,

Room R., Simpura J., and Skog O.-J. (1994) *Alcohol Policy and the Public Good.* Oxford: Oxford University Press.

Edwards G., Anderson P., Babor T.F., Casswell S., Ferrence R., Giesbrecht N., Godfrey C., Holder H.D., Lemmens P., Mäkelä K., Midanik L.T., Norström T., Österberg E., Romelsjö A., Room R., Simpura J., and Skog O.-J. (1995) *A summary of alcohol policy and the public good, a guide for action.* St Ives, UK: EUROCARE (Advocacy for the Prevention of Alcohol Related Harm in Europe) and WHO Europe Office.

Edwards G., Marshall E.J., and Cook C.C.H. (2003) *The treatment of drinking problems: A guide for the helping professions,* 4th edn. Cambridge, MA: Cambridge University Press.

Eisenberg D. (2003) Evaluating the effectiveness of policies related to drunk driving. *Journal of Policy Analysis and Management* **22**, 249–74.

Elder R.W., Shults R.A., Sleet D.A., Nichols J.L., Zaza S., and Thompson R.S. (2002) Effectiveness of sobriety checkpoints for reducing alcohol-involved crashes. *Traffic Injury Prevention* **3**, 266–74.

Elder R. W., Shults R.A., Sleet D.A., Nichols J.L., Thompson R.S., Rajab W., and the Task Force on Community Preventive Services (2004) Effectiveness of mass media campaigns for reducing drinking and driving and alcohol-involved crashes: A systematic review. *American Journal of Preventive Medicine* **27**, 57–65.

Elder, R. W., Nichols, J. L., Shults, R. A., Sleet, D. A., Barrios, L. C., Compton, R., and the Task Force on Community Preventive Services (2005) Effectiveness of school-based programs for reducing drinking and driving and riding with drinking drivers: A systematic review. *American Journal of Preventive Medicine* **28**(Suppl. 5), 288–304.

Eliany M., Giesbrecht N., Nelson M., Wellman B., and Wortley S. (1992) *Alcohol and other drug use by Canadians: A national alcohol and other drugs survey (1989) technical report.* Ottawa: Health and Welfare Canada.

Ellickson P., Collins R., Hambarsoomians K., and McCaffrey D. (2005) Does alcohol advertising promote adolescent drinking? Results from a longitudinal assessment. *Addiction* **100**, 235–46.

Engels R.C.M.E., Knibbe R.A., and Drop M.J. (1999) Visiting public drinking places: An explorative study into the functions of pub-going for late adolescents. *Substance Use and Misuse* **34**, 1261–80.

English D., Holman D., Milne E., Winter M., Hulse G., Codde G., Bower C., Corti B., de Klerk C., Lewin G., Knuiman M., Kurinczuk J., and Rayan G. (1995) *The quantification of drug caused morbidity and mortality in Australia, 1992.* Canberra: Commonwealth Department of Human Services.

Engs R.C., Diebold B.A., and Hanson D.J. (1994) Drinking patterns and problems of a national sample of college students, 1994. *Journal of Alcohol and Drug Education* **41**, 13–33.

Ennett S.T., Tobler N.S., Ringwalt C.L., and Flewelling R.L. (1994) How effective is Drug Abuse Resistance Education?: A meta-analysis of project DARE outcome evaluations. *American Journal of Public Health* **84**, 1394–1401.

Erbring L., Goldenberg E., and Miller A. (1980) Front page news and real world cues: A new look at agenda setting by the media. *American Journal of Political Science* **24**, 16–49.

Euromonitor (2005) India. Available at: http://www.euromonitor.com.

Euromonitor (2006) Alcoholic Drinks in China. Available at: http://www.euromonitor.com (accessed 20 July 2006).

European Commission (2007) Audiovisual Media Services Directive (AVMSD), Available at: http://ec.europa.eu/avpolicy/reg/avms/index_en.htm (accessed 14 April 2009).

European Commission (2009) *Excise duty tables, January 2009.* Brussels, Belgium: European Commission. Available at: http://ec.europa.eu/taxation_customs/resources/documents/taxation/excise_duties/alcoholic_beverages/rates/excise_duties-part_I_alcohol-en.pdf (accessed 6 July 2009).

Evans R.I., Rozelle R.M., Mittlemark M.B., Hansen W.B., Bane A.L., and Havis J. (1978) Deterring the onset of smoking in children: Knowledge of immediate physiological effects and coping peer pressure, media pressure, and parental modeling. *Journal of Applied Social Psychology* **8**, 126–35.

Evans W.N., Neville D., and Graham J.D. (1991) General deterrence of drunk driving: Evaluation of recent American policies. *Risk Analysis* **11**, 279–89.

Ezzati M., Lopez A.D., Rodgers A., and Murray C.J.L. (2004) *Comparative quantification of health risks: Global and regional burden of disease attributable to selected major risk factors.* Geneva: World Health Organization.

Fager J.H. and Melnyk B.M. (2004) The effectiveness of intervention studies to decrease alcohol use in college undergraduate students: An integrative analysis. *Worldviews on Evidence-Based Nursing* **1**, 102–19.

Fahrenkrug H. and Rehm J. (1995) Drinking contexts and leisure-time activities in the prephase of alcohol-related road accidents by young Swiss residents. *Sucht* **41**, 169–80.

Farrell S. (1985) Review of national policy measures to prevent alcohol-related problems. Geneva: World Health Organization.

Farrell S., Manning W.G., and Finch M.D. (2003) Alcohol dependence and the price of alcoholic beverages. *Journal of Health Economics* **22**, 117–47.

Fedler F., Philips M., Raker P., Schefsky D., and Soluri J. (1994) Network commercial promote legal drugs: Outnumber anti-drug PSAs 45-to-1. *Journal of Drug Education* **24**, 291–302.

Fell J.C. and Voas, R.B. (2009) Reducing illegal blood alcohol limits for driving: Effects on traffic safety. In: Verster J.C., Pandi-Perumal S.R., Ramaekers J.G., and de Gier J.J. (eds), *Drugs, Driving, and Traffic Safety*, pp. 414–37. Basel: Birkhäuser.

Fell J.C., Ferguson S.A., Williams A.F., and Fields M. (2003) Why are sobriety checkpoints not widely adopted as an enforcement strategy in the United States? Accident Analysis and Prevention **35**, 897–902.

Fell J.C., Fisher D.A., Voas R.B., Blackman K., and Tippetts A.S. (2009) The impact of underage drinking laws on alcohol-related fatal crashes of young drivers. *Alcoholism: Clinical and Experimental Research* **33**, 1208–19.

Felson M. (1995) Those who discourage crime. In: Eck J.E. and Weisburd D. (eds), *Crime and place: Crime prevention studies*, Vol. 4, pp. 63–6. Monsey, NY: Criminal Justice Press.

Felson M., Berends R., Richardson B., and Veno A. (1997) Reducing pub hopping and related crime. In: Homel R. (ed.), *Policing for prevention: Reducing crime, public intoxication and injury*, Vol. 7, pp. 115–32. Monsey, NY: Criminal Justice Press.

Fillmore K.M., Hartka E., Johnstone B.M., Leino E.V., Motoyoshi M., and Temple M.T. (1991a) Meta-analysis of life course variation in drinking: The Collaborative Alcohol-Related Longitudinal Project. *British Journal of Addiction* **86**, 1221–68.

Fillmore K.M., Hartka E., Johnstone B.M., Leino E.V., Motoyoshi M., and Temple M.T. (1991b) The Collaborative Alcohol-Related Longitudinal Project: Preliminary results from a meta-analysis of drinking behavior in multiple longitudinal studies. *British Journal of Addiction* **86**, 1203–10.

Fillmore K., Stockwell T.R., Kerr W., Chikritzhs T. and Bostrom A. (2006) Moderate alcohol use and reduced mortality risk: Systematic error in prospective studies. *Addiction Research and Theory* 14, 101–32.

Finney J.W., Hahn A.C., and Moos R.H. (1996) The effectiveness of inpatient and outpatient treatment for alcohol abuse: The need to focus on mediators and moderators of setting effects. *Addiction* 91, 1773–96.

Fleming M.F., Krupitsky E., Tsoy M., Zvartau E., Brazhenko N., Jakubowiak W., and McCaul M.E. (2006) Alcohol and drug use disorders: HIV status and drug resistance in a sample of Russian TB patients. *International Journal of Tuberculosis and Lung Disease* 10, 565–70.

Flora J., Maibach E., and Maccoby N. (1989) The role of the media across four levels of health promotion intervention. *Annual Review of Public Health* 10, 181–201.

Flowers N., Naimi T., Brewer R., Elder R., Shults R., and Jiles R. (2008) Patterns of alcohol consumption and alcohol-impaired driving in the United States. *Alcoholism: Clinical and Experimental Research* 32, 639–44.

Fogarty J. (2006) The nature of the demand for alcohol: understanding elasticity. *British Food Journal* 108, 316–32.

Foran H.M. and O'Leary K.D. (2008) Alcohol and intimate partner violence: A meta-analytic review. *Clinical Psychology Review* 38, 1222–34.

Fors S.W. and Rojek D.G. (1999) The effect of victim impact panels on DUI/DWI rearrest rates: A twelve month follow-up. *Journal of Studies on Alcohol* 60, 514–20.

Forsyth A.J.M. (2008) Banning glassware from nightclubs in Glasgow (Scotland): Observed impacts, compliance and patron's views. *Alcohol and Alcoholism* 43, 111–17.

Fos P.J. and Fine D.J. (2000) *Designing health care for populations*. San Francisco: Jossey-Bass.

Foss R.D., Marchetti L.J., and Holladay K.A. (2001) *Development and evaluation of a comprehensive program to reduce drinking and impaired driving*. Washington, DC: US Department of Transportation, National Highway Traffic Safety.

Foxcroft D.R. (2006) *Alcohol misuse prevention for young people: A rapid review of recent evidence*. WHO Technical Report. Geneva: World Health Organization.

Foxcroft D.R., Lister-Sharp D., and Lowe G. (1997) Alcohol misuse prevention for young people: A systematic review reveals methodological concerns and lack of reliable evidence of effectiveness. *Addiction* 92, 531–7.

Foxcroft D.R., Ireland D., Lowe G., and Breen R. (2002) Primary prevention for alcohol misuse in young people. *Cochrane Database of Systematic Reviews*. Issue 3. Art No. CD003024. doi: 10.1002?14651858.CD003024.

Foxcroft D.R., Ireland D., Lister-Sharp D., Lowe G., and Breen R. (2003) Long-term primary prevention for alcohol misuse in young people: A systematic review. *Addiction* 98, 397–411.

Franke G. and Wilcox G. (1987) Alcoholic beverage advertising and consumption in the United States, 1964–1984. *Journal of Advertising* 16, 22–30.

Freeman D.G. (2001) Beer and the business cycle. *Applied Economics Letters* 8, 51–4.

Freeman J., Liossis P., and David N. (2006) Deterrence, defiance, and deviance: An investigation into a group of recidivist drink drivers' self-reported offending behaviors. *Australian and New Zealand Journal of Criminology* 39, 1–20.

Freisthler B. and Weiss R.E. (2008) Using Bayesian space-time models to understand the substance use environment and risk for being referred to Child Protective Services. *Substance Use and Misuse* 43, 239–51.

Fromme K. and Corbin W. (2004) Prevention of heavy drinking and associated negative consequences among mandated and voluntary college students. *Journal of Consulting and Clinical Psychology* **72**, 1038–49.

Fu H. and Goldman N. (2000) Association between health-related behaviours and the risk of divorce in the USA. *Journal of Biosocial Science* **32**, 63–88.

Galanter M. (1997) Recent developments in alcoholism, Vol. 13, Alcohol and Violence. New York: Plenum Press.

Gallet C. (2007) The demand for alcohol: A meta-analysis of elasticities. *Australian Journal of Agricultural and Resource Economics* **51**, 121–36.

Gates P., Copeland J., Stevenson R., and Dillon P. (2007) The influence of product packaging on young people's palatability rating for RTDs and other alcoholic beverages. *Alcohol and Alcoholism* **42**, 138–42.

Geller E.S., Russ N.W., and Delphos W.A. (1987) Does server intervention training make a difference?: An empirical field evaluation. *Alcohol, Health and Research World* **11**, 64–9.

Gerbner G. (1995) Alcohol in American culture. In: Martin S. (ed.), *The effects of the mass media on the use and abuse of alcohol*, pp. 3–29. Bethesda, MD: NIAAA, US Department of Health and Human Services.

Germer P. (1990) Alcohol and the single market: Juridical aspects. *Contemporary Drug Problems* **17**, 481–96.

Ghalioungui P. (1979) Fermented beverages in antiquity. In: Gastineau C.F., Darby W.J., and Turner T.B. (eds), *Fermented food beverages in nutrition*, pp. 3–19. New York: Academic Press.

Giesbrecht N. (2000) Roles of commercial interests in alcohol policies: Recent developments in North America. *Addiction* **95** (Suppl. 4), 581–95S.

Giesbrecht N. (2007) Reducing alcohol-related damage in populations: Rethinking the roles of education and persuasion interventions. *Addiction* **101**, 1345–9.

Giesbrecht N. and Douglas R.R. (1990) The demonstration project and comprehensive community programming: Dilemmas in preventing alcohol-related problems. Paper presented at the International Conference on Evaluating Community Prevention Strategies: Alcohol and Other Drugs, San Diego, CA.

Giesbrecht N. and Greenfield T.K. (1999) Public opinions on alcohol policy issues: A comparison of American and Canadian surveys. *Addiction* **94**, 521–31.

Giesbrecht N. and Hammond D. (2005) *Warning labels on alcoholic beverages: An overview.* Ottawa, Canada: Health Canada.

Giesbrecht N. and Kavanagh L. (1999) Public opinion and alcohol policy: Comparison of two Canadian general population surveys. *Drug and Alcohol Review* **18**, 7–19.

Giesbrecht N., Conley P., Denniston R., Gliksman L., Holder H.D., Pederson A., Room R., and Shain M. (eds) (1990) *Research, action, and the community: Experiences in the prevention of alcohol and other drug problems.* Rockville, MD: Office for Substance Abuse Prevention.

Giesbrecht N., Ialomiteanu A., Room R., and Anglin L. (2001) Trends in public opinion on alcohol policy measures: Ontario 1989–1998. *Journal of Studies on Alcohol* **62**, 142–9.

Giesbrecht N., Demers A., Ogborne A., Room R., Stoduto G., and Lindquist E. (eds) (2006) *Sober reflections: Commerce, public health, and the evolution of alcohol policy in Canada, 1980–2000.* Montreal, Canada: McGill-Queen's University Press.

Ginsburg E.S. (1999) Estrogen, alcohol and breast cancer risk. *Journal of Steroid Biochemistry and Molecular Biology* **69**, 299–306.

Ginsburg E.S., Mello N.K., and Mendelson J.H. (1996) Effects of alcohol ingestion on estrogens in postmenopausal women. *Journal of the American Medical Association* **276**, 1747–51.

Gliksman L., McKenzie D., Single E., Douglas R., Brunet S., and Moffatt K. (1993) The role of alcohol providers in prevention: An evaluation of a server intervention programme. *Addiction* **88**, 1189–97.

Gliksman L., Douglas R.R., Rylett M., and Narbonne-Fortin C. (1995) Reducing problems through municipal alcohol policies: The Canadian experiment in Ontario. *Drugs: Education, Prevention and Policy* **2**, 105–18.

Gliksman L., Demers A., Adlaf E.M., Newton-Taylor B., and Schmidt K. (2000) *Canadian campus survey, 1998.* Toronto, Canada: Centre for Addiction and Mental Health.

Global Road Safety Partnership (2007) *Drinking and driving: A road safety manual for decision-makers and practitioners.* Geneva: Global Road Safety Partnership.

Gmel G., Rehm J., and Ghazinouri A. (1998) Alcohol and suicide in Switzerland: An aggregate-level analysis. *Drug and Alcohol Review* **17**, 27–37.

Gmel G., Rehm J., Room R., and Greenfield T.K. (2000) Dimensions of alcohol-related social harm in survey research. *Journal of Substance Abuse* **12**, 113–38.

Gmel G., Klingemann S., Müller R., and Brenner D. (2001) Revisiting the preventive paradox: The Swiss case. *Addiction* **96**, 273–84.

Gmel G., Wicki M., Rehm J., and Heeb J.-L. (2008) Estimating regression to the mean and true effects of an intervention in a four-wave panel study. *Addiction* **103**, 32–41.

Godfrey C. (1988) Licensing and the demand for alcohol. *Applied Economics* **20**, 1541–58.

Goerdt A., Koplan J.P., Robine J.M., Thuriaux M.C., and van Ginneken J.K. (1996) Non-fatal health outcomes: Concepts, instruments and indicators. In: Murray C.J.L. and Lopez A.D. (eds), *The global burden of disease: A comprehensive assessment of mortality and disability from diseases, injuries and risk factors in 1990 and projected to 2020*, pp. 201–46. Boston: Harvard School of Public Health.

Gómez-Talegón M. and Alvarez F. (2006) Road traffic accidents among alcohol-dependent patients: The effect of treatment. *Accident Analysis and Prevention* **38**, 201–7.

Gonzalez G.M. and Clement V.V. (eds) (1994) *Research and intervention: Preventing substance abuse in higher education.* Washington, DC: US Department of Education.

Goodman A.C., Nishiura E., and Humphreys R.S. (1997) Cost and usage impacts of treatment initiation: A comparison of alcoholism and drug abuse treatments. *Alcoholism: Clinical and Experimental Research* **21**, 931–8.

Goodstadt M. and Flynn L. (1993) Protecting oneself and protecting others: Refusing service, providing warnings, and other strategies for alcohol warnings. *Contemporary Drug Problems* **20**, 277–91.

Gordon R., McDermott L., Stead M. and Angus K. (2006) The effectiveness of social marketing interventions for health improvement: What's the evidence? *Public Health* **120**, 1133–9.

Gorman D.M. (1995) Are school-based resistance skills training programs effective in preventing alcohol abuse? *Journal of Alcohol and Drug Education* **41**, 74–98.

Gorman D.M. (1996) Do school-based social skills training programs prevent alcohol use among young people? *Addiction Research* **4**, 191–210.

Gorman D.M. (1998) The irrelevance of evidence in the development of school-based drug prevention policy, 1986–1996. *Evaluation Review* **22**, 118–46.

Gossop M. (1995) The treatment mapping survey: A descriptive study of drug and alcohol treatment responses in 23 countries. *Drug and Alcohol Dependence* **39**, 7–14.

Graham J.W., Collins L.M., Wulgalter S.E., Chung N.K., and Hansen W.B. (1991) Modeling transitions in latent stage-sequential processes: A substance use prevention example. *Journal of Clinical and Consulting Psychology* **59**, 48–57.

Graham K. (1999) *Safer bars: Assessing and reducing risks of violence*. Toronto, Canada: Centre for Addiction and Mental Health.

Graham K. (2000) Preventive interventions for on-premise drinking: A promising but underresearched area of prevention. *Contemporary Drug Problems* **27**, 593–668.

Graham K. (2009) They fight because we let them!: Applying a situational crime prevention model to barroom violence. *Drug and Alcohol Review* **28**, 103–9.

Graham K. and Bernards S. (2009) Canada. In: P. Hadfield (ed.), *Nightlife and crime: Social order and governance in international perspective*, pp. 237–60. Oxford: Oxford University Press.

Graham K. and Homel R. (2008) *Raising the bar: Preventing aggression in and around bars, pubs and clubs*. Cullompton, UK: Willan.

Graham K. and Wells S. (2001) Aggression among young adults in the social context of the bar. *Addiction Research* **9**, 193–219.

Graham K. and Wells S. (2003) "Somebody's gonna get their head kicked in tonight!" Aggression among young males in bars: A question of values. *British Journal of Criminology* **43**, 546–66.

Graham K., Schmidt G., and Gillis K. (1996) Circumstances when drinking leads to aggression: An overview of research findings. *Contemporary Drug Problems* **23**, 493–557.

Graham K., Leonard K.E., Room R., Wild T.C., Pihl R.O., Bois C., and Single E. (1998) Current directions in research in understanding and preventing intoxicated aggression. *Addiction* **93**, 659–76.

Graham K., West P., and Wells S. (2000) Evaluating theories of alcohol-related aggression using observations of young adults in bars. *Addiction* **95**, 847–63.

Graham K., Osgood D.W., Zibrowski E., Purcell J., Gliksman L., Leonard K., Perkanen K., Saltz R.F., and Toomey T.L. (2004) The effect of the Safer Bars programme on physical aggression in bars: Results of a randomized controlled trial. *Drug and Alcohol Review* **23**, 31–41.

Graham K., Bernards S., Osgood D.W., Homel R., and Purcell J. (2005a) Guardians and handlers: The role of bar staff in preventing and managing aggression. *Addiction* **100**, 755–66.

Graham K., Jelley J., and Purcell J. (2005b) Training bar staff in preventing and managing aggression in licensed premises. *Journal of Substance Use* **10**, 48–61.

Graham K., Bernards S., Osgood D.W., and Wells S. (2006a) Bad nights or bad bars? Multilevel analysis of environmental predictors of aggression in late-night large-capacity bars and clubs. *Addiction* **101**, 1569–80.

Graham K., Osgood D. W., Wells S., and Stockwell T. (2006b) To what extent is intoxication associated with aggression in bars? A multilevel analysis. *Journal of Studies on Alcohol* **67**, 382–90.

Graham K. and Braun, K., with Bois C., et al. (2008) *Safer bars trainer's guide*, 2nd edn. Toronto: Centre for Addiction and Mental Health.

Grant B.F., Dawson D.A., Stonson F.s., Chou S.P., Dufour M.C., and Pickering R.P. (2004) The 12-month prevalence and trends in DSM-IV alcohol abuse and dependence: United States, 1991–1992 and 2001–2002. *Drug and Alcohol Dependence* **74**, 223–34.

Graves K. (1993) Evaluation of the alcohol warning label: A comparison of the United States and Ontario, Canada in 1990 and 1991. *Journal of Public Policy and Marketing* **12**, 19–29.

Gray D., Saggers S., Atkinson D., Sputore B., and Bourbon D. (1998) *Evaluation of the Tennant Creek liquor licensing restrictions.* Perth, Australia: National Centre for Research into the Prevention of Drug Abuse, Curtin University of Technology.

Greater London Authority (2002) *Late night London: Planning and managing the late-*night *economy.* SDS Technical Report 6. London, UK: Greater London Authority.

Greenfield T. (1995) What's in a problem?: Type and seriousness of harmful effects of drinking on health, based on a pilot US national telephone survey. Paper presented at the 21st annual Alcohol Epidemiology Symposium, Kettil Bruun Society, Porto, June 5–9.

Greenfield T.K. (1997) Warning labels: Evidence of harm-reduction from long-term American surveys. In: Plant M., Single E., and Stockwell T. (eds), *Alcohol: Minimizing the Harm,* pp. 105–25. London: Free Association Books.

Greenfield T.K. and Kaskutas L.A. (1998) Five years' exposure to alcohol warning label messages and their impacts: Evidence from diffusion analysis. *Applied Behavioral Science Review* **6**, 39- 68.

Greenfield T.K. and Rogers J.D. (1999) Who drinks most of the alcohol in the US?: The policy implications. *Journal of Studies on Alcohol* **60**, 78–89.

Greenfield T.K. and Zimmerman R. (eds) (1993) *Second international research symposium on experiences with community action projects for the prevention of alcohol and other drug problems.* Washington, DC: US Department of Health and Human Services.

Greenfield T.K., Giesbrecht N., Johnson S.P., Kaskutas L.A., Anglin L.T., Kavanagh L., Room R., and MacKenzie B. (1999) *US federal alcohol control policy development: A manual.* Berkeley, CA: Alcohol Research Group.

Greenfield T.K., Graves K.L., and Kaskutas L.A. (1993) Alcohol warning labels for prevention: National survey results. *Alcohol, Health and Research World* **17**, 67–75.

Gregory B. (2001) College alcohol and life skills study with student-athletes. Doctoral dissertation. Boca Raton: Florida Atlantic University.

Grieshaber-Otto J., Sinclair S., and Schacter N. (2000) Impacts of international trade, services and investment treaties on alcohol regulation. *Addiction* **95**, S491–504.

Grieshaber-Otto J. and Schacter N. (2002) The GATS: Impacts of the international 'services' treaty on health based alcohol regulation. *Nordisk alcohol- & narkotikatidskrift* **19**, 50–68.

Grieshaber-Otto J., Schacter N., and Sinclair S. (2006) Dangerous cocktail: International trade treaties, alcohol policy, and public health. Draft report prepared for the World Health Organization.

Grossman M. and Markowitz S. (1999) *Alcohol regulation and violence on college campuses.* NBER Working Paper 7129. Cambridge, MA: National Bureau of Economic Research.

Grossman M., Chaloupka F.J., Saffer H., and Laixuthai A. (1994) Effects of alcohol price policy on youth: A summary of economic research. *Journal of Research on Adolescence* **4**, 347–64.

Grossman M., Kaestner R., and Markowitz S. (2004) *An investigation of the effects of alcohol policies on youth STDs.* NBER Working Paper W10949. New York: National Bureau of Economic Research.

Grube J.W. (1993) Alcohol portrayals and alcohol advertising on television. *Alcohol, Health and Research World* **17**, 61–6.

Grube J.W. (1995) Television alcohol portrayals, alcohol advertising and alcohol expectancies among children and adolescents. In: Martin S.E. (ed.), *The effects of the mass media on the use and abuse of alcohol*, pp. 105–21. Bethesda, MD: US Dept of Health & Human Sciences.

Grube J.W. (1997) Preventing sales of alcohol to minors: Results from a community trial. *Addiction* **92** (Suppl. 2), S251–60.

Grube J.W. (2007) Alcohol regulation and traffic safety: An overview. In: *Transportation Research Circular, E-C123*, pp. 13–30. Available at: http://onlinepubs.trb.org/onlinepubs/circulars/ec123.pdf (accessed 13 July 2009).

Grube J.W. (in press) Environmental approaches to preventing adolescent drinking. In: Scheier L. (ed.), *Handbook of drug use etiology: Theory, methods, and empirical findings*. Washington, DC: American Psychological Association.

Grube J.W. and Nygaard P. (2001) Adolescent drinking and alcohol policy. *Contemporary Drug Problems* **28**, 87–131.

Grube J.W. and Nygaard P. (2005) Alcohol policy and youth drinking: Overview of effective interventions for young people. In: Stockwell T., Gruenewald P.J., Tournbourou J., and Loxley W. (eds), *Preventing harmful substance use: The evidence base for policy and practice*, pp. 113–27. New York: Wiley.

Grube J.W. and Stewart K. (2004) Preventing impaired driving using alcohol policy. *Traffic Injury Prevention* **5**, 199–207.

Grube J.W. and Wallack L. (1994) Television beer advertising and drinking knowledge, beliefs and intentions among school children. *American Journal of Public Health* **84**, 254–9.

Gruenewald P.J. (2007) The spatial ecology of alcohol problems: Niche theory and assortative drinking. *Addiction* **102**, 870–8.

Gruenewald P.J. (2008) Why do alcohol outlets matter anyway? A look into the future. *Addiction* **103**, 1585–7.

Gruenewald P.J. and Ponicki W.R. (1995) Relationship of the retail availability of alcohol and alcohol sales to alcohol-related traffic crashes. *Accident Analysis and Prevention* **27**, 249–59.

Gruenewald P.J. and Remer L. (2006) Changes in outlet densities affect violence rates. *Alcoholism: Clinical and Experimental Research* **30**, 1184–93.

Gruenewald, P.J., Madden, P. and Janes, K. (1992) Alcohol availability and the formal power and resources of state alcohol beverage control agencies. *Alcoholism: Clinical and Experimental Research* **16**, 591–7.

Gruenewald P.J., Ponicki W.R., and Holder H.D. (1993) The relationship of outlet densities to alcohol consumption: A time series cross-sectional analysis. *Alcoholism: Clinical and Experimental Research* **17**, 38–47.

Gruenewald P.J., Mitchell P.R., and Treno A.J. (1996) Drinking and driving: Drinking patterns and drinking problems. *Addiction* **91**, 1637–49.

Gruenewald P.J., Stockwell T., Beel A., and Dyskin E.V. (1999) Beverage sales and drinking and driving: The role of on-premise drinking places. *Journal of Studies on Alcohol* **60**, 47–53.

Gruenewald P.J., Millar A.B., Ponicki W.R., and Brinkley G. (2000) Physical and economic access to alcohol: The application of geostatistical methods to small area analysis in community settings. In: Wilson R. and Dufour M. (eds), Small Area Analysis and the Epidemiology of Alcohol Problems, pp. 163–212. NIAAA Research Monograph #36. Rockville, MD: NIAAA.

Gruenewald P.J., Johnson F.W., and Treno A. (2002) Outlets, drinking and driving: A multi-level analysis of availability. *Journal of Studies on Alcohol* **63**, 460–8.

Gruenewald P.J., Ponicki W.R., Holder H.D., and Romelsjö A. (2006) Alcohol prices, beverage quality, and the demand for alcohol: Quality substitutions and price elasticities. *Alcoholism Clinical and Experimental Research* **30**, 96–105.

Gual A. and Colom J. (1997) Why has alcohol consumption declined in countries of southern Europe? *Addiction* **92** (Suppl. 1), 21–31S.

Gual A. and Colom J. (2001) From Paris to Stockholm: Where does the European Alcohol Action Plan lead to? *Addiction* **96**, 1093–6.

Gunter B., Hansen A., and Touri M. (2008) *The representation of meaning in alcohol advertising and young people's drinking.* Leicester, UK: Department of Media and Communication, University of Leicester.

Gururaj G., Girish N., and Benegal V. (2006) Burden and socio-economic impact of alcohol— The Bangalore study. Bangalore: National Institute of Mental Health and Neurosciences/ WHO-SEARO.

Gustafson R. (1993) What do experimental paradigms tell us about alcohol-related aggressive responding? *Journal of Studies on Alcohol Suppl.* **11**, 20–29S.

Gutjahr E. and Gmel G. (2001a) The social costs of alcohol consumption. In: Klingemann H. and Gmel G. (eds) *Mapping the Social Consequences of Alcohol Consumption,* pp. 133–43. Dordrecht: Kluwer.

Gutjahr E. and Gmel G. (2001b) *Die sozialen kosten des alkoholkonsums in der Schweiz: Epidemiologische grundlagen 1995–1998* (The social costs of alcohol consumption in Switzerland: epidemiological foundations 1995–1998). Forschungsbericht Nr. 36 im Auftrag des Bundesamtes für Gesundheit, Vertrag Nr. 98.000794 (8120). Lausanne, Switzerland: SFA (Schweizerische Fachstelle für Alkohol- und andere Drogenprobleme).

Gutjahr E., Gmel G., and Rehm J. (2001) The relation between average alcohol consumption and disease: An overview. *European Addiction Research* **7**, 117–27.

Gutzke D.W. (2006) *Pubs and progressives: Reinventing the public house in England 1896–1960.* Dekalb, IL: Northern Illinois UP.

Hadfield P. (2006) *Bar wars: Contesting the night in contemporary British cities.* Oxford: Oxford University Press.

Haines M.P. (1996) *Social norms approach to preventing binge drinking at colleges and universities.* Newton, MA: Higher Education Center for Alcohol and Other Drug Prevention, Department of Education.

Haines M.P. (1998) Social norms in a wellness model for health promotion in higher education. *Wellness Management* **14**, 1–10.

Haines M.P. and Spear S.F. (1996) Changing the perception of the norm: A strategy to decrease binge drinking among college students. *Journal of American College Health* **45**, 134–40.

Hajema K.-J., Knibbe R.A., and Drop M.A. (1997) Changes in alcohol consumption in a general population in The Netherlands: A 9-year follow-up study. *Addiction* **92**, 49–60.

Hall W. (1995) Changes in public perceptions of the health benefits of alcohol use, 1989 to 1994. *Australian and New Zealand Journal of Public Health* **20**, 93–5.

Hall W., Saunders J.B., Babor T.F., Aasland O.G., Amundsen A., Hodgson R., and Grant M. (1993) The structure and correlates of alcohol dependence: WHO collaborative project on the early detection of persons with harmful alcohol consumption: III. *Addiction* **88**, 1627–36.

Hamajima N, Hirose K, Tajima K, et al. (2002) Alcohol, tobacco and breast cancer—collaborative reanalysis of individual data from 53 epidemiological studies, including 58,515 women with breast cancer and 95,067 women without the disease. *British Journal of Cancer* **87**, 1234–45.

Hammurabi (2000) Code of Hammurabi. Translated by L.W. King. Available at: http://www.fordham.edu/halsall/ancient/hamcode.html (accessed 6 July 2009).

Hanewinkel R., Tanski S., and Sargent J. (2007) Exposure to alcohol use in motion pictures and teen drinking in Germany. *International Journal of Epidemiology* **36**, 1068–77.

Hansen D.J. (1992) School-based substance abuse prevention: A review of the state of the art in curriculum, 1980–1990. *Health Education Research* **7**, 403–30.

Hansen D.J. (1993) School-based alcohol prevention programmes. *Alcohol, Health and Research World* **17**, 54–61.

Hansen D.J. (1994) Prevention of alcohol use and abuse. *Preventive Medicine* **23**, 683–7.

Hansen D.J. and Graham J.W. (1991) Preventing alcohol, marijuana, and cigarette use among adolescents: Peer pressure resistance training versus establishing conservative norms. *Preventive Medicine* **20**, 414–30.

Hao W., Su Z., Liu B., Zhang K., Yang H., Chen S., Biao M. and Cui C. (2004) Drinking and drinking patterns and health status in the general population of five areas of China. *Alcohol and Alcoholism* **39**, 43–52.

Harding W.M., Caudill B.D, Moore B.A., and Frissell K.C. (2001) Do drivers drink more when they use a safe ride? *Journal of Substance Abuse* **13**, 283–90.

Harrison P.A., Fulkerson J.A., and Park E. (2000) The relative importance of social versus commercial sources in youth access to tobacco, alcohol, and other drugs. *Preventive Medicine* **31**, 39–48.

Hartling L., Wiebe N., Russell K., Petruk J., Spinola C., and Klassen T.P. (2004) Graduated driver licensing for reducing motor vehicle crashes among young drivers. *Cochrane Database Systematic Reviews*, Issue 2. Art. No. CD003300. doi: 10.1002/14651858. CD003300.pub2.

Hastings G. and Haywood A. (1991) Social marketing and communication in health promotion. *Health Promotion International* **6**, 135–45.

Hastings G., Stead M., McDermott L., Forsyth A., MacKintosh A.M., Rayner M., Godfrey C., Caraher M., and Angus K. (2003) Review of research on the effects of food promotion to children. Glasgow, UK: Centre for Social Marketing, University of Strathclyde.

Hastings G., Anderson S., Cooke E., and Gordon R. (2005) Alcohol marketing and young people's drinking: A review of the research. *Journal of Public Health Policy* **26**, 296–311.

Hauritz M., Homel R., McIlwain G., Burrows T., and Townsley M. (1998a) Reducing violence in licensed venues through community safety action projects: The Queensland experience. *Contemporary Drug Problems* **25**, 511–51.

Hauritz M., Homel R., Townsley M., Burrows T., and McIlwain G. (eds) (1998b) *An evaluation of the local government safety action projects in Cairns, Townsville and Mackay: A report to the Queensland Department of Health and the Criminology Research Council.* Australia: Griffith University, Centre for Crime Policy and Public Safety; School of Justice Administration.

Haustein S., Pohlmann U., and Schreckenberg D. (2004) *Inhalts- und zielgruppenanalyse von alkoholwerbung im Deutschen fernsehen* (Content and target group analysis of alcohol advertising in German television). Bonn, Germany: Bundesministeriums für Gesundheit und Soziale Sicherung (Federal Ministry of Health).

Hawkins T.E., Dreyer C.B., and Cooper E.J. (1977) *Analysis of public information and education 1975–1976*. Analytic Study No. 7. San Antonio, TX: San Antonio Alcohol Safety Action Project.

Hawks D. (1990) The watering down of Australia's health policy on alcohol. *Drug and Alcohol Review* 9, 91–5.

Hawks D. (1993) The formulation of Australia's National Health Policy on Alcohol. *Addiction* 88 (Suppl.), 19–26S.

Hawks D., Rydon P., Stockwell T., White M., Chikritzhs T., and Heale P. (1999) *The evaluation of the Fremantle police—Licensee accord: Impact on serving practices, harm and the wider community*. Perth, Australia: National Drug Research Institute; Curtin University of Technology.

Hawthorne G. (1996) The social impact of Life Education: Estimating drug use prevalence among Victorian primary school students and the statewide effect of the Life Education programme. *Addiction* 91, 1151–9.

Hayward K. and Hobbs D. (2007) Beyond the binge in 'booze Britain': Market-led liminalization and the spectacle of binge drinking. *British Journal of Sociology* 58, 437–56.

Hearst M.O., Fulkerson J.A., Maldonado-Molina M.M., Perry C.L., and Komro K.A. (2007) Who needs liquor stores when parents will do? The importance of social sources of alcohol among young urban teens. *Preventive Medicine* 44, 471–6.

Heath D.B. (1983) Alcohol use among North American Indians. In: Smart R.G., Glasser F., and Israel Y. (eds), *Research advances in alcohol and drug problems*, Vol. 7, pp. 343–96. New York: Plenum Press.

Heath D.B. (1984) Cross-cultural studies of alcohol use. In: Galanter M. (ed.), *Recent Developments in alcoholism*, Vol. 2, pp. 405–15. New York: Plenum Press.

Heeb J.-L., Gmel G., Zurbrügg C., Kuo M., and Rehm J. (2003) Changes in alcohol consumption following a reduction in the price of spirits: A natural experiment in Switzerland. *Addiction* 98, 1433–46.

Hemström Ö. (2001) Per capita alcohol consumption and ischaemic heart disease. *Addiction* 96 (Suppl. 1), 93–112S.

Henderson-Yates L., Wagner S., Parker H., and Yates D. (2008) *Fitzroy Valley liquor restriction report: An evaluation of the effects of a six month restriction on take-away alcohol relating to measurable health and social benefits and community perceptions and behaviours*. Perth: Drug and Alcohol Office of Western Australia.

Henriksen L., Feighery E.C., Schleicher, N.C., and Fortmann S.P. (2008) Receptivity to alcohol marketing predicts initiation of alcohol use. *Journal of Adolescent Health* 42, 28–35.

Henstridge J., Homel R.J., and Mackay P. (1997) *The long-term effects of random breath testing in four Australian states: A time series analysis*. Canberra: Federal Office of Road Safety.

Her M. and Rehm J. (1998) Alcohol and all-cause mortality in Europe 1982–1990: A pooled cross-section time-series analysis. *Addiction* 93, 1335–40.

Her M., Giesbrecht N., Room R. and Rehm J. (1999) Privatizing alcohol sales and alcohol consumption: Evidence and implications. *Addiction* 94, 1125–39.

Herd D. (2005) Changes in the prevalence of alcohol use in rap song lyrics, 1970–1997. *Addiction* 100, 1258–69.

Herring R., Thom B., Foster J., Franey C., and Salazar C. (2008) Local responses to the Alcohol Licensing Act 2003: The case of Greater London. *Drugs: Education, Prevention and Policy* 15, 251–65.

Herttua K., Mäkelä P., and Martikainen P. (2008) Changes in alcohol-related mortality and its socioeconomic differences after a large reduction in alcohol prices: A natural experiment based on register data. *American Journal of Epidemiology* 168, 1110–18.

Hettige S. and Paranagama H. (2005) Gender, alcohol and culture in Sri Lanka. In: Obot I.S. and Room R. (eds), *Alcohol, gender and drinking problems. perspectives from low and middle income countries*, pp. 176–88. Geneva: World Health Organization.

Heuveline P. and Slap G.B. (2002) Adolescent and young adult mortality by cause: Age, gender, and country, 1955 to 1994. *Journal of Adolescent Health* 30, 29–34.

Hibell B. (1984) Mellanölets borttagande och indikationer på alkoholskadeutvecklingen [The withdrawal of medium beer and indications on alcohol damages]. In: Nilsson T. (ed.) *När Mellanölet Försvann* [When the medium beer was withdrawn], pp. 121–172. Linköping, Sweden: Samhällsvetenskapliga institutionen, Universitet i Linköping.

Hibell B., Andersson B., Ahlström S., Balakireva O., Bjarnason T., Kokkevi A., and Morgan M. (2000) *The 1999 ESPAD report: Alcohol and other drug use among students in 30 European countries*. Stockholm: Swedish Council for Information on Alcohol and Other Drugs (CAN).

Hibell B., Andersson B., Bjarnason T., Ahlström S., Balakireva O., Kokkevi A., and Morgan M. (2004) *The ESPAD report 2003: Alcohol and other drug use among students in 35 European countries*. Stockholm: Swedish Council for Information on Alcohol and Other Drugs (CAN) and The Pompidou Group at the Council of Europe. Available at: http://www.espad.org/documents/Espad/ESPAD_reports/The_2003_ESPAD_report.pdf (accessed 6 July 2009).

Hibell B., Guttormsson U., Ahlström S., Balakireva O., Bjarnason T., Kokkevi A., and Kraus L. (2009) The 2007 ESPAD report: Substance use among students in 35 European countries. Stockholm, Sweden: The Swedish Council for Information on Alcohol and Other Drugs. Available at: http://www.espad.org/documents/Espad/ESPAD_reports/2007/The_2007_ESPAD_Report-FULL_090617.pdf (accessed 6 July 2009).

Hill L. (2008) The alcohol industry. In: Heggenhougen H.K. and Quah S. (eds), *International Encyclopedia of Public Health*, pp. 124–35. San Diego, CA: Academic Press.

Hill L. and Casswell S. (2004) Alcohol advertising and sponsorship: Commercial freedom or control in the public interest? In: Heather N. and Stockwell T. (eds), *The Essential Handbook of Treatment and Prevention of Alcohol Problems*. Chichester, UK: Wiley.

Hill L. and Stewart L. (1996) The Sale of Liquor Act 1989: Reviewing regulatory practices. *Social Policy Journal of New Zealand* 7, 174–90.

Hingson R.W., Heeren T., and Winter M. (1994) Effects of lower legal blood alcohol limits for young and adult drivers. *Alcohol, Drugs and Driving* 10, 243–52.

Hingson R., McGovern T., Howland J., Heeren T., Winter M., and Zakoes R. (1996) Reducing alcohol-impaired driving in Massachusetts: The Saving Lives Program. *American Journal of Public Health* 86, 791–7.

Hingson R., Heeren T., Zakocs R., Kopstein A., and Wechsler, H. (2002) Magnitude of alcohol-related morbidity, mortality, and alcohol dependence among US college students age 18–24. *Journal of Studies on Alcohol* 63, 136–44.

Hobbs D., Lister S., Hadfield P.,Winlow S., and Hall S. (2000) Receiving shadows: Governance and criminality in the night-time economy. *British Journal of Sociology* **51**, 701–17.

Hobbs D., Hadfield P., Lister S., Winlow S., and Hall S. (2002) "Door loor:" The art and economics of intimidation. *British Journal of Criminology* **42**, 352–70.

Hobbs D., Hadfield P., Lister S., and Winlow S. (2003) *Bouncers: Violence and governance in the night-time economy*. Oxford: Oxford University Press.

Hobbs, D., Hadfield P., Lister S., and Winlow S. (2005) Violence and control in the night-time economy. *European Journal of Crime, Criminal Law and Criminal Justice* **13**, 89–102.

Hobbs D., O'Brien K., and Westmarland L. (2007) Connecting the gendered door: Women, violence and doorwork. *The British Journal of Sociology* **58**, 21–38.

Hoek J. (2004) Tobacco promotion restrictions: Ironies and unintended consequences. *Journal of Business Research* **57**, 1250–7.

Hogan E., Boffa J., Rosewarne C., Bell S. and Chee D.A.H. (2006) What price do we pay to prevent alcohol-related harms in Aboriginal communities?: The Alice Springs trial of liquor licensing restrictions. *Drug and Alcohol Review* **25**, 207–12.

Holder H.D. (1987) Alcoholism treatment and potential health care cost saving. *Medical Care* **25**, 52–71.

Holder H.D. (1994a) Mass communication as an essential aspect of community prevention to reduce alcohol-involved traffic crashes. *Alcohol, Drugs and Driving* **10**, 3–4.

Holder H.D. (1994b) Alcohol availability and accessibility as part of the puzzle: Thoughts on alcohol problems and young people. In: *The Development of Alcohol Problems: Exploring the Biopsychosocial Matrix of Risk*, pp. 249–54. NIAAA Research Monograph #26. Rockville, MD: National Institute on Alcohol Abuse and Alcoholism.

Holder H.D. (2000) The supply side initiative as an international collaboration to study alcohol supply, drinking, and consequences: Current knowledge, policy issues, and research opportunities. *Addiction* **95**, S461–3.

Holder H.D. and Blose J.O. (1987) Impact of changes in distilled spirits availability on apparent consumption: A time series analysis of liquor-by-the-drink. *Addiction* **82**, 623–31.

Holder H.D. and Edwards G. (eds) (1995) *Alcohol and public policy: Evidence and issues*. Oxford: Oxford University Press.

Holder H.D. and Parker R.N. (1992) Effect of alcoholism treatment on cirrhosis mortality: A 20-year multivariate time series analysis. *British Journal of Addiction* **87**, 1263–74.

Holder H.D. and Treno A.J. (1997) Media advocacy in community prevention: News as a means to advance policy change. *Addiction* **92** (Suppl. 2), 189–99S.

Holder H.D. and Wagenaar A.C. (1994) Mandated server training and reduced alcohol-involved traffic crashes: A time series analysis of the Oregon experience. *Accident Analysis and Prevention* **26**, 89–97.

Holder H.D., Longabaugh R., Miller W.R., and Rubonis A.V. (1991) The cost of effectiveness of treatment of alcoholism: A first approximation. *Journal of Studies on Alcohol* **52**, 517–40.

Holder H.D., Janes K., Mosher J., Saltz R., Spurr S., and Wagenaar A.C. (1993) Alcoholic beverage server liability and the reduction of alcohol-involved problems. *Journal of Studies on Alcohol* **54**, 23–36.

Holder H.D, Saltz R.F., Grube J.W., Treno A.J., Reynolds R.I., Voas R.B., and Gruenewald P.J. (1997) Summing up: Lessons from a comprehensive community prevention trial. *Addiction* **92** (Suppl. 2), 293–301S.

Holder H.D., Kühlhorn E., Nordlund S., Österberg E., Romelsjö A., and Ugland T. (1998) *European integration and Nordic alcohol policies. Changes in alcohol controls and consequences in Finland, Norway and Sweden, 1980–1997.* Aldershot, UK: Ashgate.

Holder H.D., Agardh E., Högberg P., Miller T., Norström T., Österberg E., Ramstedt M., Rossow I., and Stockwell T. (2008) *If retail alcohol sales in Sweden were privatized, what would be the potential consequences?* Östersund, Sweden: Swedish National Institute of Public Health.

Holder H.D., Gruenewald P.J., Ponicki W.R., Treno A.J., Grube J.W., Saltz R.F., Voas R.B., Reynolds R., Davis J., Sanchez L., Gaumont G., and Roeper P. (2000) Effect of community-based interventions on high-risk drinking and alcohol-related injuries. *Journal of the American Medical Association* **284**, 2341–7.

Hollingworth W., Ebel E., McCarty C., Garrison M., Christakis G., and Rivara F. (2006) Prevention of deaths from harmful drinking in the United States: The potential effects of tax increases and advertising bans on young drinkers. *Journal of Studies on Alcohol* **67**, 300–8.

Holmila M. and Raitasalo K. (2005) Gender differences in drinking: Why do they still exist? *Addiction* **100**, 1763–9.

Home Office (2008) *A practical guide to dealing with alcohol problems: What you need to know.* London: Home Office.

Homel R. (1993) Random breath testing in Australia: Getting it to work according to specifications. *Addiction* **88** (Suppl. 1), 27–33S.

Homel R. and Clark J. (1994) The prediction and prevention of violence in pubs and clubs. *Crime Prevention Studies* **3**, 1–46.

Homel R., Tomsen S., and Thommeny J. (1992) Public drinking and violence: Not just an alcohol problem. *Journal of Drug Issues* **22**, 679–97.

Homel R., Hauritz M.A., Wortley R.K., McIlwain G., and Carvolth R. (1997) Preventing alcohol-related crime through community action: The Surfers Paradise Safety Action Project. *Crime Prevention Studies* **7**, 35–90.

Homel R., Carvolth R., Hauritz M., McIlwain G., and Teague R. (2004) Making licensed venues safer for patrons: What environmental factors should be the focus of interventions? *Drug and Alcohol Review* **23**, 19–29.

Horverak Ø. (2008) The transition from over-the-counter to self-service sales of alcoholic beverages in Norwegian monopoly outlets: Implications for sales and customer satisfaction. *Nordisk alkohol och narkotikatidskrift* **25**, 77–99.

Horverak Ø. and Bye E.K. (2007) *Det Norske drikkemønsteret: En studie basert på intervjudata fra 1973–2004* (The Norwegian drinking pattern: A study based on surveys from 1973 to 2004). Oslo: Norwegian Institute for Alcohol and Drug Research.

Hough M. and Hunter G. (2008) The 2003 Licensing Act's impact on crime and disorder: An evaluation. *Criminology and Criminal Justice* **8**, 239–60.

Howard-Pitney B., Johnson M.D., Altman D.G., Hopkins R., and Hammond N. (1991) Responsible alcohol service: A study of server, manager, and environmental impact. *American Journal of Public Health* **81**, 197–9.

Huang C.D. (2003) *Econometric models of alcohol demand in the UK.* Government Economic Service, Working Paper 140. London: UK Customs and Excise.

Huckle T. and Huakau J. (2006) *Exposure and response of young people to marketing of alcohol in New Zealand.* Auckland, New Zealand: Centre for Social and Health Outcomes Research and Evaluation (SHORE), Massey University.

Huckle T., Pledger M., and Casswell S. (2006) Trends in alcohol-related harms and offences in a liberalized alcohol environment. *Addiction* **101**, 232–40.

Huckle T., Huakau J., Sweetsur P., Huisman O., and Casswell S. (2008a) Density of alcohol outlets and teenage drinking: Living in an alcogenic environment is associated with higher consumption in a metropolitan setting. *Addiction* **103**, 1614–21.

Huckle T., Sweetsur P., Moyes S., and Casswell S. (2008b) Ready to drinks are associated with heavier drinking patterns among young females. *Drug and Alcohol Review* **27**, 398–403.

Hughes K., Anderson Z., Morleo M., and Bellis M.A. (2008) Alcohol, nightlife and violence: The relative contributions of drinking before and during nights out to negative health and criminal justice outcomes. *Addiction* **103**, 60–5.

Huitfeldt B. and Jorner U. (1972) *Efterfrågan på rusdrycker i Sverige* (The demand for alcoholic beverages in Sweden). Statens offentliga utredningar (Government Official Reports) 91. Stockholm: Alcohol Policy Commission.

Humphreys K. (2004) *Circles of recovery: Self-help organizations for addictions.* Cambridge, UK: Cambridge UP.

Hunt G. and Dong Sun A.X. (1998) The drug treatment system in the United States: A panacea for the drug war? In: Klingemann H. and Hunt G. (eds), *Drug treatment systems in an international perspective: Drugs, demons and delinquents,* pp. 3–19. London: Sage.

Hunter E.M., Hall W.D., and Spargo R.M. (1992) Patterns of alcohol consumption in the Kimberley Aboriginal population. *Medical Journal of Australia* **156**, 764–8.

Hurst P.M., Harte D., and Frith W.J. (1994) The Grand Rapids dip revisited. *Accident Analysis and Prevention* **26**, 647–54.

Hurst S. (2006) Alcohol advertising and youth: Themes, appeals and future directions. *International Journal of Advertising* **25**, 541–8.

Hurst W., Gregory, E., and Gussman T. (1997) *International survey: Alcoholic beverage taxation and control policies,* 9th edn. Ottowa: Brewers Association of Canada.

Hurtz S.Q., Henriksen L., Wang Y., Feighery E.C., and Fortmann S.P. (2007) The relationship between exposure to alcohol advertising in stores, owning alcohol promotional items, and adolescent alcohol use. *Alcohol and Alcoholism* **42**, 143–9.

Impact Databank (2007) *The global drinks market.* New York: M. Shanken Communications.

Imrie C.W. (1997) Acute pancreatitis: Overview. *European Journal of Gastroenterology and Hepatology* **9**, 103–5.

International Center for Alcohol Policies (2001) *Self-regulation of beverage alcohol advertising.* ICAP Reports No. 9. Washington, DC: ICAP. Available at: http://www.icap.org/LinkClick.a spx?fileticket=IZBG%2Fehb9GE%3D&tabid=75 (accessed 14 July 2009).

International Center for Alcohol Policies (2005) *ICAP blue book: Practical guides for alcohol policy and prevention approaches.* Washington, DC: ICAP.

International Center for Alcohol Policies (2006) *The structure of the beverage alcohol industry.* ICAP Report 17. Washington, DC: ICAP.

International Center for Alcohol Policies (2008) Noncommercial alcohol in three regions. ICAP Review 3. Washington, DC: ICAP.

Institute of Medicine (1989) *Prevention and treatment of alcohol problems: Research opportunities.* Washington, DC: National Academy Press.

Institute of Medicine (1990) *Broadening the base of treatment for alcohol problems.* Washington, DC: National Academy Press.

International Labour Organization (1949) *Protection of Wages Convention, C95*. Geneva: ILO.

IOGT International (2006) Money from misery. News story from 15 March 2006. Available at: http://www.iogt.org/viewarticle.php?id=330&type=sub&t=home (accessed 17 July 2009).

Ireland C.S. and Thommeny J.L. (1993) The crime cocktail: Licensed premises, alcohol and street offences. *Drug and Alcohol Review* 12, 143–50.

Ivanets N.N. and Lukomskaya M.I. (1990) USSR's new alcohol policy. *World Health Forum* 11, 246–52.

Jackson M.C., Hastings G., Wheeler C., Eadie D., and MacKintosh A.M. (2000) Marketing alcohol to young people: Implications for industry regulation and research policy. *Addiction* 95 (Suppl. 4), 597–608.

Jacobson J.M. (1992) Alcoholism and tuberculosis. *Alcohol Health and Research World* 16, 39–45.

Jahiel R. and Babor T.F. (2007) Industrial epidemics, public health advocacy and the alcohol industry: Lessons from other fields. *Addiction* 102, 1335–9.

Jakubowiak W.M., Bogorodskaya E.M., Borisov E.S., Danilova D.I., and Kourbatova E.K. (2007) Risk factors associated with default among new pulmonary TB patients and social support in six Russian regions. *International Journal of Tuberculosis and Lung Disease* 11, 46–53.

Jeffrey L.R. (2000) *The New Jersey Higher Education Consortium Social Norms Project: Decreasing binge drinking in New Jersey colleges and universities by correcting student misperceptions of college drinking Norms*. Glassboro, NJ: Center for Addiction Studies, Rowan University.

Jeffs B.W. and Saunders W.M. (1983) Minimizing alcohol related offences by enforcement of the existing licensing legislation. *British Journal of Addiction* 78, 67–77.

Jensen G.F. (2000) Prohibition, alcohol, and murder: Untangling countervailing mechanisms. *Homicide Studies* 4, 18–36.

Jernigan D.H. (1999) Country profile on alcohol in Zimbabwe. In: Riley L. and Marshall M. (eds) *Alcohol and Public Health in 8 Developing Countries*, pp. 157–75. Publication WHO/HSC/SAB/99.9. Geneva, Switzerland: WHO Substance Abuse Department.

Jernigan D.H. (2000a) Applying commodity chain analysis to changing modes of alcohol supply in a developing country. *Addiction* 95 (Suppl. 4), 465–75S.

Jernigan D.H. (2000b) Implications of structural changes in the global alcohol supply. *Contemporary Drug Problems* 27, 163–87.

Jernigan D.H. (2005) Globalisation of alcohol markets in Central and South America. Presentation to the CISA Conference, Brasilia, 28–30 November.

Jernigan D.H. (2006) *The extent of global alcohol marketing and its impact on youth*. A paper prepared for the World Health Organization. Washington, DC: Center on Alcohol Marketing and Youth.

Jernigan D.H. (2009) The global alcohol industry: An overview. *Addiction* 104 (Suppl. 1), 6–12.

Jernigan D.H. and O'Hara J. (2004) Alcohol advertising and promotion. In: O'Connell M. (ed.) *Reducing Underage Drinking: A Collective Responsibility*, pp. 625–53. Washington, DC: National Academies Press.

Jernigan D. and Wright P. (1996) Media advocacy: Lessons from community experiences. *Journal of Public Health Policy* 17, 306–30.

Jernigan D., Monteiro M., Room R., and Saxena S. (2000) Towards a global alcohol policy: Alcohol, public health and the role of WHO. *Bulletin of the World Health Organization* 78, 491–9.

Jernigan D.H., Ostroff J., Ross C., and O'Hara J.A. (2004) Sex differences in adolescent exposure to alcohol advertising in magazines. *Archives of Pediatrics and Adolescent Medicine* **158**, 629–34.

Jernigan D.H., Ostroff J., and Ross C. (2005) Alcohol advertising and youth: A measured approach. *Journal of Public Health Policy* **26**, 312–25.

Johannessen K., Collins C., Mills-Novoa B., and Glider P.A. (1999) *A practical guide to alcohol abuse prevention: A campus case study in implementing social norms and environmental management approaches.* Tucson, AZ: Campus Health Services, University of Arizona.

Johansen P.O. (1994) *Markedet som ikke ville dø: Forbudstiden og de illegale alkoholmarkedene i Norge og USA* [The market that would not die: Times of prohibition and the illegal alcohol markets in Norway and the United States of America]. Oslo: National Directorate for Prevention of Alcohol and Drug Use.

Johansson E., Böckerman P., Prättälä R., and Uutela A. (2006) Alcohol-related mortality, drinking behavior, and business cycles. *European Journal of Health Economics* **7**, 212–17.

John R.M. (2005) Price elasticity estimates for tobacco and other addictive goods in India. Working Paper Series No. WP-2005–003. Mumbai, India: Indira Gandhi Institute of Development Research. Available at: http://www.igidr.ac.in/pdf/publication/WP-2005–003. pdf (accessed 9 July 2009).

Johnson C.A., Pentz M.A., Weber M.D., Dwyer J.H., Baer N. MacKinnon D.P., Hansen W.B., and Flay B.R. (1990) Relative effectiveness of comprehensive community programming for drug abuse prevention with high risk and low risk adolescents. *Journal of Consulting and Clinical Psychology* **58**, 447–56.

Johnson K.O. and Berglund M. (2003) Education of key personnel in student pubs leads to a decrease in alcohol consumption among the patrons: A randomized controlled trial. *Addiction* **98**, 627–33.

Johnston P. (2001) Trends in negligence and public liability: The evolving liability of licensees and servers of alcohol to their patrons and third parties. Occasional paper. Melbourne, Australia: Drugs and Crime Prevention Committee, Parliament of Victoria. Available at: http://www.parliament.vic.gov.au/dcpc/Reports%20in%20PDF/Occ%20Rpt%20amended_ v2.pdf (accessed 12 July 2009).

Jones N.E., Pieper C.F., and Robertson L.S. (1992) Effect of legal drinking age on fatal injuries of adolescents and young adults. *American Journal of Public Health* **82**, 112–15.

Jones S. and Donovan R. (2001) Messages in alcohol advertising targeted to youth. *Australian and New Zealand Journal of Public Health* **25**, 126–31.

Jones S., Casswell S., and Zhang J. (1995) Economic costs of alcohol-related absenteeism and reduced productivity among the working population of New Zealand. *Addiction* **90**, 1455–61.

Jones S., Hall D., and Munro G. (2008) How effective is the revised regulatory code for alcohol advertising in Australia? *Drug and Alcohol Review* **27**, 29–38.

Jones S.C. and Lynch M. (2007) Non-advertising alcohol promotions in licensed premises: Does the Code of Practice ensure responsible promotion of alcohol? *Drug and Alcohol Review* **26**, 477–85.

Jones-Webb R., Toomey T., Miner K., Wagenaar A.C., Wolfson M., and Poon R. (1997) Why and in what context adolescents obtain alcohol from adults: A pilot study. *Substance Use and Misuse* **32**, 219–28.

Joossens L. (2000) From public health to international law: Possible protocols for inclusion in the Framework Convention on Tobacco Control. *Bulletin of the World Health Organization* **78**, 930–7.

Kairouz S., Gliksman L., Demers A. and Adlaf E.M. (2002) For all these reasons, I do . . . drink: A multilevel analysis of contextual reasons for drinking among Canadian undergraduates. *Journal of Studies on Alcohol* **63**, 600–8.

Kaplan S. and Prato C. (2007) Impact of BAC limit reduction on different population segments: A Poisson fixed effect analysis. *Accident Analysis and Prevention* **39**, 1146–54.

Karlsson T. and Österberg E. (2001) A scale of formal alcohol control policy in 15 European countries. *Nordisk alcohol- & narkotikatidskrift* **18**, 117–31.

Karlsson T. and Österberg E. (2007) Scaling alcohol policies across Europe. *Drugs: Education, Prevention and Policy* **14**, 499–511.

Karlsson T. and Österberg E. (2009) The Nordic borders are not alike. *Nordisk alcohol- & narkotikatidskrift* **26**, in press.

Kaskutas L.A. (1995) Interpretations of risk: The use of scientific information in the development of the alcohol warning label policy. *International Journal of the Addictions* **30**, 1519–48.

Kaskutas L.A. and Greenfield T.K. (1992) First effects of warning labels on alcoholic beverage containers. *Drug and Alcohol Dependence* **31**, 1–14.

Kaskutas L.A. and Greenfield T.K. (1997a) Behavior change: The role of health consciousness in predicting attention to health warning messages. *American Journal of Health Promotion* **11**, 183–93.

Kaskutas L.A. and Greenfield T.K. (1997b) The role of health consciousness in predicting attention to health warning messages. *American Journal of Health Promotion*, **11**, 186–93.

Kaskutas L.A., Greenfield T.K., Lee M., and Cote J. (1998) Reach and effects of health messages on drinking during pregnancy. *Journal of Health Education* **29**, 11–17.

Keller M., McCormick H., and Efron V. (1982) *A dictionary of words about alcohol*. New Brunswick, NJ: Rutgers Center of Alcohol Studies.

Kelly K., Slater M., and Karan D. (2002) Image advertisements' influence on adolescents' perceptions of the desirability of beer and cigarettes. *Journal of Public Policy and Marketing* **21**, 295–304.

Kelsey J. (2008) *Serving whose interests? The political economy of trade in service agreements.* Abingdon, UK: Routledge Cavendish.

Kendell R.E., de Roumanie M., and Ritson E.B. (1983) Effect of economic changes on Scottish drinking habits, 1978–82. *British Journal of Addiction* **78**, 365–79.

Kennedy B.P., Isaac N.E., Nelson T.F., and Graham J.D. (1997) Young male drinkers and impaired driving intervention: results of a US telephone survey. *Accident Analysis and Prevention* **29**, 707–13.

Kerr W.C., Greenfield T.K., and Midanik L.T. (2006) How many drinks does it take you to feel drunk? Trends and predictors for subjective drunkenness. *Addiction* **101**, 1428–37.

Kerr-Correa F., Hegedus A.M., Trinca L.A., Tucci A.M., Kerr-Pontes L.R.S., Sanches A.F. and Floripes T.M.F. (2005) Differences in drinking patterns between men and women in Brazil. In: Obot I.S. and Room R. (eds), *Alcohol, Gender and Drinking Problems: Perspectives from Low and Middle Income Countries*, pp. 49–68. Geneva: World Health Organization.

Kinney A.Y., Millikan R.C., Lin Y.H., Moorman P.G., and Newman B. (2000) Alcohol consumption and breast cancer among black and white women in North Carolina (United States). *Cancer Causes and Control* 11, 345–57.

Kirin Research Institute of Drinking and Lifestyle (2004) Beer consumption in major countries in 2004. Report No. 29. Tokyo. Available at: http://www.kirinholdings.co.jp/english/ir/news_release051215_4.html (accessed 3 July 2009).

Klein N. (2000) *No space, no choice, no jobs, no logo*. London: HarperCollins.

Klepp K.I., Kelder S.H., and Perry C.L. (1995) Alcohol and marijuana use among adolescents: Long-term outcomes of the Class of 1989 Study. *Annals of Behavioral Medicine* 17, 19–24.

Klepp K.I., Schmid L.A., and Murray D.M. (1996) Effects of the increased minimum drinking age law on drinking and driving behavior among adolescents. *Addiction Research* 4, 237–44.

Klingemann H. and Gmel G. (2001) Introduction: Social consequences of alcohol—the forgotten dimension? In: Klingemann H. and Gmel G. (eds), *Mapping the social consequences of alcohol consumption*, pp. 1–9. Dordrecht, The Netherlands: Kluwer.

Klingemann H. and Hunt G. (eds) (1998) *Drug treatment systems in an international perspective: Drugs, demons, and delinquents*. London: Sage publications.

Klingemann H. and Klingemann H.D. (1999) National treatment systems in global perspective. *European Addiction Research* 5, 109–17.

Klingemann H., Takala J.P., and Hunt G. (1992) *Cure, care or control: Alcoholism treatment in sixteen countries*. Albany, NY: State University of New York Press.

Klingemann H., Takala J.P., and Hunt G. (1993) The development of alcohol treatment systems: An international perspective. *Alcohol Health and Research World* 3, 221–7.

Kloeden C.N. and McLean A.J. (1994) *Late night drink driving in Adelaide two years after the introduction of the 05 limit*. Adelaide: NHMRC Road Accident Research Unit.

Knupfer G. (1987) Drinking for health: The daily light drinker fiction. *British Journal of Addiction* 82, 547–55.

Kohlmeier L. and Mendez M. (1997) Controversies surrounding diet and breast cancer. *Proceedings of the Nutrition Society* 56, 369–82.

Komro K.A., Perry C.L., Murray D.M., Veblen-Mortenson S., Williams C.L., and Anstine P.S. (1996) Peer-planned social activities for preventing alcohol use among young adolescents. *Journal of School Health* 66, 328–34.

Komro K.A., Perry C.L., Veblen-Mortenson S., Farbakhsh K., Toomey T.L., Stigler M.H., Jones-Webb R., Kugler K.C., Pasch K.E., and Williams C.L. (2008) Outcomes from a randomized controlled trial of multi-component alcohol use preventive intervention for urban youth: Project Northland Chicago. *Addiction* 103, 606–18.

Kortteinen T. (ed.) (1989) *State monopolies and alcohol prevention: Report and working papers of a collaborative international study*. Helsinki, Finland: Social Research Institute of Alcohol Studies.

Koski A., Sirén R., Vuori E., and Poikolainen K. (2007) Alcohol tax cuts and increase in alcohol-positive sudden deaths: A time-series intervention analysis. *Addiction* 102, 362–8.

Kotakorpi K. (2008) The incidence of sin taxes. *Economics Letters* 98, 95–9.

KPMG (2008a) *Evaluation of the Temporary Late Night Entry Declaration Final Report*. Melbourne: Department of Justice, State of Victoria.

KPMG (2008b) *Review of the social responsibility standards for the production and sale of alcoholic drinks*, Vol. 1. London: Home Office.

Kranzler H.R. and Van Kirk J. (2001) Naltrexone and acamprosate in the treatment of alcoholism: A meta-analysis. *Alcoholism: Clinical and Experimental Research* **25**, 1335–41.

Krass I. and Flaherty B. (1994) The impact of Responsible Beverage Service training on patron and server behaviour: A trial in Waverly (Sydney). *Health Promotion Journal of Australia* **4**, 51–8.

Kreft I.G.G. (1997) The interactive effect of alcohol prevention programs in high school classes: An illustration of item homogeneity scaling and multilevel analysis techniques. In: Bryant K.J., Windle M., and West S.G. (eds), *The Science of Prevention: Methodological Advances from Alcohol and Substance Abuse Research*, pp. 251–77. Washington, DC: American Psychological Association.

Kreitman N. (1986) Alcohol consumption and the preventive paradox. *British Journal of Addiction* **81**, 353–63.

Kriebel D. and Tickner J. (2001) Reenergizing public health through precaution. *American Journal of Public Health* **91**, 1351–5.

Krüger N.A. and Svensson M. (2008) Good times are drinking times: Empirical evidence on business cycles and alcohol sales in Sweden 1861–2000. *Applied Economics Letters* (Online early access). doi: 10.1080/13504850802167215

Kunitz S.J., Levy J.E., Andrews T., DuPuy C., Gabriel K.R., and Russell S. (1994) *Drinking careers: A twenty-five year study of three Navajo populations*. New Haven, CT: Yale UP.

Kunitz S.J., Woodall W.G., Zhao H., Wheeler D.R., Lillis R., and Rogers E. (2002) Rearrest rates after incarceration for DWI: A comparative study in a southwestern US county. *American Journal of Public Health* **92**, 1826–31.

Kuo M., Heeb J.-L., Gmel G., and Rehm J. (2003a) Does price matter? The effect of decreased price on spirits consumption in Switzerland. *Alcoholism: Clinical and Experimental Research* **27**, 720–5.

Kuo M., Wechsler H., Greenberg P., and Lee H. (2003b) The marketing of alcohol to college students: The role of low prices and specials promotions. *American Journal of Preventative Medicine* **25**, 204–11.

Kypri K., Saunders J.B., Williams, S.M., McGee R.O., Langley J.D., Cashell-Smitth M.J., and Gallagher S.J. (2004) Web-based screening and brief intervention for hazardous drinking: A double-blind randomized controlled trial. *Addiction* **99**, 1410–17.

Kypri K., Voas R.B., Langley J.D., Stephenson S.C.R., Begg D.J., Tippetts A.S., and Davie G.S. (2006) Minimum purchasing age for alcohol and traffic crash injuries among 15-to 19-year-olds in New Zealand. *American Journal of Public Health* **96**, 126–31.

Kypri K., Bell M.L., Hay G.C., and Baxter J. (2008) Alcohol outlet density and university student drinking: A national study. *Addiction* **103**, 1131–8.

Labrie J.W. (2002) Weighing the pros and cons: A brief motivational intervention reduces risk associated with drinking and unsafe sex. Doctoral dissertation. Los Angeles: University of Southern California.

Lacey J.H., Ferguson S., Kelley-Baker T., and Rider R. (2006) Low-manpower checkpoints: Can they provide effective DUI enforcement in small communities? *Traffic Injury Prevention* **7**, 213–18.

Lacey J.H., Kelley-Baker T., Furr-Holden D., Brainard K., and Moore C. (2007) *Pilot test of new roadside survey methodology for impaired driving.* NHTSA Publication No. DOT HS 810 704. Washington, DC: National Highway Traffic safety Administration.

LaChance H. (2004) Group motivational intervention for underage college student drinkers in mandated university-based programming. Doctoral dissertation. Boulder, CO: University of Colorado.

Lachenmeier D.W. and Rehm J. (2009) Unrecorded alcohol: A threat to public health? *Addiction* **104**, 875–7.

Laixuthai A. and Chaloupka F.J. (1993) Youth alcohol use and public policy. *Contemporary Economic Policy* **11**, 70–81.

Lakins N.E., Williams G.D., and Yi H (2007) Apparent per capita alcohol consumption: National, state, and regional trends, 1977–2005. Surveillance report #82. Arlington, VA: CSR Inc.

Lal Pai U. (2008) Alcohol industry in India: High-spirited growth. Available at: http://www.investorideas.com/IiI/News/011607.asp (accessed 6 April 2008).

Land Transport Safety Authority (2003) *Road safety to 2010.* Available at: http://www.ltsa.govt.nz/strategy-2010/docs/2010-strategy.pdf (accessed 13 July 2009).

Landis B.Y. (1952) Some economic aspects of inebriety. In: *Alcohol, science and society, Quarterly Journal of Studies on Alcohol*, pp. 201–21.

Lang E. and Rumbold G. (1997) The effectiveness of community-based interventions to reduce violence in and around licensed premises: A comparison of three Australian models. *Contemporary Drug Problems* **24**, 805–26.

Lang E., Stockwell T.R., Rydon P., and Beel A.C. (1998) Can training bar staff in responsible serving practices reduce alcohol-related harm? *Drug and Alcohol Review* **17**, 39–50.

Lange J.E., Reed M.B., Johnson M.B., and Voas R.B. (2006) The efficacy of experimental interventions designed to reduce drinking among designated drivers. *Journal of Studies on Alcohol* **67**, 261–8.

Lapham S.C, C'de Baca J., McMillan G.P., and Lapidus J. (2006a) Psychiatric disorders in a sample of repeat impaired-driving offenders. *Journal of Studies on Alcohol* **67**, 707–13.

Lapham S.C., Kapitula L.R., C'de Baca J., and McMillan G.P. (2006b) Impaired-driving recidivism among repeat offenders following an intensive court-based intervention. *Accident Analysis and Prevention* **38**, 162–9.

Lapham S.C., C'de Baca J., Lapidus J., and McMillan G. (2007) Randomized sanctions to reduce re-offense among repeat impaired-driving offenders. *Addiction* **102**, 1618–25.

Larimer M.E. and Cronce J.M. (2002) Identification, prevention and treatment: a review of individual-focused strategies to reduce problematic alcohol consumption by college students. *Journal of Studies on Alcohol* Suppl. 14, 148–63.

Larimer M.E. and Cronce J.M. (2007) Identification, prevention, and treatment revisited: Individual-focused college drinking prevention strategies 1999–2006. *Addictive Behaviors* **32**, 2439–68.

Larimer M.E., Turner A.P., Anderson B.K., Fader J.S., Kilmer J.R., Palmer R.S., and Cronce J.M. (2001) Evaluating a brief alcohol intervention with fraternities. *Journal of Studies on Alcohol* **62**, 370–80.

Larimer M.E., Lee C.M., Kilmer J.R., Fabiano P.M., Stark C.B., Geisner I.M., Mallett K.A., Lostutter T.W., Cronce J.M., Feeney M., and Neighbors C. (2007) Personalized mailed feedback for college drinking prevention: A randomized clinical trial. *Journal of Consulting and Clinical Psychology* **75**, 285–93.

Larsen S. and Saglie J. (1996) Alcohol use in Saami and non-Saami areas in northern Norway. *European Addiction Research* 2, 78–82.

Larsson S. and Hanson B.S. (1999) Prevent alcohol problems in Europe by community actions: Various national and regional contexts. In: Larsson S. and Hanson B.S. (eds), *Community-based alcohol prevention in Europe: Research and evaluations*, pp. 220–39. Lund, Sweden: Lunds Universitet.

LaScala E.A., Johnson F.W., and Gruenewald P.J. (2001) Neighborhood characteristics of alcohol-related pedestrian injury collisions: A geostatistical analysis. *Prevention Science* 2, 123–34.

Latimer J., Dowden C., and Muise D. (2001) *The effectiveness of restorative justice practices: A meta*-analysis. Ottawa: Research and Statistics Division, Department of Justice.

Lavoie M., Godin G. and Valois P. (1999) Understanding the use of the community-based drive-home service after alcohol consumption among young adults. *Journal of Community Health* 24, 171–86.

Lee B. and Tremblay V.J. (1992) Advertising and the US market demand for beer. *Applied Economics* 24, 69–77.

Lee K. and Chinnock P. (2006) Interventions in the alcohol server setting for preventing injuries. *Cochrane Database of Systematic Reviews*, Issue 2, Art. No.: CD005244.pub2. doi: 10.1002/14651858.CD005244.pub2.

Legge J.S. Jr, and Park J. (1994) Policies to reduce alcohol-impaired driving: Evaluating elements of deterrence. *Social Science Quarterly* 75, 594–606.

Lieber C.S. (1988) Biochemical and molecular basis of alcohol-induced injury to liver tissues. *New England Journal of Medicine* 319, 1639–50.

Leifman H. (1996) Perspectives on alcohol prevention. Dissertation. Stockholm: Almquist & Wiksell International.

Leifman H. (2001) Homogenization in alcohol consumption in the European Union. *Nordic Studies on Alcohol and Drugs* 18 (English Suppl.), 15–30.

Leifman H. (2002) A comparative analysis of drinking patterns in 6 EU countries in the year 2000. *Contemporary Drug Problems* 29, 501–48.

Lemmens P.H. (1991) Measurement and distribution of alcohol consumption. Dissertation. Maastricht, The Netherlands: University of Limburg.

Lenke L. (1990) *Alcohol and criminal violence: Time series analysis in a comparative perspective.* Stockholm Sweden: Almquist & Wiksell International.

Leon D.A., Chenet L., Shkolnikov V.M., Zakharov S., Shapiro J., Rakhmanova G., Vassin S., and McKee M. (1997) Huge variation in Russian mortality rates 1984--94: Artefact, alcohol, or what? *Lancet* 350, 383–8.

Leonard K.E. (1990) Marital functioning among episodic and steady alcoholics. In: Collins R.L., Leonard K.E., and Searless J.S. (eds), *Alcohol and the Family: Research and Clinical Perspectives*, pp. 220–43. New York: Guilford Press.

Leonard K.E. and Rothbard J.C. (1999) Alcohol and the marriage effect. *Journal of Studies on Alcohol* Suppl. 13, 139–46S.

Leonard K.E., Quigley B.M., and Collins R.L. (2002) Physical aggression in the lives of young adults: Prevalence, location, and severity among college and community samples. *Journal of Interpersonal Violence* 17, 533–50.

Leppänen K., Sullström R., and Suoniemi I. (2001) *The consumption of alcohol in fourteen European countries: A comparative econometric analysis.* Helsinki: STAKES.

Levy D.T. and Miller T.R. (1995) A cost-benefit analysis of enforcement efforts to reduce serving intoxicated patrons. *Journal of Studies on Alcohol* **56**, 240–7.

Lewis M.A. and Neighbors C. (2006) Social norms approaches using descriptive drinking norms education: A review of the research on personalized normative feedback. *Journal of American College Health* **54**, 213–18.

Lindstrom P. and Svensson R. (1998) Attitudes toward drugs among youths: An evaluation of the Swedish DARE programme. *Nordisk alcohol- & nartkotikatidskrift* **15** (English Suppl.), 7–23.

Lipsey M.W., Wilson D.B., Cohen M.A., and Derzon J.H. (1997) Is there a causal relationship between alcohol use and violence? In: Galanter M. (ed.), *Recent developments in alcoholism, Vol. 13: Alcohol and violence*, pp. 245–82. New York: Plenum Press.

Lishman W.A. (1998) *Organic psychiatry: the psychological consequences of cerebral disorder.* Oxford: Blackwell.

Lister S., Hobbs D., Hall S., and Winslow S. (2000) Violence in the night-time economy. Bouncers: The reporting, recording and prosecution of assaults. *Policing and Society* **10**, 383–402.

Lister S., Hadfield P., Hobbs D., and Winlow S. (2001) Accounting for bouncers: Occupational licensing as a mechanism for regulation. *Criminology and Criminal Justice* **1**, 363–84.

Little B. and Bishop M. (1998) Minor drinkers/major consequences: Enforcement strategies for underage alcoholic beverage violators. *Impaired Driving Update II*, **88**.

Little H.J. (2000) Behavioral mechanisms underlying the link between smoking and drinking. *Alcohol Research and Health* **24**, 215–24.

Little J.W. (1975) *Administration of justice in drunk driving cases.* Gainesville, FL: University Presses of Florida.

Livingston M. (2008) A longitudinal analysis of alcohol outlet density and assault. *Alcoholism: Clinical and Experimental Research* **32**, 1074–9.

Livingston M., Chikritzhs T., and Room R. (2007) Changing the density of alcohol outlets to reduce alcohol-related problems. *Drug and Alcohol Review* **26**, 553–62.

Livingston M., Laslett A.M., and Dietze P. (2008) Individual and community correlates of young people's high-risk drinking in Victoria, Australia. *Drug and Alcohol Dependence* **98**, 241–8.

Longest B.B. (1998) *Health policymaking in the United States.* Chicago: Health Administration Press.

Lönnroth, K., Williams, B., Stadlin, S., Jaramillo, E., and Dye, C. (2008) Alcohol use as a risk factor for tuberculosis—a systematic review. *BMC Public Health* **8**, 289.

Lopez A.D., Mathers C.D., Ezzati M., Jamison D.T., and Murray D.J.L. (2006) *Global burden of disease and risk factors.* New York: Oxford University Press/World Bank.

Lovato C., Linn G., Stead L., and Best A. (2003) Impact of tobacco advertising and promotion on increasing adolescent smoking behaviours. *Cochrane Database of Systematic Reviews* Issue 3, Art. No. CD003439. doi: 10.1002/14651858.CD003439.

Lovato C., Linn G., Stead L., and Best A. (2004) *Impact of tobacco advertising and promotion on increasing adolescent smoking behaviours.* Chichester, UK: Wiley.

Lubek I. (2005) Cambodian 'beer promotion women' and corporate caution: Recalcitrance or worse? *Psychology of Women Section Review* **7**, 2–11.

Ludwig M.J. (1994) Mass media and health education: A critical analysis and reception study of a selected anti-drug campaign. *Dissertation Abstracts International* **55**, 1479A.

Lyon A.B. and Schwab R.M. (1995) Consumption taxes in a life-cycle framework: Are sin taxes regressive? *Review of Economics and Statistics* **77**, 389–406.

MacAndrew, C. and Edgerton, R. (1969). *Drunken comportment: A social explanation.* London: Thomas Nelsen & Sons.

Macdonald S., Wells S., Giesbrecht N., and Cherpitel C.J. (1999) Demographic and substance use factors related to violent and accidental injuries: results from an emergency room study. *Drug and Alcohol Dependence* **55**, 53–61.

Mackay G. (2003) Chief executive's review. *SABMiller Annual report.* Available at: http://www.sabmiller.com/files/reports/ar2003/index.html (accessed 3 July 2009).

MacKinnon D.P. and Nohre L. (2006) *Alcohol and tobacco warnings.* Mahwah, NJ: Erlbaum.

MacKinnon D.P., Johnson C.A., Pentz M.A., Dwyer J.H., Hansen W.B., Flay B.R., and Wang E.Y.-I. (1991) Mediating mechanisms in a school-based drug prevention program: First-year effects of the Midwestern Prevention Project. *Health Psychology* **10**, 164–72.

MacKinnon D.P., Pentz M.A., and Stacy A.W. (1993) The alcohol warning label and adolescents: The first year. *American Journal of Public Health* **83**, 585–7.

Maclure M. (1993) Demonstration of deductive meta-analysis: Ethanol intake and risk of myocardial infarction. *Epidemiologic Reviews* **15**, 328–51.

Madden P.A. and Grube J.W. (1994) The frequency and nature of alcohol and tobacco advertising in televised sports, 1990 through 1992. *American Journal of Public Health* **84**, 297–9.

Madrigal E. (1998) Drug policies and tradition: Implications for the care of addictive disorders in two Andean countries. In: Klingemann H. and Hunt G. (eds), *Drug treatment systems in an international perspective: Drugs, demons and delinquents*, pp. 195–200. London: Sage Publications.

Maguire M. and Nettleton H. (2003) *Reducing alcohol-related violence and disorder: An evaluation of the 'TASC' project* (No. 265). London: Home Office Research, Development and Statistics Directorate.

Majnoni d'Intignano B. (1998) Industrial epidemics. In: Chinitz D. and Cohen J. (eds), *Governments and health systems: Implications of differing involvement*, pp. 585–96. Chichester, UK: Wiley.

Mäkelä K. (1970) Dryckegångernas frekvens enligt de konsumerade drykerna och mängden före och efter lagreformen (The frequency of drinking occasions according to type of beverage and amount consumed before and after the new alcohol law). *Alkoholpolitik* **33**, 144–53.

Mäkelä K. (1983) The uses of alcohol and their cultural regulation. *Acta Sociologica* **1**, 21–31.

Mäkelä P. (2002) Whose drinking does a liberalization of alcohol policy increase?: Change in alcohol consumption by the initial level in the Finnish panel survey in 1968 and 1969. *Addiction* **97**, 701–6.

Mäkelä P. and Österberg E. (2009) Weakening of one more alcohol control pillar: A review of the effects of alcohol tax cuts in Finland in 2004. *Addiction* **104**, 554–63.

Mäkelä K., Österberg E., and Sulkunen P. (1981a) Drink in Finland: Increasing alcohol availability in a monopoly state. In: Single E., Morgan P., and deLint J. (eds), *Alcohol, society and the state II: The social history of control policy in seven countries*, pp. 31–59. Toronto: Addiction Research Foundation.

Mäkelä K., Room R., Single E.R., Sulkunen P. and Walsh B., with Bunce R., Cahannes M., Cameron T., Giesbrecht N., de Lint J., Mäkinen H., Morgan P., Mosher J., Moskalewicz J., Müller R., Österberg E., Wald I. and Walsh D. (1981b) Alcohol, society, and the state, Vol. 1, *A comparative study of alcohol control*. Toronto: Addiction Research Foundation.

Mäkelä P., Fonager K., Hibell B., Nordlund S., Sabroe S., and Simpura J. (1999) *Drinking habits in the Nordic countries*. SIFA Rapport 2/99. Oslo, Norway: National Institute for Alcohol and Drug Research.

Mäkelä P., Tryggvesson K., and Rossow I. (2002) Who drinks more or less when policies change? The evidence from 50 years of Nordic studies. In: Room R. (ed.), *The Effects of Nordic alcohol policies: Analyses of changes in control systems*, pp. 17–70. Publication No. 42. Helsinki, Finland: Nordic Council for Alcohol and Drug Research.

Mäkelä P., Mustonen H., and Österberg E. (2007) Does beverage type matter? *Nordisk alkohol- & narkotikatidskrift* [Nordic Studies on Alcohol and Drugs] 24, 617–31.

Mäkelä P., Bloomfield K., Gustafsson N.-K., Huhtanen P., and Room R. (2008) Changes in volume of drinking after changes in alcohol taxes and travellers' allowances: Results from a panel study. *Addiction* 103, 181–91.

Makowsky C. and Whitehead P.C. (1991) Advertising and alcohol studies: A legal impact study. *Journal of Studies on Alcohol* 52, 555–67.

Males M. (2007) California's graduated driver license law: Effect on teenage drivers' deaths through 2005. *Journal of Safety Research* 38, 651–9.

Mangeloja E. and Pehkonen J. (2009) Availability and consumption of alcoholic beverages: Evidence from Finland. *Applied Economics Letters* 16, 425–9.

Mangione T.W., Howland J., Amick B., Cote J., Lee M., Bell N., and Levine S. (1999) Employee drinking practices and work performance. *Journal of Studies on Alcohol* 60, 261–70.

Mann R.E., Smart R., Anglin L., and Rush B. (1988) Are decreases in liver cirrhosis rates a result of increased treatment for alcoholism? *British Journal of Addiction* 83, 683–8.

Mann R.E., Vingilis E.R., Gavin D., Adlaf E. and Anglin L. (1991) Sentence severity and the drinking driver: Relationships with traffic safety outcome. *Accident Analysis and Prevention* 23, 483–91.

Mann R.E., MacDonald S., Stoduto G., Bondy S., Jonah B., and Shaikh A. (2001) The effects of introducing or lowering legal *per se* blood alcohol limits for driving: An international review. *Accident Analysis and Prevention* 33, 569–83.

Manning W.G., Blumberg L., and Moulton L.H. (1995) The demand for alcohol: The differential response to price. *Journal of Health Economics* 14, 123–48.

Margolis L.H., Masten S.V., and Foss R.D. (2007) The effects of graduated driver licensing on hospitalization rates and charges for 16-and 17-year-olds in North Carolina. *Traffic Injury Prevention* 8, 35–8.

Marin Institute (2008a) *Why big alcohol can't police itself: A review of advertising self-regulation in the distilled spirits industry*. San Rafael, CA: Marin Institute. Available at: http://www.marininstitute.org/site/index.php?option=com_content&view=article&id=118:why-big-alcohol-cant-police-itself&catid=18:reports&Itemid=15 (accessed 14 July 2009).

Marin Institute (2008b) *You get what you pay for: California's alcohol lobby*. San Rafael, CA: Marin Institute.

Markowitz S. (2000) *Criminal violence and alcohol beverage control: Evidence from an international study*. National Bureau of Economic Research Working Paper Series No. 7481. New York: National Bureau of Economic Research.

Markowitz S. and Grossman M. (1998) Alcohol regulation and domestic violence towards children. *Contemporary Economic Policy* **16**, 309–20.

Markowitz S. and Grossman M. (2000) The effects of beer taxes on physical child abuse. *Journal of Health Economics* **19**, 271–82.

Markowitz S., Chatterji P. and Kaestner R. (2003) Estimating the impact of alcohol policies on youth suicides. *Journal of Mental Health Policy and Economics* **6**, 37–46.

Markowitz S., Kaestner R., and Grossman M. (2005) An investigation of the effects of alcohol consumption and alcohol policies on youth risky sexual behaviors. *American Economic Review* **95**, 263–6.

Marmot M.G. (2001) Alcohol and coronary heart disease. *International Journal of Epidemiology* **30**, 724–9.

Marques P. R. (2009) The alcohol ignition interlock and other technologies for the prediction and control of impaired drivers. In: Verster J.C., Pandi-Perumal S.R., Ramaekers J.G., and de Gier J.J. (eds), *Drugs, driving, and traffic safety*, pp. 457–76. Basel: Birkhäuser.

Marques P.R. and Voas R.B. (1995) Case-managed alcohol interlock programs: A bridge between the criminal and health systems. *Journal of Traffic Medicine* **23**, 77–85.

Marques P.R. and Voas R.B. (1998) Using the alcohol safety interlock data logger to track the drinking of convicted drunk drivers. Supplement to Alcoholism: Clinical and Experimental Research. 1998 Scientific Meeting of the Research Society on Alcoholism, Hilton Head Island, South Carolina, 20–25 June. 41A.

Marques P.R. and Voas R.B. (2005) Interlock BAC tests, alcohol biomarkers, and motivational interviewing: Methods for detecting and changing high-risk offenders. In: Marques P.R. (ed.), Alcohol ignition interlock devices, Vol. II, *Research, policy, and program status 2005*, pp. 25–41. Oosterhout, The Netherlands: International Council on Alcohol, Drugs and Traffic Safety.

Marsden Jacob Associates (2005) Identifying a framework for regulation in packaged liquor retailing. Report prepared for the National Competition Council as part of the NCC Occasional Series. Melbourne: Marsden Jacob Associates. Available at: http://www.ncc.gov.au/pdf/PIReMJ-003.pdf (accessed 8 Oct 2008).

Martin C., Wyllie A., and Casswell S. (1992) Types of New Zealand drinkers and their associated problems. *Journal of Drug Issues* **22**, 773–96.

Martin S., Grube J.W., Voas R.B., Baker J., and Hingson R. (1996) Zero tolerance laws: Effective policy? *Alcoholism: Clinical and Experimental Research* **20**, 147–50a.

Martin S., Snyder L., Hamilton M., Fleming-Milici F., Slater M., Stacy A., Chen M.-J., and Grube J. (2002) Alcohol advertising and youth. *Alcoholism: Clinical and Experimental Research* **26**, 900–6.

Mast B.D., Benson B.L., and Rasmussen D.W. (1999) Beer taxation and alcohol-related fatalities. *Southern Economic Journal* **66**, 214–49.

Masten S.V. and Hagge R.A. (2004) Evaluation of California's graduated driver licensing program. *Journal of Safety Research* **35**, 523–35.

Mazzocchi M. (2006) Time patterns in UK demand for alcohol and tobacco: An application of the EM algorithm. *Computational Statistics and Data Analysis* **50**, 2191–205.

McBride N., Farringdon F., Midford R., Meuleners L., and Philip M. (2004) Harm minimisation in school drug education: Final results of the School Health and Alcohol Harm Reduction Project (SHAHRP). *Addiction* **99**, 278–91.

McCarthy P. (2007) *Accords: Are they an effective means of mitigating alcohol-related harm?* Melbourne: DrinkWise Australia.

McCarthy P.S. (2003) Effects of alcohol and highway speed policies on motor vehicle crashes involving older drivers. *Journal of Transportation and Statistics* **6**, 51–65.

McCartt A.T. and Northrup V.S. (2004) Effects of enhanced sanctions for high BAC DWI offenders on case dispositions and rates of recidivism. *Traffic Injury Prevention* **5**, 270–7.

McCartt A.T. and Williams A.F. (2004) Characteristics of fatally injured drivers with high blood alcohol concentrations (BACs). In: *Proceedings of the 17th International Conference on Alcohol, Drugs, and Traffic Safety.* Glasgow: The International Council on Alcohol, Drugs & Traffic Safety. Available at: http://www.icadts.org/t2004/O105.html (accessed 13 July 2009).

McCartt A.T., Blackman K., and Voas R. (2007) Implementation of Washington state's zero tolerance law: Patterns of arrests, dispositions, and recidivism. *Traffic Injury Prevention* **8**, 339–45.

McCartt A.T., Mayhew D.R., Braitman K.A, Ferguson S.A., and Simpson H.M. (2008) *Effects of age and experience on young driver crashes: Review of recent literature.* Arlington, VA: Insurance Institute for Highway Safety.

McCombs M. and Shaw D. (1972) The agenda-setting function of the mass media. *Public Opinion Quarterly* **36**, 176–87.

McCreanor T., Casswell S., and Hill L. (2000) ICAP and the perils of partnership. (Editorial.) *Addiction* **95**, 179–85.

McCreanor T., Moewaka Barnes H., Gregory M., Kaiwai H., and Borell S. (2005) Consuming identities: Alcohol marketing and the commodification of youth experience. *Addiction Research and Theory* **13**, 579–90.

McCreanor T., Moewaka Barnes H., Kaiwai H., Borell S., and Gregory A. (2008) Creating intoxigenic environments: Marketing alcohol to young people in Aotearoa New Zealand. *Social Science and Medicine* **67**, 938–46.

McGuiness T. (1980) An econometric analysis of total demand for alcoholic beverages in the UK, 1956–1975. *Journal of Industrial Economics* **29**, 85–109.

McKilip J., Lockhart D.C., Eckert P.S., and Phillips J. (1985) Evaluation of a responsible alcohol use media campaign on a college campus. *Journal of Alcohol and Drug Education* **30**, 88–97.

McKinlay J.B. (1992) Health promotion through healthy public policy: The contribution of complementary research methods. *Canadian Journal of Public Health* **83** (Suppl.), 11–19S.

McKnight A.J. (1990) Intervention with alcohol-impaired drivers by peers, parents and purveyors of alcohol. *Health Education Research: Theory and Practice* **5**, 225–36.

McKnight A.J. (1991) Factors influencing the effectiveness of server-intervention education. *Journal of Studies on Alcohol* **52**, 389–97.

McKnight A.J. and Streff F.M. (1994) The effect of enforcement upon service of alcohol to intoxicated patrons of bars and restaurants. *Accident Analysis and Prevention* **26**, 79–88.

McKnight A.J. and Voas R.B. (2001) Prevention of alcohol-related road crashes. In: Heather N., Peters T.J., and Stockwell T. (eds), *International Handbook of Alcohol Dependence and Problems*, pp. 741–70. Chichester, UK: John Wiley & Sons.

McMillan G.P. and Lapham S. (2006) Effectiveness of bans and laws in reducing traffic deaths: Legalized Sunday packaged alcohol sales and alcohol-related traffic crashes and crash fatalities in New Mexico. *American Journal of Public Health* **96**, 1944–8.

McMillan G.P., Hanson T.E., and Lapham S.C. (2007) Geographic variability in alcohol-related crashes in response to legalized Sunday packaged alcohol sales in New Mexico. *Accident Analysis and Prevention* **39**, 252–7.

McNally A.M. and Palfai T.P. (2003) Brief group alcohol intervention with college students: Examining motivational components. *Journal of Drug Education* **33**, 159–76.

Meier P., Booth A., Stockwell T., Sutton A., Wilkinson A., and Wong R. (2008a) *Independent Review of the Effects of Alcohol Pricing and Promotion: Part A: Systematic Reviews.* Sheffield, UK: ScHARR, University of Sheffield. Available at: http://www.dh.gov.uk/en/Publichealth/Healthimprovement/Alcoholmisuse/DH_4001740 (accessed 9 July 2009).

Meier P., Brenna A., Purshouse R., Taylor K., Rafia R., Booth A., Stockwell T., Sutton A., Wilkinson A., and Wong R. (2008b) *Independent review of the effects of alcohol pricing and promotion: Part B—Modelling the potential impact of pricing and promotion policies for alcohol in England: Results from the Sheffield Alcohol Policy Model.* Sheffield, UK: ScHARR, University of Sheffield. Available at: http://www.dh.gov.uk/en/Publichealth/Healthimprovement/Alcoholmisuse/DH_4001740 (accessed 9 July 2009).

Meilman P.W. and Haygood-Jackson D. (1996) Data on sexual assault from the first 2 years of a comprehensive campus prevention program. *Journal of American College Health* **44**, 157–65.

Meilman P.W., Burwell C., Smith K.E., Canterbury R.J., Gressard C.G., Pryor J.H., Fleming R.L., Gaylor M.S., Nelson G.C., and Turco J.H. (1993) Using survey data to capture students'attention: Three institutions look at alcohol-induced sexual behavior. *Journal of College Student Development* **34**, 72–3.

Mendoza M.M., Medina-Mora E.M., Villatoro J., and Durand A. (2005) Alcohol consumption among Mexican women: Implications in a syncretic culture. In: Obot I.S. and Room R. (eds), *Alcohol, gender and drinking problems: Perspectives from low and middle income countries*, pp. 125–42. Geneva: World Health Organization.

Metzner C. and Kraus L. (2008) The impact of alcopops on adolescent drinking: A literature review. *Alcohol and Alcoholism* **43**, 230–9.

Miczek K.A., Weerts E.M., and DeBold J.F. (1993) Alcohol, benzodiazepine-GABA receptor complex and aggression: Ethological analysis of individual differences in rodents and primates. *Journal of Studies on Alcohol* Suppl. 11, 170–9S.

Miczek K.A., DeBold J.F., van Erp A.M.M., and Tornatzky W. (1997) Alcohol, GABAA: benzodiazepine receptor complex, and aggression. In: Galanter M. (ed.) *Recent Developments in Alcoholism.* Vol. 13: *Alcohol and Violence*, pp. 139–71. New York, NY: Plenum Press.

Midanik L. (1999) Drunkenness, feeling the effects, and 5+ measures: Meaning and predictiveness. *Addiction* **94**, 887–97.

Midanik L.T., Tam T.W., Greenfield T., and Caetano R. (1996) Risk functions for alcohol-related problems in a 1988 U.S. national sample. *Addiction* **91**, 1427–37.

Midford R. and McBride N. (2004) Alcohol education in schools. In: Heather N. and Stockwell T. (eds), *The essential handbook of treatment and prevention of alcohol problems*, pp. 298–319. Chichester, UK: Wiley.

Milio N. (1988) Making healthy public policy: Developing the science by learning the art: An ecological framework for policy studies. *Health Promotion* **2**, 263–74.

Miller P.G., Kypri K., Chikritzhs T.N., Skov S.J., and Rubin G. (2009) Health experts reject industry-backed funding for alcohol research. *Medical Journal of Australia* **190**, 713–14.

Miller T., Snowden C., Birckmayer J., and Hendrie D. (2006) Retail alcohol monopolies, underage drinking, and youth impaired driving deaths. *Accident Analysis and Prevention* **38**, 1162–7.

Miller T.R., Lestina D.C., and Spicer R.S. (1998) Highway crash costs in the United States by driver age, blood alcohol level, victim age, and restraint use. *Accident Analysis and Prevention* **30**, 137–50.

Miller T.R., Blewden M., and Zhang J.-F. (2004) Cost savings from a sustained compulsory breath testing and media campaign in New Zealand. *Accident Analysis and Prevention* **36**, 783–94.

Miller W.R., Brown J.M., Simpson T.L., Handmaker N.S., Bien T.H., Luckie L.F., Montgomery H.A., Hester R.K., and Tonigan J.S. (1995) What works?: A methodological analysis of the alcohol treatment outcome literature. In: Hester R.K. and Miller W.R. (eds), *Handbook of alcoholism treatment approaches: effective alternatives*, 2nd edn, pp. 12–44. Boston: Allyn & Bacon.

Miron J.A. and Tetelbaum E. (2007) *Does the minimum legal drinking age save lives?* NBER Working Paper No. 13257. Cambridge, MA: National Bureau of Economic Research.

Mohan D. (2002) Road safety in less motorized environments: Future concerns. *International Journal of Epidemiology* **31**, 527–32.

Møller L. (2002) Legal restrictions resulted in a reduction of alcohol consumption among young people in Denmark. In: Room R. (ed.), *The effects of Nordic alcohol policies: analyses of changes in control systems*, pp. 155–66. Publication No. 42. Helsinki: Nordic Council for Alcohol and Drug Research.

Molof J.J., Dresser J., Ungerleider S., Kimball C., and Schaefer J. (1995) *Assessment of year-round and holiday ride service programs*. DOT HS 808 203. Springfield, VA: National Technical Information Service.

Monaghan L.F. (2002) Regulating 'unruly' bodies: Work tasks, conflict and violence in Britain's night-time economy. *British Journal of Sociology* **53**, 403–29.

Monteiro M.G. (2007) *Alcohol and public health in the Americas: A case for action*. Washington, DC: Pan American Health Organization.

Montgomery K. (1997) Alcohol and tobacco on the web: New threats to young. Executive summary. Washington, DC: Center for Media Education.

Morgenstern H. (1998) Ecologic studies. In: Rothman K.J. and Greenland S. (eds), *Modern Epidemiology*, pp. 459–80. Philadelphia: Lippincott–Raven.

Morrisey M.A., Grabowski D.C., Dee T.S., and Campbell C. (2006) The strength of graduated drivers licensing programs and fatalities among teen drivers and passengers. *Accident Analysis and Prevention* **38**, 135–41.

Morrison L., Begg D.J., and Langley J.D. (2002) Personal and situational influences on drink driving and sober driving among a cohort of young adults. *Injury Prevention* **8**, 111–15.

Mosher J., Toomey T.L., Good C., Harwood E., and Wagenaar A.C. (2002) State laws mandating or promoting training programs for alcohol servers and establishment managers: An assessment of statutory and administrative procedures. *Journal of Public Health Policy* **23**, 90–113.

Mosher J.F. (1990) *Community responsible beverage service programs: An implementation handbook*. San Rafael, CA: Marin Institute for Prevention of Alcohol and Other Drug-Related Problems.

Mosher J.F. (ed.) (2002) *Liquor liability law*. Albany, NY: Bender.

Mosher J.F. (2005) Transcendental alcohol marketing: Rap music and the youth market. *Addiction* **100**, 1203–4.

Mosher J.F. and Johnsson D. (2005) Flavored alcoholic beverages: An international marketing campaign that targets youth. *Journal of Public Health Policy* **26**, 326–42.

Moskalewicz J. (1993) Lessons to be learnt from Poland's attempt at moderating its consumption of alcohol. *Addiction* **88** (Suppl.), 135–42S.

Moskalewicz J. (2000) Alcohol in the countries in transition: The Polish experience and the wider context. *Contemporary Drug Problems* **27**, 561–92.

Moskalewicz J. and Swiatkiewicz G. (2000) Alcohol consumption and its consequences in Poland in the light of official statistics. In: Leifman H. and Edgren Henrichsen N. (eds), *Statistics on alcohol, drugs and crime in the Baltic Sea region*, pp. 143–161. Publication No. 37. Helsinki: Nordic Council for Alcohol and Drug Research.

Moskowitz H. and Fiorentino D. (2000) A review of the literature on the effects of low doses of alcohol on driving related skills. NHTSA Publication No. DOT HS-809–028. Washington, DC: National Highway Traffic Safety Administration.

Moskowitz H., Blomberg R., Burns M., Fiorentino D., and Peck R. (2002) Methodological issues in epidemiological studies of alcohol crash risk. In: Mayhew D.R. and Dussault C. (eds), *Proceedings of the 16th International Conference on Alcohol, Drugs and Traffic Safety, Montreal, Canada, 4–9 August 2002*, pp. 45–50. Québec, Canada: Société de l'automobile du Québec. Available at: http://www.saaq.gouv.qc.ca/t2002/actes/pdf/%2806a%29.pdf (accessed 13 July 2009).

Moskowitz J.M. (1989) Primary prevention of alcohol problems: A critical review of the research literature. *Journal of Studies on Alcohol* **50**, 54–88.

Mugford S. (1984) *Experiment in price manipulation of low alcohol beer*. Sydney: New South Wales Drug and Alcohol Authority.

Mukamal K.J. and Rimm E.B. (2001) Alcohol's effects on the risk for coronary heart disease. *Alcohol Research and Health* **25**, 255–61.

Mulder M., Ranchor A.V., Sanderman R., Bouma J., and van den Heuvel W.J. (1998) Stability of lifestyle behaviour. *International Journal of Epidemiology* **27**, 199–207.

Mulford H.A., Ledolter J., and Fitzgerald J.L. (1992) Alcohol availability and consumption: Iowa sales data revisited. *Journal of Studies on Alcohol* **53**, 487–94.

Mumenthaler M.S., Taylor J.L., O'Hara R., and Yesavage J.A. (1999) Gender differences in moderate drinking effects. *Alcohol Research and Health* **23**, 55–64.

Munro G. (2004) An addiction agency's collaboration with the drinks industry: Moo Joose as a case study. *Addiction* **99**, 1370–4.

Murphy G.E. (2000) Psychiatric aspects of suicidal behaviour: Substance abuse. In: Hawton K. and van Heeringen K. (eds), *The International Handbook of Suicide and Attempted Suicide*, pp. 135–46. Chichester, UK: Wiley.

Murphy J.G., Duchnick J.J., Vuchinich R.E., Davison J.W., Karg R.S., Olson A.M., Smith A.F., and Coffey T.T. (2001) Relative efficacy of a brief motivational intervention for college student drinkers. *Psychology of Addictive Behaviors* **15**, 373–9.

Murray C.J.L. and Lopez A. (1996a) Quantifying the burden of disease and injury attributable to ten major risk factors. In: Murray C.J.L. and Lopez A. (eds), *The global burden of disease: A comprehensive assessment of mortality and disability from diseases, injuries and risk factors in 1990 and projected to 2020*, pp. 295–324. Cambridge, MA: Harvard University Press.

Murray C.J.L. and Lopez A.D. (eds) (1996b) *The global burden of disease: A comprehensive assessment of mortality and disability from diseases, injuries and risk factors in 1990 and projected to 2020*. Global Burden of Disease and Injury Series, Vol. I. Cambridge, MA: Harvard School of Public Health on behalf of the World Health Organization and the World Bank.

Murray C.J.L. and Lopez A. (1997) Mortality by cause for eight regions of the world: Global Burden of Disease study. *The Lancet* **349**, 1269–76.

Murray C.J.L. and Lopez A. (1999) On the comparable quantification of health risks: Lessons from the Global Burden of Disease study. *Epidemiology* **10**, 594–605.

Murray C.J.L., Salomon J.A., and Mathers C. (2000) A critical examination of summary measures of population health. *Bulletin of the World Health Organization* **78**, 981–94.

Murray J.P., Jr, Stam A., and Lastovicka J.L. (1996) Paid- versus donated-media strategies for public service announcement campaigns. *Public Opinion Quarterly* **60**, 1–29.

Murray L.F. and Belenko S. (2005) CASASTART: A community-based, school-centered intervention for high-risk youth. *Substance Use and Misuse* **40**, 913–33.

Murray R.P., Rehm J., Shaten J., and Connett J.E. (1999) Does social integration confound the relation between alcohol consumption and mortality in the Multiple Risk Factor Intervention Trial (MRFIT)? *Journal of Studies on Alcohol* **60**, 740–5.

Musgrave S. and Stern N. (1988) Alcohol: Demand and taxation under monopoly and oligopoly in South India in the 1970s. *Journal of Development Economics* **28**, 1–41.

Mustonen H. and Mäkelä K. (1999) Relationships between characteristics of drinking occasions and negative and positive experiences related to drinking. *Drug and Alcohol Dependence* **56**, 79–84.

Nagata T., Setoguchi S., Hemenway D., and Perry M. (2008) Effectiveness of a law to reduce alcohol-impaired driving in Japan. *Injury Prevention: Journal of the International Society for Child and Adolescent Injury Prevention* **14**, 19–23.

Naimi T.S., Brewer R.D., Miller J.W., Okoro C., and Mehrotra C. (2007) What do binge drinkers drink?: Implications for alcohol control policy. *American Journal of Preventive Medicine* **30**, 188–93.

National Health and Medical Research Council (2009) *Australian guidelines to reduce health risks from drinking alcohol*. Canberra: National Health and Medical Research Council. Available at: http://www.nhmrc.gov.au/publications/synopses/ds10syn.htm (accessed 15 July 2009).

National Highway Traffic Safety Administration (1998) *Traffic safety facts, 1997*. Washington, DC: US Government Printing Office.

National Highway Traffic Safety Administration (2008) *Traffic safety facts 2006*. NHTSA Publication No. DOT HS 810 818. Washington, DC: National Highway Traffic Safety Administration. Available at: http://www-nrd.nhtsa.dot.gov/Pubs/TSF2006FE.PDF (accessed 13 July 2009).

National Institute for Alcohol and Drug Research (2001) *Alcohol and drugs in Norway*. Oslo: National Institute for Alcohol and Drug Research.

Neighbors C., Lewis M.A., Bergstrom R.L., and Larimer M.E. (2006) Being controlled by normative influences: Self-determination as a moderator of a normative feedback alcohol intervention. *Health Psychology* **25**, 571–9.

Nelson J. (2003) Advertising bans, monopoly, and alcohol demand: testing for substitution effects using state panel data. *Review of Industrial Organization* **22**, 1–25.

Nelson J. (2008a) Alcohol advertising bans, consumption and control policies in seventeen OECD countries, 1975–2000. *Applied Economics*. doi: 10.1080/00036840701720952

Nelson J.P. (2008b) How similar are youth and adult alcohol behaviors?: Panel results for excise taxes and outlet density. *Atlantic Economic Journal* **36**, 89–104.

Nelson J. and Moran J. (1995) Advertising and U.S. alcoholic beverage demand: System-wide estimates. *Applied Economics* **27**, 1225–36.

Nelson J. and Young D. (2001) Do advertising bans work? An international comparison. *International Journal of Advertising* **20**, 273–96.

Nemtsov A.V. (1998) Alcohol-related harm and alcohol consumption in Moscow before, during and after a major anti-alcohol campaign. *Addiction* **93**, 1501–10.

Nemtsov A.V. (2005) Russia: Alcohol yesterday and today. *Addiction* **100**, 146–9.

Nemtsov A.V. and Krasovsky C.S. (1996) An overview of national and local alcohol-related problems in the CIS. *Drugs: Education, Prevention and Policy* **3**, 21–8.

Newman I.M., Anderson C.S., and Farrell K.A. (1992) Role rehearsal and efficacy: Two 15-month evaluations of a ninth-grade alcohol education program. *Journal of Drug Education* **22**, 55–67.

Newton A., Sarker S.J., Pahal G.S., van den Bergh E., and Young C. (2007) Impact of the new UK licensing law on emergency hospital attendances: A cohort study. *British Medical Journal* **24**, 532–4.

Niederer R., Korn K., Lussmann D., and Kölliker M. (2008) *Marktstudie und Befragung junger Erwachsener zum Konsum alkoholhaltiger Mischgetränke (Alcopops)*. Olten, Switzerland: Direktionsbereich Öffentliche Gesundheit.

Nordlund S. (1985) *Effects of Saturday closing of wine and spirits shops in Norway*. SIFA Mimeograph No. 5/85. Oslo: National Institute of Alcohol Research.

Nordlund S. and Österberg E. (2000) Unrecorded alcohol consumption: Its economics and its effects on alcohol control in the Nordic countries. *Addiction* **12**, 551–64.

Nordwall S.P. (2000) Homemade alcohol kills 121 in Kenya. Arlington, VA. *USA Today*, 20 November.

Norström T. (1987) Abolition of the Swedish rationing system: Effects on consumption distribution and cirrhosis mortality. *British Journal of Addiction* **82**, 633–41.

Norström T. (1988) Alcohol and suicide in Scandinavia. *British Journal of Addiction* **83**, 553–9.

Norström T. (1993) Family violence and total consumption of alcohol. *Nordisk Alkoholtidskrift* **10**, 311–18.

Norström T. (1995) Alcohol and suicide: A comparative analysis of France and Sweden. *Addiction* **90**, 1463–9.

Norström T. (1996) Per capita consumption and total mortality: An analysis of historical data. *Addiction* **91**, 339–44.

Norström T. (1997) Assessment of the impact of the 0.02% BAC-limit in Sweden. *Studies on Crime and Crime Prevention* **6**, 245–58.

Norström T. (1998) Effects on criminal violence of different beverage types and private and public drinking. *Addiction* **93**, 689–99.

Norström T. (2000) Outlet density and criminal violence in Norway, 1960–1995. *Journal of Studies on Alcohol* **61**, 907–11.

Norström T. (2005) The price elasticity for alcohol in Sweden 1984–2003. *Nordisk alkohol- & narkotikatidskrift* [Nordic Studies on Alcohol and Drugs] **22** (English Suppl.), 87–101.

Norström T. and O.-J. Skog. (2005) Saturday opening of alcohol retail shops in Sweden: An experiment in two phases. *Addiction* **100**, 767–76.

Northbridge D.B., McMurray J., and Lawson A.A. (1986) Association between liberalization of Scotland's liquor licensing laws and admissions for self poisoning in West Fife. *British Medical Journal (Clinical Research Edition)* **293**, 1466–8.

Noval S. and Nilsson T. (1984) Mellanölets effekt på konsumtionsnivån och tillväxten hos den totala alkoholkonsumtionen [The effects of medium beer on consumption levels and the rise in overall alcohol consumption]. In: Nilsson T. (ed.), *När Mellanölet Försvann* [When the medium beer was withdrawn], pp. 77–93. Linköping, Sweden: Samhällsvetenskapliga institutionen, Universitetet i Linköping.

Nygaard P., Waiters E.D., Grube J.W., and Keefe D. (2003) Why do they do it?: A qualitative study of adolescent drinking and driving. *Substance Use and Misuse* **38**, 835–63.

O'Brien K.S. and Kypri K. (2008) Alcohol industry sponsorship and hazardous drinking among sportspeople. *Addiction* **103**, 1961–6.

O'Connor R.E., Lin L., Tinkoff G.H., and Ellis H. (2007) Effect of a graduated licensing system on motor vehicle crashes and associated injuries involving drivers less than 18 years-of-age. *Prehospital Emergency Care* **11**, 389–93.

O'Donnell M. (1985) Research on drinking locations of alcohol-impaired drivers: Implications for prevention policies. *Journal of Public Health Policy* **6**, 510–25.

Ofcom (2007) *Young people and alcohol advertising: An investigation of alcohol advertising following changes to the advertising code.* London: Office of Communications. Available at: http://www.ofcom.org.uk/research/tv/reports/alcohol_advertising/alcohol_advertising.pdf (accessed 9 March 2009).

Ogborne A.C. and Smart. R.G. (1980) Will restrictions on alcohol advertising reduce alcohol consumption? *British Journal of Addiction* **75**, 293–329.

Ogden E.J. and Moskowitz H. (2004) Effects of alcohol and other drugs on driver performance. *Traffic Injury Prevention* **5**, 185–98.

Ohsfeldt R.L. and Morrisey M.A. (1997) Beer taxes, workers' compensation, and industrial injury. *Review of Economics and Statistics* **79**, 155–60.

Okello A.K. (2001) *An analysis of excise taxation in Kenya.* African Economic Policy Discussion Paper No. 73. Arlington, VA: Equity and Growth through Economic Research.

Olsson B., Ólafsdóttir H., and Room R. (2002) Introduction: Nordic traditions of studying the impact of alcohol policies. In: Room R. (ed.), *The effects of Nordic alcohol policies: what happens to drinking and problems when alcohol controls change?*, pp. 5–11. NAD Publication No. 42. Helsinki: Nordic Council for Alcohol and Drug Research. Available at: http://www.nad.fi/pdf/NAD_42.pdf (accessed 9 July 2009).

O'Malley P.M. and Wagenaar A.C. (1991) Effects of minimum drinking age laws on alcohol use, related behaviors and traffic crash involvement among American youth: 1976–1987. *Journal of Studies on Alcohol* **52**, 478–91.

O'Neill B. and Mohan D. (2002) Reducing motor vehicle crash deaths and injuries in newly motorizing countries. *British Medical Journal* **324**, 1142–5.

Ornstein S.I. and Hanssens D.M. (1985) Alcohol control laws and the consumption of distilled spirits and beer. *Journal of Consumer Research* **12**, 200–13.

Osoro N., Mpango P., and Mwinyimvua H. (2001) *An analysis of excise taxation in Tanzania.* African Economic Policy Discussion Paper No. 72. Arlington, VA: Equity and Growth through Economic Research.

Österberg E. (1979) *Recorded consumption of alcohol in Finland, 1950–1975.* Report No. 125. Helsinki: Social Research Institute of Alcohol Studies.

Österberg E. (1985) From home distillation to the state alcohol monopoly. *Contemporary Drug Problems* **12**, 31–51.

Österberg E. (1995) Do alcohol prices affect consumption and related problems? In: Holder H.D. and Edwards G. (eds), *Alcohol and public policy: Evidence and issues*, pp. 145–63. Oxford: Oxford University Press.

Österberg E. and Haavisto K. (1997) Alkoholsmugglingen till Finland under 1990-talet [Smuggling of alcoholic beverages into Finland in the 1990s]. *Nordisk alkohol- and narkotikatidskrift* **14**, 290–303.

Österberg E. and Karlsson T. (eds) (2003) *Alcohol policies in EU member states and Norway: A collection of country reports*. Helsinki: STAKES.

Ouimette P.C., Finney J.W., Gima K., and Moos R.H. (1999) A comparative evaluation of substance abuse treatment: examining mechanisms underlying patient-treatment matching hypotheses for 12-step and cognitive-behavioral treatments for substance abuse. *Alcoholism: Clinical and Experimental Research* **23**, 545–51.

Özgüven C. (2004) *Analysis of demand and pricing policies in Turkey beer market. [Dissertation.]* Ankara: Graduate School of Natural and Applied Sciences, Middle East Technical University. Available at: http://etd.lib.metu.edu.tr/upload/3/12605208/index.pdf (accessed 9 July 2009).

Paasma R., Hovda K.E., Tikkerberi A., and Jacobsen D. (2007) Methanol mass poisoning in Estonia: Outbreak in 154 patients. *Clinical Toxicology* **45**, 152–7.

Paglia A. and Room R. (1999) Preventing substance use problems among youth: A literature review and recommendations. *Journal of Primary Prevention* **20**, 3–50.

Pan-European Designated Driver Campaign 2006 (2007). Available at: http://ec.europa.eu/ transport/roadsafety_library/publications/eurobob_final_report.pdf (accessed 16 July 2009).

Paradis C., Demers A., Picard E., and Graham K. (2009) The importance of drinking frequency in evaluating individuals' drinking patterns: Implications for the development of national drinking guidelines. *Addiction* **104**, 1179–84.

Parker R.N. (2004) Alcohol and violence: Connections, evidence and possibilities for prevention. *Journal of Psychoactive Drugs* Suppl. 2, 157–63.

Parker R.N. and Cartmill R.S. (1998) Alcohol and homicide in the United States 1934–1995— or one reason why US rates of violence may be going down. *Journal of Criminal Law and Criminology* **88**, 1369–98.

Parry C.D.H. (1998) *Alcohol policy and public health in South Africa*. Cape Town: Oxford University Press.

Parry C., Rehm J., Poznyak V., and Room R. (2009) Alcohol and infectious diseases: An overlooked causal linkage? *Addiction* **104**, 331–2.

Partanen J. (1975) On the role of situational factors in alcohol research: Drinking in restaurants vs. drinking at home. *Drinking and Drug Practices Surveyor* **10**, 14–16.

Partanen J. (1991) *Sociability and intoxication: Alcohol and drinking in Kenya, Africa, and the modern world*. Helsinki: Finnish Foundation for Alcohol Studies.

Pasch K., Komro K., Perry C., Hearst M., and Farbakhsh K. (2007) Outdoor alcohol advertising near schools: What does it advertise and how is it related to intentions and use of alcohol among young adolescents? *Journal of Studies on Alcohol and Drugs* **68**, 587–96.

Paschall M.J., Grube J.W., Black C.A., and Ringwalt C.L. (2007) Is commercial alcohol availability related to adolescent alcohol sources and alcohol use? Findings from a multi-level study. *Journal of Adolescent Health* **41**, 168–74.

Paulson R.E. (1973) *Women's suffrage and prohibition: A comparative study of equality and social control.* Glenview, IL: Scott, Foresman & Co.

Peden M., Scurfield R., Sleet D., Mohan D., Hyder A.A., Jarawan E., and Mathvers C. (eds) (2004) *World report on road traffic injury prevention.* Geneva: World Health Organization.

Pedersen M.U., Vind L., Milter M., and Grønbæk M. (2004) *Alkoholbehandlingsindsatsen i Danmark—semmenlignet med Sverige* (The alcohol treatment efforts in Denmark— compared with Sweden). Aarhus, Denmark: Center for Rusmiddelforskning.

Peek-Asa C. (1999) The effect of random alcohol screening in reducing motor vehicle crash injuries. *American Journal of Preventative Medicine* **16** (Suppl. 1), 57–67.

Peele S. and Brodsky A. (2000) Exploring psychological benefits associated with moderate alcohol use: Necessary corrective to assessments of drinking outcomes? *Drug and Alcohol Dependence* **60**, 221–47.

Pentz M.A., Dwyer J.H., MacKinnon D.P., Flay B.R., Hansen W.B., Wang E.Y.-I., and Johnson C.A. (1989) A multi-community trial for primary prevention of drug abuse: Effects on drug use prevalence. *Journal of the American Medical Association* **261**, 3259–66.

Perdrix J., Bovet P., Larue D., Yersin B., Burnand B., and Paccaud F. (1999) Patterns of alcohol consumption in the Seychelles Islands (Indian Ocean). *Alcohol and Alcoholism* **34**, 773–85.

Perez R.L. (2000) Fiesta as tradition, fiesta as change: Ritual, alcohol and violence in a Mexican community. *Addiction* **95**, 365–73.

Perkins H.W. (2002) Social norms and the prevention of alcohol misuse in collegiate contexts. *Journal of Studies on Alcohol* Suppl. 14, 164–72.

Perkins H.W. and Craig D.W. (2003) *A multifaceted social norms approach to reduce high-risk drinking: Lessons from Hobart and William Smith Colleges.* Newton, MA: Higher Education Center for Alcohol and other Drug Prevention, Department of Education.

Pernanen K. (1991) *Alcohol in human violence.* New York: Guilford Press.

Pernanen K. (1996) *Sammenhengen alkohol-vold* (The relationship between alcohol and violence). Oslo: National Institute for Alcohol and Drug Research.

Pernanen K. (2001) What is meant by 'alcohol-related' consequences? In: Klingemann H. and Gmel G. (eds), *Mapping the social consequences of alcohol consumption*, pp. 21–31. Dordrecht: Kluwer.

Perry C.L., Williams C.L., Forster J.L., Wolfson M., Wagenaar A.C., Finnegan J.R., McGovern P.G., Veblen-Mortenson S., Komro K.A., and Anstine P.S. (1993) Background, conceptualization and design of a community-wide research program on adolescent alcohol use: Project Northland. *Health Education Research: Theory and Practice* **8**, 125–36.

Perry C.L., Williams C.L., Veblen-Mortenson S., Toomey T.L., Komro K.A., Anstine P.S., McGovern P.G., Finnegan J.R., Forster J.L., Wagenaar A.C., and Wolfson M. (1996) Project Northland: Outcomes of a community-wide alcohol use prevention program during early adolescence. *American Journal of Public Health* **86**, 956–65.

Perry C.L., Williams C.L., Komro K.A., Veblen-Mortenson S., Forster J.L., Bernsten-Lachter R., Pratt L.K., Munson K.A., and Farbakhsh K. (1998) Project Northland—phase II: Community action to reduce adolescent alcohol use. Paper presented at the Kettil Bruun Society Thematic Meeting, February, Russell, Bay of Islands, New Zealand.

Peters T. (ed.) (1998) *Alcohol and cardiovascular diseases.* Novartis Foundation Symposium 216. Chichester, UK: Wiley.

Peterson J.B., Rothfleisch J., Zelazo P., and Pihl R.O. (1990) Acute alcohol intoxication and neuropsychological functioning. *Journal of Studies on Alcohol* **51**, 114–22.

Petrie J., Bunn F., and Byrne G. (2007) Parenting programmes for preventing tobacco, alcohol or drugs misuse in children <18: A systematic review. *Health Education Research* **22**, 177–191.

Pierce J. (2007) Tobacco industry marketing, population-based tobacco control, and smoking behavior. *American Journal of Preventive Medicine* **33** (Suppl.), S327–34.

Pihl R.O., Peterson J.B., and Lau M.A. (1993) A biosocial model of the alcohol-aggression relationship. *Journal of Studies on Alcohol* Suppl. 11, 128–39S.

Pindyck R.S., Rubinfeld D.L., and Eastin R.V. (1989) *Microeconomics*. New York: Macmillan.

Pinsky I. and Laranjeira R. (2007) Ethics of an unregulated alcohol market. *Addiction* **102**, 1038–9.

Pissochet P., Biache P., and Paille F. (1999) Alcool, publicité et prévention: Le régard des jeunes (Alcohol, advertising and prevention: Young people's point of view). *Alcoologie* **21**, 15–24.

Poikolainen K. (1980) Increase in alcohol-related hospitalizations in Finland 1969–1975. *British Journal of Addiction* **75**, 281–91.

Poikolainen K. (2002) Alcohol sales and fatal alcohol poisonings. *Addiction* **97**, 1037–40.

Poikolainen K., Paljärvi T., and Mäkelä P. (2007) Alcohol and the preventive paradex: Serious harms and drinking patterns. *Addiction* **102**, 571–8.

Polacsek M., Rogers E.M., Woodall W.G., Delaney H., Wheeler D., and Rao N. (2001) MADD victim impact panels and stages of change in drunk driving prevention. *Journal of Studies on Alcohol* **62**, 344–50.

Pollack C.E., Cubbin C., Ahn D., and Winkleby M. (2005) Neighbourhood deprivation and alcohol consumption: Does the availability of alcohol play a role? *International Journal of Epidemiology* **34**, 772–80.

Pomerleau J., McKee M., Rose R., Haerpfer C.W., Rotman D., and Tumanov S. (2005) Drinking in the Commonwealth of Independent States: Evidence from eight countries. *Addiction* **100**, 1647–68.

Pomerleau J., McKee M., Rose R., Haerpfer C.W., Rotman D., and Tumanov S. (2008) Hazardous alcohol drinking in the former Soviet Union: A cross-sectional study of eight countries. *Alcohol and Alcoholism* **43**, 351–9.

Ponicki W.R., Gruenewald P.J., and LaScala E.A. (2007) Joint impacts of minimum legal drinking age and beer taxes on US youth traffic fatalities, 1975 to 2001. *Alcoholism: Clinical and Experimental Research* **31**, 804–13.

Prasad R. (2009) Alcohol use on the rise in India. *Lancet* **373**, 17–18.

Pratten J. and Greig B. (2007) Can Pubwatch address the problems of binge drinking?: A case study from the North West of England. *International Journal of Contemporary Hospitality Management* **17**, 252–60.

Pridemore W.A. (2002) Vodka and violence: Alcohol consumption and homicide rates in Russia. *American Journal of Public Health* **92**, 1921–30.

Puddey I.B., Rakic V., Dimmitt S.B., and Beilin L.J. (1999) Influence of pattern of drinking on cardiovascular disease and cardiovascular risk factors: A review. *Addiction* **94**, 649–63.

Puffer R. and Griffith G.W. (1967) *Patterns of urban mortality*. Scientific Publication No. 151. Washington, DC: Pan American Health Organization.

Putnam S.L., Rockett I.R.H., and Campbell M.K. (1993) Methodological issues in community-based alcohol-related injury prevention projects: Attribution of program effects. In: Greenfield T.K. and Zimmerman R. (eds), *Experiences with community action projects:*

New research in the prevention of alcohol and other drug problems, pp. 31–9. Rockville, MD: Center for Substance Abuse Prevention.

Quigley B.M. and Leonard K.E. (1999) Husband alcohol expectancies, drinking, and marital conflict styles as predictors of severe marital violence among newlywed couples. *Psychology of Addictive Behaviors* **13**, 49–59.

Rabinovich L., Brutscher P.B., de Vries H., Tiessen J., Clift J., and Reding A. (2009) *The affordability of alcoholic beverages in the European Union: Understanding the link between alcohol affordability, consumption and harms*. Rand Technical Report. Cambridge: Rand Europe. Available at: http://www.rand.org/pubs/technical_reports/2009/RAND_TR689.pdf (accessed 9 July 2009).

Rae J. (1991) Too many ifs and buts on alcohol. (Letter.) *The Times*, 26 December.

Ragnarsdóttir T., Kjartansdóttir A., and Davidsdóttir S. (2002) Effect of extended alcohol serving-hours in Reykjavik. In: Room R. (ed.), *The effects of Nordic alcohol policies: analyses of changes in control systems*, pp. 145–54. Publication No. 42. Helsinki: Nordic Council for Alcohol and Drug Research.

Rahman L. (2002) *Alcohol prohibition and addictive consumption in India*. London: London School of Economics.

Raistrick D., Hodgson R., and Ritson B. (1999) *Tackling alcohol together: The evidence base for a UK alcohol policy*. London: Free Association Books.

Ramful P. and Zhao X. (2008) Individual heterogeneity in alcohol consumption: The case of beer, wine and spirits in Australia. *Economic Record* **84**, 207–22.

Ramstedt M. (2001) Alcohol and suicide in 14 European countries. *Addiction* **96** (Suppl. 1), 59–75S.

Ramstedt M. (2002a) Alcohol-related mortality in 15 European countries in the postwar period. *European Journal of Population* **18**, 307–23.

Ramstedt M. (2002b) The repeal of medium strength beer in grocery stores in Sweden: The impact on alcohol-related hospitalizations in different age groups. In: Room R. (ed.), *The effects of Nordic alcohol policies: analyses of changes in control systems*, pp. 69–78. Publication No. 42. Helsinki: Nordic Council for Alcohol and Drug Research.

Ramstedt M. (2006) Is alcohol good or bad for Canadian hearts? A time-series analysis of the link between alcohol consumption and IHD mortality. *Drug and Alcohol Review* **25**, 315–20.

Ramstedt M. (2009) Fluctuations in male ischaemic heart disease mortality in Russia 1959–1998: Assessing the importance of alcohol. *Drug and Alcohol Review* **28**, 390–5.

Rearck Research (1991) *A study of attitudes towards alcohol consumption, labelling and advertising*. Canberra: Department of Community Services and Health.

Reed D.S. (1981) Reducing the costs of drinking and driving. In: Moore M.H. and Gerstein D.R. (eds), *Alcohol and public policy: Beyond the shadow of prohibition*, pp. 336–87. Washington DC: National Academy Press.

Rehm J.T. (2000) Alcohol consumption and mortality: What do we know and where should we go? *Addiction* **95**, 989–95.

Rehm J.T. and Eschmann S. (2002) Global monitoring of average volume of alcohol consumption. *Sozial- und Präventivmedizin* **47**, 48–58.

Rehm J.T. and Fischer B. (1997) Measuring harm: Implications for alcohol epidemiology. In: Plant M., Single E., and Stockwell T. (eds), *Alcohol: minimising the harm: What works?*, pp. 248–61. London: Free Association Books.

Rehm J.T. and Gmel G. (2000a) Gaps and needs in international alcohol epidemiology. *Journal of Substance Use* 5, 6–13.

Rehm J.T. and Gmel G. (2000b) Aggregating dimensions of alcohol consumption to predict medical and social consequences. *Journal of Substance Abuse* 12, 155–68.

Rehm J.T. and Rossow I. (2001) The impact of alcohol consumption on work and education. In: Klingemann H. and Gmel G. (eds), *Mapping the social consequences of alcohol consumption*, pp. 67–77. Dordrecht: Kluwer.

Rehm J.T. and Sempos C.T. (1995a) Alcohol Consumption and mortality—questions about causality, confounding and methodology. *Addiction* 90, 493–8.

Rehm J.T. and Sempos C.T. (1995b) Alcohol consumption and all-cause mortality. *Addiction* 90, 471–80.

Rehm J.T., Bondy S., Sempos C.T., and Vuong C.V. (1997) Alcohol consumption and coronary heart disease morbidity and mortality. *American Journal of Epidemiology* 146, 495–501.

Rehm J.T., Frick U., and Bondy S. (1999) A reliability and validity analysis of an alcohol-related harm scale for surveys. *Journal of Studies on Alcohol* 60, 203–8.

Rehm J.T., Gmel G., Room R., Monteiro M., Gutjahr E., Graham K., Jernigan D. and Sempos C. (2001a) Alcohol as a risk factor for burden of disease. In: Ezzati M., Lopez A.D., Rodgers A., and Murray C.J.L. (eds), *Comparative quantification of health risks: Global and regional burden of disease due to selected major risk factors*. Geneva: World Health Organization.

Rehm J.T., Greenfield T.K., and Rogers J.D. (2001b) Average volume of alcohol consumption, patterns of drinking and all-cause mortality: Results from the US National Alcohol Survey. *American Journal of Epidemiology* 153, 64–71.

Rehm J.T., Gutjahr E., and Gmel G. (2001c) Alcohol and all-cause mortality: A pooled analysis. *Contemporary Drug Problems* 28, 337–61.

Rehm J.T., Monteiro M., Room R., Gmel G., Jernigan D., Frick U., and Graham K. (2001d) Steps towards constructing a global comparative risk analysis for alcohol consumption: Determining indicators and empirical weights for patterns of drinking, deciding about the theoretical minimum, and dealing with differential consequences. *European Addiction Research* 7, 138–47.

Rehm J.T., Room R., Monteiro M., Gmel G., Graham K., Rehn N., Sempos C.T., and Jernigan D. (2003a) Alcohol as a risk factor for global burden of disease. *European Addiction Research* 9, 157–64.

Rehm J.T., Sempos C.T., and Trevisan M. (2003b) Average volume of alcohol consumption, patterns of drinking and risk of coronary heart disease: A review. *Journal of Cardiovascular Risk* 10, 15–20.

Rehm J.T., Room R., Monteiro M., Gmel G., Graham K., Rehn N., Sempos C.T., Frick U., and Jernigan D. (2004) Alcohol use. In: Ezzati M., Lopez A.D., Rodgers A., and Murray C.J.L. (eds), *Comparative quantification of health risks: Global and regional burden of disease attributable to selected major risk factors*, Vol. 1, pp. 959–1108. Geneva: World Health Organization.

Rehm J.T., Patra J., Baliunas D., Popova S., Roerecke M., and Taylor B. (2006) *Alcohol consumption and the global burden of disease 2002*. Geneva: WHO, Department of Mental Health and Substance Abuse, Management of Substance Abuse.

Rehm J.T., Mathers C., Popova S., Thavorncharoensap M., Teerawattananon Y., and Patra J. (2009) Global burden of disease and injury and economic cost attributable to alcohol use and alcohol use disorders. *Lancet* 373, 2223–33.

Reiling D.M. and Nusbaumer M.R. (2007) An exploration of the potential impact of the designated driver campaign on bartenders' willingness to over-serve. *International Journal of Drug Policy* **18**, 458–63.

Reitan T.C. (2000) Does alcohol matter? Public health in Russia and the Baltic countries before, during, and after the transition. *Contemporary Drug Problems* **27**, 511–60.

Rigaud A. and Craplet M. (2004) The 'Loi Évin': A French exception. *The Globe* 1/2, 33–4.

Rimm E.B., Klatsky A.L., Grobbe D., and Stampfer M. (1996) Review of moderate alcohol consumption and reduced risk of coronary heart disease: Is the effect due to beer, wine, or spirits? *British Medical Journal* **312**, 731–6.

Ripatti S. and Mäkelä P. (2008) Conditional models accounting for regression to the mean in observational multi-wave panel studies on alcohol consumption. *Addiction* **103**, 24–31.

Rise J., Natvig H., and Storvoll E.E. (2005) Evaluering av alkoholkampanjen 'Alvorlig talt'(Evaluation of the alcohol campaign 'Seriously talking'). Oslo: Norwegian Institute for Alcohol and Drug Research.

Rivara F.P., Relyea-Chew A., Wang J., Riley S., Boisvert D., and Gomez T. (2007) Drinking behaviors in young adults: The potential role of designated driver and safe ride home programs. *Injury Prevention* **13**, 168–72.

Roberts M. (2004) *Good practice in managing the evening and late night economy: A literature review from an environmental perspective.* London: Office of the Deputy Prime Minister.

Roberts A.J. and Koob G.F. (1997) The neurology of addiction: An overview. *Alcohol Health and Research World* **21**, 101–43.

Robinson S.E., Roth S.L., Gloria A.M., Keim J., and Sattler H. (1993) Influence of substance abuse education on undergraduates' knowledge, attitudes and behaviors. *Journal of Alcohol and Drug Education* **39**, 123–30.

Rogers J.D. and Greenfield T.K. (1999) Beer drinking accounts for most of the hazardous alcohol consumption reported in the United States. *Journal of Studies on Alcohol* **60**, 732–9.

Rohrbach L.A., Howard-Pitney B., Unger J.B., Dent C.W., Howard K.A., Cruz T.B., Ribis K.M., Norman G.J., Fishbein H., and Johnson C.A. (2002) Independent evaluation of the California Tobacco Control program: Relationships between program exposure and outcomes, 1996–1998. *American Journal of Public Health* **92**, 975–83.

Roizen R. (1981) *The world health organization study of community responses to alcohol-related problems: A review of cross-cultural findings.* Geneva: World Health Organization.

Romanus G. (2000) Alcopops in Sweden: A supply-side initiative. *Addiction* **95** (Suppl. 4): S609–19.

Romelsjö A. (1987) Decline in alcohol-related in-patient care and mortality in Stockholm County. *British Journal of Addiction* **82**, 653–63.

Romelsjö A. and Andersson T. (1999) Emergence of community alcohol and drug prevention programs in municipalities and communities during a transition phase for alcohol policy in Sweden. In: Larsson S. and Hanson B.S. (eds), *Community-based alcohol prevention in Europe: Research and Evaluations*, pp. 208–19. Lund: Lunds Universitet.

Roncek D.W. and Maier P.A. (1991) Bars, blocks, and crimes revisited: Linking the theory of routine activities to the empiricism of "hot spots". *Criminology* **29**, 725–53.

Room R. (1984a) The World Health Organization and alcohol control. *British Journal of Addiction* **79**, 85–92.

Room R. (1984b) Alcohol control and public health. *Annual Review of Public Health* **5**, 293–317.

Room R. (1993) Evolution of alcohol monopolies and their relevance for public health. *Contemporary Drug Problems* **20**, 169–87.

Room R. (1996) Alcohol consumption and social harm: conceptual issues and historical perspectives. *Contemporary Drug Problems* **23**, 373–88.

Room R. (1998) Thirsting for attention. (Editorial.) *Addiction* **93**, 797–8.

Room R. (1999) The idea of alcohol policy. *Nordic Studies on Alcohol and Drugs* **16**, 7–20.

Room R. (2000a) Alcohol monopolies as instruments for alcohol control policies. In: Österberg E. (ed.), *International seminar on alcohol retail monopolies*, pp. 7–16. Helsinki: National Research and Development Centre for Welfare and Health, Themes 5/2000.

Room R. (2000b) Concepts and items in measuring social harm from drinking. *Journal of Substance Abuse* **12**, 93–111.

Room R. (2001) Intoxication and bad behaviour: Understanding cultural differences in the link. *Social Science and Medicine* **53**, 189–98.

Room R. (2004) Disabling the public interest: Alcohol strategies and policies for England. *Addiction* **99**, 1083–9.

Room R. (2006a) International control of alcohol: Alternative paths forward. *Drug and Alcohol Review* **25**, 581–95.

Room R. (2006b) Advancing industry interests in alcohol policy: The double game. *Nordic Studies on Alcohol and Drugs* **23**, 389–92.

Room R. and Jernigan D. (2000) The ambiguous role of alcohol in economic and social development. *Addiction* **95**, S523–35.

Room R. and Mäkelä K. (2000) Typologies of the cultural position of drinking. *Journal of Studies on Alcohol* **61**, 475–83.

Room R. and Paglia A. (1999) The international drug control system in the post-Cold War era: Managing markets or fighting a war? *Drug and Alcohol Review* **18**, 305–15.

Room R. and Rossow I. (2001) The share of violence attributable to drinking. *Journal of Substance Use* **6**, 218–28.

Room R., Bondy S., and Ferris J. (1995a) The risk of harm to oneself from drinking, Canada 1989. *Addiction* **90**, 499–513.

Room R., Graves K., Giesbrecht N., and Greenfield T. (1995b) Trends in public opinion about alcohol policy initiatives in Ontario and the US: 1989–91. *Drug and Alcohol Review* **14**, 35–47.

Room R., Janca A., Bennett L.A., Schmidt L., and Sartorius N., with 15 others (1996) WHO cross-cultural applicability research on diagnosis and assessment of substance use disorders: An overview of methods and selected results. *Addiction* **91**, 199–220.

Room R., Rehm J., Trotter R.T., II, Paglia A., and Üstün T.B. (2001) Cross-cultural views on stigma, valuation, parity, and societal values towards disability. In: Üstün T.B., Chatterji S., Bickenbach J.E., Trotter R.T., II, Room R., Rehm J., and Saxena S. (eds), *Disability and culture: Universalism and diversity*, pp. 247–91. Seattle: Higrefe & Huber.

Room R., Jernigan D., Carlini-Marlatt B., Gureje O., Mäkelä K., Marshall M., Medina Mora M.E., Monteiro M., Parry C., Partanen J., Riley L., and Saxena S. (2002) *Alcohol in developing societies: A public health approach*. Helsinki: Finnish Foundation for Alcohol Studies.

Room R., Österberg E., Ramstedt M., and Rehm J. (2009) Explaining change and stasis in alcohol consumption. *Addiction Research and Theory [online access]*, doi: 10.1080/16066350802626966.

Rose G. (2001) Sick individuals and sick populations. *International Journal of Epidemiology* **30**, 427–32.

Ross H.L. (1982) *Deterring the drinking driver: Legal policy and social control.* Lexington, MA: Lexington Books.

Ross H.L. (1992) *Confronting drunk driving: Social policy for saving lives.* New Haven, CT: Yale University Press.

Ross H.L. (1993) Prevalence of alcohol-impaired driving: An international comparison. *Accident Analysis and Prevention* **25**, 777–9.

Ross H.L. and Klette H. (1995) Abandonment of mandatory jail for impaired drivers in Norway and Sweden. *Accident Analysis and Prevention* **27**, 151–7.

Ross H.L. and Voas R.B. (1989) *The new Philadelphia story: The effects of severe penalties for drunk driving.* Washington, DC: AAA Foundation for Traffic Safety.

Rossow I. (1996) Alcohol related violence: The impact of drinking pattern and drinking context. *Addiction* **91**, 1651–61.

Rossow I. (2000) Suicide, violence and child abuse: Review of the impact of alcohol consumption on social problems. *Contemporary Drug Problems* **27**, 397–434.

Rossow I. (2001) Drinking and violence: A cross-cultural comparison of the relationship between alcohol consumption and homicide in 14 European countries. *Addiction* **96** (Suppl. 1), 77–92S.

Rossow I. and Romelsjö A. (2006) The extent of the 'prevention paradox' in alcohol problems as a function of population drinking patterns. *Addiction* **101**, 84–90.

Rossow I. and Wichstrøm L. (1994) Parasuicide and use of intoxicants among Norwegian adolescents. *Suicide and Life-Threatening Behavior* **24**, 174–83.

Rossow I., Pape H., and Wichstrøm L. (1999) Young, wet and wild? Associations between alcohol intoxication and violent behaviour in adolescence. *Addiction* **94**, 1017–31.

Rossow I., Pernanen K., and Rehm J. (2001) Alcohol, suicide and violence. In: Klingemann H. and Gmel G. (eds), *Mapping the social consequences of alcohol consumption*, pp. 93–112. Dordrecht: Kluwer.

Rossow I., Pape H., and Storvoll E.E. (2005) Beruselsens kilder: hvordan ungdom skaffer seg alkohol [Sources of intoxication: How do adolescents get hold of alcohol?]. *Tidsskr Nor Laegeforen* **125**, 1160–2.

Rossow I., Karlsson T., and Raitasalo K. (2008) Old enough for a beer?: Compliance with minimum legal age for alcohol purchases in monopoly and other off-premise outlets in Finland and Norway. *Addiction* **103**, 1468–73.

Roth R., Voas R., and Marques P. (2007) Mandating interlocks for fully revoked offenders: The New Mexico experience. *Traffic Injury Prevention* **8**, 20–25.

Rothe J.P. (2005) *Impaired driving as lifestyle for 18–29-year-old Alberta drivers: Focus group analysis.* Alberta: Alberta Centre for Injury Control and Research. Available at: http://www.acicr.ualberta.ca/pages/documents/ABTransGroupAnalysisFINALReport.pdf (accessed 13 July 2009).

Rothman K.J., Greenland S., and Lash T.L. (2008) *Modern epidemiology*, 3rd edn. Philadelphia: Lippincott Williams & Wilkins.

Royal D. (2003) *2001 National survey of drinking and driving. Volume I: Summary report.* NHTSA Publication No. DOT HS 809 549. Washington, DC: National Highway Traffic

Safety Administration. Available at: http://www.nhtsa.dot.gov/staticfiles/DOT/NHTSA/ Traffic%20Injury%20Control/Articles/Associated%20Files/DD2001v1.pdf (accessed 13 July 2009).

Ruhm C.J. (1995) Economic conditions and alcohol problems. *Journal of Health Economics* **14**, 583–603.

Ruhm C.J. (1996) Acohol policies and highway vehicle fatalities. *Journal of Health Economics* **15**, 435–54.

Ruhm C.J. and Black W.E. (2002) Does drinking really decrease in bad times? *Journal of Health Economics* **21**, 659–78.

Rush B. (1785) *An inquiry into the effects of ardent spirits upon the human body and mind, with an account of the means of preventing, and of the remedies for curing them.* 8th edn. Reprint. Exeter: N.H. Richardson.

Russ N.W. and Geller E.S. (1987) Training bar personnel to prevent drunken driving: A field evaluation. *American Journal of Public Health* **77**, 952–4.

SABMiller (2007). SABMiller Annual report. Available at: http://www.sabmiller.com/files/ reports/ar2007/index.html (accessed 3 July 2009).

Saffer H. (1991) Alcohol advertising bans and alcohol abuse: An international perspective. *Journal of Health Economics* **10**, 65–79.

Saffer H. (1997) Alcohol advertising and highway fatalities. *Review of Economics and Statistics* **79**, 431–42.

Saffer H. (1998) Economic issues in cigarette and alcohol advertising. *Journal of Drug Issues* **28**, 781–93

Saffer H. (2002) Alcohol advertising and youth. *Journal of Studies on Alcohol* Suppl. 14, 173–81.

Saffer H. and Chaloupka F. (2000) The effect of tobacco advertising bans on tobacco consumption. *Journal of Health Economics* **19**, 1117–37.

Saffer H. and Dave D. (2002) Alcohol consumption and alcohol advertising bans. *Applied Economics* **30**, 1325–34.

Saffer H. and Dave D. (2006) Alcohol advertising and alcohol consumption by adolescents. *Health Economics* **15**, 617–37.

Saffer H. and Grossman M. (1987a) Beer taxes, the legal drinking age, and youth motor vehicle fatalities. *Journal of Legal Studies* **16**, 351–74.

Saffer H. and Grossman M. (1987b) Drinking age laws and highway mortality rates: Cause and effect. *Economic Inquiry* **25**, 403–17.

Saltz R.F. (1987) The roles of bars and restaurants in preventing alcohol-impaired driving: An evaluation of server intervention. *Evaluation and the Health Professions* **10**, 5–27.

Saltz R.F. and Stanghetta P. (1997) A community-wide responsible beverage service program in three communities: Early findings. *Addiction* **92** (Suppl. 2), 237–49S.

San José B., van Oers J.A.M., van de Mheen H., Garretsen H.F.L., and Mackenbach J.P. (2000) Drinking patterns and health outcomes: Occasional versus regular drinking. *Addiction* **95**, 865–72.

Sarkar S., Andreas M., and de Faria F. (2005) Who uses safe ride programs: An examination of the dynamics of individuals who use a safe ride program instead of driving home while drunk. *American Journal of Drug and Alcohol Abuse* **31**, 305–25.

Saunders B. and Yap E. (1991) Do our guardians need guarding? An examination of the Australian system of self-regulation of alcohol advertising. *Drug and Alcohol Review* **10**, 15–17.

Saunders J.B., Kypri K., Walters S.T., Laforge R.G., and Larimer M.E. (2004) Approaches to brief intervention for hazardous drinking in young people. *Alcoholism: Clinical and Experimental Research* **28**, 322–9.

Sayette M.A., Wilson T., and Elias M.J. (1993) Alcohol and aggression: A social information processing analysis. *Journal of Studies on Alcohol* **54**, 399–407.

Schaap M., Kunst A., Leinsalu M., Regidor E., Ekholm O., Dzurova D., Helmert U., Klumbiene J., Santana P., and Mackenbach J.P. (2008) Effect of nationwide tobacco control policies on smoking cessation in high and low educated groups in 18 European countries. *Tobacco Control* **17**, 248–55.

Schechter E. (1986) Alcohol rationing and control systems in Greenland. *Contemporary Drug Problems* **13**, 587–620.

Schroeder C.M. and Prentice D.A. (1998) Exposing pluralistic ignorance to reduce alcohol use among college students. *Journal of Applied Social Psychology* **28**, 2150–80.

Schwartz M.D. and Kennedy W.S. (1997) Factors associated with male peer support for sexual assault on the college campus. In: Schwartz M.D. and DeKeseredy W.S. (eds), *Sexual assault on the college campus: The role of male peer support*, pp. 97–136. Thousand Oaks, CA: Sage.

Scott L., Donnelly N., Poynton S., and Weatherburn D. (2007) Young adults' experience of responsible service practice in NSW: An update. *Alcohol Studies Bulletin* **9**, 1–8.

Scottish Government (2009) Tackling alcohol misuse. [News release] Edinburgh: Scottish Government. Available at: http://www.scotland.gov.uk/News/Releases/2009/03/02085300 (accessed 9 July 2009).

Scottish Health Action on Alcohol Problems (2007) *Alcohol—price, policy and public health*. Edinburgh: SHAAP.

Scribner R.A., MacKinnon D.P., and Dwyer J.H. (1994) Alcohol outlet density and motor vehicle crashes in Los Angeles County cities. *Journal of Studies on Alcohol* **55**, 447–53.

Scribner R.A., Cohen D.A., and Fisher W. (2000) Evidence of a structural effect for alcohol outlet density: A multilevel analysis. *Alcoholism: Clinical and Experimental Research* **24**, 188–95.

Scribner R.A., Mason K., Theall K., Simonsen N., Schneider S.K., Towvim G.L., and DeJong W. (2008) The contextual role of alcohol outlet density in college drinking. *Journal of Studies on Alcohol and Drugs* **69**, 112–20.

Searles H., Bernard J.P., and Johnson C.D. (1996) Alcohol and the pancreas. In: Peters T.J. (ed.), *Alcohol misuse: A European perspective*, pp. 145–162. Amsterdam: Harwood.

Seeley J.R. (1960) Death by liver cirrhosis and the price of beverage alcohol. *Canadian Medical Association Journal* **83**, 1361–6.

Seeley J.R. (1988) Death by liver cirrhosis and the price of beverage alcohol. In: Buck C. (ed.), *The challenge of epidemiology: issues and selected readings*, pp. 350–357. Washington, DC: Pan American Health Organization. (Originally published Canadian Medical Association Journal 83, 1361–6, 1960.)

Selvanathan E. (1989) Advertising and alcohol demand in the U.K.: Further results. *International Journal of Advertising* **8**, 181–8.

Selvanathan E.A. (1991) Cross-country alcohol consumption comparison: An application of the Rotterdam demand system. *Applied Economics* **23**, 1613–22.

Selvanathan S. and Selvanathan E.A. (2005a) *The demand for alcohol, tobacco and marijuana: International evidence*. Burlington VT: Ashgate Publishing.

Selvanathan S. and Selvanathan E.A. (2005b) Empirical regularities in cross-country alcohol consumption. *The Economic Record* **81** (Suppl. 1), 128–42.

Sen B. (2006) The relationship between beer taxes, other alcohol policies, and child homicide deaths. *Topics in Economic Analysis and Policy* **6**, 1–17.

SHAAP. See Scottish Health Action on Alcohol Problems.

Shamblen S.R. and Derzon J.H. (2009) A preliminary study of the population-adjusted effectiveness of substance abuse prevention programming: towards making IOM program types comparable. *Journal of Primary Prevention* **30**, 89–107.

Shaper A.G. (1990a) Alcohol and mortality: A review of prospective studies. *British Journal of Addiction* **85**, 837–47.

Shaper A.G. (1990b) A response to commentaries: The effects of self-selection. *British Journal of Addiction* **85**, 859–61.

Shaper A.G., Wannamethee S.G., and Walker M. (1988) Alcohol and mortality in British men: Explaining the U-shaped curve. *Lancet* **2**, 1267–73.

Sheldon T. (1996) Dutch anti-alcohol campaign is under attack. *British Medical Journal* **313**, 1349.

Sheldon T. (2000) Dutch tighten their rules on advertising of alcohol. *British Medical Journal* **320**, 1094.

Sherman D.J.N. and Williams R. (1994) Liver damage: Mechanisms and management. *British Medical Bulletin* **50**, 124–38.

Sherman L.W., Strang H., and Woods D.J. (2000) *Recidivism patterns in the Canberra Reintegrative Shaming Experiment (RISE)*. Canberra: Centre for Restorative Justice, Research School of Social Sciences, Australian National University.

Shinar D. and Compton R.P. (1995) Victim impact panels: Their impact on DWI recidivism. *Alcohol, Drugs and Driving* **11**, 73–87.

Shkolnikov V., McKee M., and Leon D.A. (2001) Changes in life expectancy in Russia in the mid-1990s. *Lancet* **357**, 917–921.

Shkolnikov V.M and Nemtsov A. (1997) The anti-alcohol campaign and variations in Russian mortality. In: Bobadilla J.L., Costello C.A., and Mitchell F. (eds), *Premature death in the new Independent States*, pp. 239–61. Washington, DC: National Academy Press.

Shope J.T. (2007) Graduated driver licensing: Review of evaluation results since 2002. *Journal of Safety Research* **38**, 165–75.

Shope J.T. and Molnar L.J. (2003) Graduated driver licensing in the United States: Evaluation results from the early programs. *Journal of Safety Research* **34**, 63–9.

Shope J.T., Dielman T.E., Butchart A.T., Campanelli P.C., and Kloska D.D. (1992) An elementary school-based alcohol misuse program: A follow-up evaluation. *Journal of Studies on Alcohol* **53**, 106–21.

Shope J.T., Kloska D.D., Dielman T.E., and Maharg R. (1994) Longitudinal evaluation of an enhanced Alcohol Misuse Prevention Study (AMPS) curriculum for grades six-eight. *Journal of School Health* **64**, 160–6.

Shope J.T., Copeland L.A., Maharg R., and Dielman T.E. (1996a) Effectiveness of a high school alcohol misuse prevention program. *Alcoholism: Clinical and Experimental Research* **20**, 791–8.

Shope J.T., Copeland L.A., Marcoux B.C., and Kamp M.E. (1996b) Effectiveness of a school-based substance abuse prevention program. *Journal of Drug Education* **26**, 323–37.

Shults R.A., Elder R.W., Sleet D.A., Nicholas J.L., Alao M.O., Carande-Kulis V.G., Zaza S., Sosin D.M., Thompson R.S., and the Task Force on Community Preventive Services (2001) Reviews of evidence regarding interventions to reduce alcohol-impaired driving. *American Journal of Preventive Medicine* **21**, 66–88.

Shults R.A., Sleet D.A. Elder R.W., Ryan G.W., and Sehgal M. (2002) Association between state level drinking and driving countermeasures and self reported alcohol impaired driving. *Injury Prevention* **8**, 106–10.

Sim M., Morgan E., and Batchelor J. (2005) *The impact of enforcement on intoxication and alcohol related harm.* Wellington, New Zealand: Accident Compensation Corporation.

Simpson H.M., Beirness D.J., Robertson R.D., Mayhew D.R. and Hedlund J.H. (2004) Hard core drinking drivers. *Traffic Injury Prevention* **5**, 261–9.

Simpura J. (1995) Alcohol in Eastern Europe: market prospects, prevention puzzles. *Addiction* **90**, 467–70.

Simpura J. (1998) Mediterranean mysteries: Mechanisms of declining alcohol consumption. *Addiction* **93**, 1301–4.

Simpura J. and Karlsson T. (2001) Trends in drinking patterns among adult population in 15 European countries, 1950 to 2000: A review. *Nordic Studies on Alcohol and Drugs* **15** (English Suppl.), 31–53.

Simpura J., Levin B., and Mustonen H. (1997) Russian drinking in the 1990s: Patterns and trends in international comparison. In: Simpura J. and Levin B. (eds), *Demystifying Russian drinking: comparative studies from the 1990s*, pp. 79–107. Helsinki: STAKES.

Singh A. (1993) Evaluation of four films on drinking and driving known as 'One for the Road' series. *Journal of Traffic Medicine* **21**, 65–72.

Single E. (1993) Public drinking. In: Galanter M. (ed.), *Recent developments in alcoholism*, Vol. 11, *Ten years of progress*, pp. 143–52. New York: Plenum Press.

Single E. and McKenzie D. (1992) The epidemiology of impaired driving stemming from licensed establishments. Presented at 18th Annual Alcohol Epidemiology Symposium, Toronto, 1–5 June.

Single E. and Wortley S. (1993) Drinking in various settings as it relates to demographic variables and level of consumption: Findings from a national survey in Canada. *Journal of Studies on Alcohol* **54**, 590–9.

Single E., Beaubrun M., Mauffret M., Minoletti A., Moskalewicz J., Moukolo A., Plange N.K., Saxena S., Stockwell T., Sulkunen P., Suwaki H., Hoshigoe K., and Weiss S. (1997) Public drinking, problems and prevention measures in twelve countries: Results of the WHO project on public drinking. *Contemporary Drug Problems* **24**, 425–48.

Single E., Robson L., Xie X., and Rehm J. (1998) The economic costs of alcohol, tobacco and illicit drugs in Canada, 1992. *Addiction* **93**, 991–1006.

Single E., Robson L., Rehm J., and Xie X. (1999) Morbidity and mortality attributable to alcohol, tobacco, and illicit drug use in Canada. *American Journal of Public Health* **89**, 385–90.

Singletary K.W. and Gapstur S.M. (2001) Alcohol and breast cancer: Review of epidemiologic and experimental evidence and potential mechanisms. *Journal of the American Medical Association* **286**, 2143–51.

Sivarajasingam V., Matthews K., and Shepherd J. (2006) Price of beer and violence-related injury in England and Wales. *Injury* **37**, 388–94.

Skager R. (2007) Replacing ineffective early alcohol/drug education in the United States with age-appropriate adolescent programmes and assistance to problematic users. *Drug and Alcohol Review* **26**, 577–84.

Skara S. and Sussman S. (2003) A review of 25 long-term adolescent tobacco and other drug use prevention program evaluations. *Preventive Medicine* **37**, 451–74.

Skog O.-J. (1985) The collectivity of drinking cultures: A theory of the distribution of alcohol consumption. *British Journal of Addiction* **80**, 83–99.

Skog O.-J. (1988) Effect of introducing a new light beer in Norway: Substitution or addition? *British Journal of Addiction* **83**, 665–8.

Skog O.-J. (1991a) Alcohol and suicide: Durkheim revisited. *Acta Sociologica* **34**, 193–206.

Skog O.-J. (1991b) Drinking and the distribution of alcohol consumption. In: Pittman D.J. and Raskin H. (eds), *White society, culture, and drinking patterns reexamined*, pp. 135–56. New Brunswick, NJ: Alcohol Research Documentation.

Skog O.-J. (1996) Public health consequences of the J-curve hypothesis of alcohol problems. *Addiction* **91**, 325–37.

Skog O.J. (1999) The prevention paradox revisited. *Addiction*, 94, 751–7.

Skog O.-J. (2000) An experimental study of a change from over-the-counter to self-service sales of alcoholic beverages in monopoly outlets. *Journal of Studies on Alcohol* **61**, 95–100.

Skog O.-J. (2001a) Alcohol consumption and mortality rates from traffic accidents, accidental falls, and other accidents in 14 European countries. *Addiction* **96** (Suppl. 1), 49–58S.

Skog O.-J. (2001b) Commentary on Gmel and Rehm's interpretation of the theory of collectivity in drinking culture. *Drug and Alcohol Review* **20**, 325–31.

Skog O.-J. and Bjørk E. (1988) *Alkohol og voldskriminalitet: En analyse av utviklingen i Norge 1931–1982* (Alcohol and violent crimes: An analysis of the 1931–1982 trends in Norway). Oslo, Norway: SIFO.

Skog O.-J. and Melberg H.O. (2006) Becker's rational addiction theory: An empirical test with price elasticities for distilled spirits in Denmark 1911–31. *Addiction* **101**, 1444–50.

Slater M.D., Kelly K.J., Edwards R.W., Thurman P.J., Plested B.A., Keefe T.J., Lawrence F.R., and Henry K.L. (2006) Combining in-school and community-based media efforts: Reducing marijuana and alcohol intake among younger adolescents. *Health Education Research* **21**, 157–67.

Slater M.D., Rouner D., Murphy K., Beauvais F., Van Leuven J.K., and Domenech-Rodriguez M.M. (1996) Adolescents counterarguing of TV beer advertisements: Evidence for effectiveness of alcohol education and critical viewing discussions. *Journal of Drug Education* **26**, 143–58.

Sloan F.A., Reilly B.A., and Schenzler C. (1994a) Effects of prices, civil and criminal sanctions and law enforcement on alcohol-related mortality. *Journal of Studies on Alcohol* **55**, 454–65.

Sloan F.A., Reilly B.A., and Schenzler C.M. (1994b) Tort liability versus other approaches for deterring careless driving. *International Review of Law and Economics* **14**, 53–71.

Sloan F.A., Stout E.M., Whetten-Goldstein K., and Liang L. (2000) *Drinkers, drivers, and bartenders: Balancing private choices and public accountability*. Chicago: University of Chicago Press.

Smart R.G. (1996a) Behavioral and social consequences related to the consumption of different beverage types. *Journal of Studies on Alcohol* **57**, 77–84.

Smart R.G. (1996b) Happy hour experiment in North America. *Contemporary Drug Problems* **23**, 291–300.

Smart R.G. and Adlaf E.M. (1986) Banning happy hours: The impact on drinking and impaired driving charges in Ontario, Canada. *Journal of Studies on Alcohol* **47**, 256–8.

Smart R.G. and Cutler R.E. (1976) The alcohol advertising ban in British Colombia: Problems and effects on beverage consumption. *British Journal of Addiction* **71**, 13–21.

Smart R.G. and Mann R.E. (2000) The impact of programs for high-risk drinkers on population levels of alcohol problems. *Addiction* **95**, 37–52.

Smith C.A., Wolynetz M.S. and Wiggins T.R.I. (1976) *Drinking drivers in Canada: A national roadside survey of the blood alcohol concentrations in nighttime Canadian drivers.* Ottawa: Transport Canada, Road and Motor Vehicle Traffic Safety Branch.

Smith D.I. (1986a) Comparison of patrons of hotels with early opening and standard hours. *International Journal of the Addictions* **21**, 155–63.

Smith D.I. (1986b) Effect on non-traffic accident hospital admissions of lowering the drinking age in two Australian states. *Contemporary Drug Problems* **13**, 621–39.

Smith D.I. and Burvill P. (1986) Effect on traffic safety of lowering the drinking age in three Australian states. *Journal of Drug Issues* **16**, 183–98.

Smith D.I. and Burvill P. (1987) Effect on juvenile crime of lowering the drinking age in three Australian states. *Addiction* **82**, 181–8.

Smith L. and Foxcroft D. (2009) The effect of alcohol advertising and marketing on drinking behaviour in young people: A systematic review. *BMC Public Health* 9:51, doi:10.1186/1471-2458-9-51.

Smith R., Beaglehole R., Woodward D., and Drager N. (eds) (2003) *Global public goods for health: Health, economic and public health perspectives.* Oxford: Oxford University Press.

Smith S., Atkin C., and Roznowski J. (2006) Are "drink responsibly" alcohol campaigns strategically ambiguous? *Health Communication* **20**, 1–111.

Smith W.R., Frazee S.G., and Davison E.L. (2000) Furthering the integration of routine activity and social disorganization theories: Small units of analysis and street robbery as a diffusion process. *Criminology* **38**, 489–524.

Smith-Warner S.A., Spiegelman D., Yaun S.-S., Van den Brandt P.A., Folsom A.R., Goldbohm R.A., Graham S., Holmberg L., Howe G.R., Marshall J.R., Miller A.B., Potter J.D., Speizer F.E., Willett W.C., Wolk A., and Hunter D.J. (1998) Alcohol and breast cancer in women: A pooled analysis of cohort studies. *Journal of the American Medical Association* **279**, 535–40.

Snow R.W. and Landrum J.W. (1986) Drinking locations and frequency of drunkenness among Mississippi DUI offenders. *American Journal of Drug and Alcohol Abuse* **12**, 389–402.

Snyder L., Milici F., Slater M., Sun H., and Strizhakova Y. (2006) Effects of advertising exposure on drinking among youth. *Archives of Pediatrics and Adolescent Medicine* **160**, 18–24.

Snyder L.B. and Blood D.J. (1992) Caution: Alcohol advertising and the Surgeon General's alcohol warning may have adverse effects on young adults. *Journal of Applied Communication Research* **20**, 37–53.

Solomon R. and Payne J. (1996) Alcohol liability in Canada and Australia: Sell, serve and be sued. *Tort Law Review* **4**, 188–241.

Spaite D.W., Meislin H.W., Valenzuela T.D., Criss E.A., Smith R., and Nelson A. (1990) Banning alcohol in a major college stadium: Impact on the incidence and patterns of injury and illness. *Journal of American College Health* **39**, 125–8.

Spoth R., Redmond C., and Lepper H. (1999) Alcohol initiatiation outcomes of universal family-focused prevention interventions: One- and two-year follow-ups of a controlled study. *Journal of Studies on Alcohol* **13**, 103–11.

Spoth R., Redmond C., and Shin C. (2001) Randomized trial of brief family interventions for general populations: Adolescent substance use outcomes four years following baseline. *Journal of Consulting and Clinical Psychology* **69**, 627–42.

Spoth R., Redmond C., Trudeau L., and Shin C. (2002) Longitudinal substance initiation outcomes for a universal prevention intervention combining family and school programs. *Psychology of Addictive Behavior* **16**, 129–34.

Spoth R., Redmond C., Shin C., and Azevedo K. (2004) Brief family intervention effects on adolescent substance initiation school-level growth curve analyses 6 years following baseline. *Journal of Consulting and Clinical Psychology* **72**, 535–42.

Spoth R., Randall K.G., Shin C., and Redmond C. (2005) Randomized study of combined universal family and school prevention interventions: Patterns of long-term effects on initiation, regular use, and weekly drunkenness. *Psychology of Addictive Behaviors* **19**, 372–81.

Stacy A., Zogg J., Ungar M., and Dent C. (2004) Exposure to televised alcohol ads and subsequent adolescent alcohol use. *American Journal of Health Behavior* **28**, 498–509.

Steffian G. (1999) Correction of normative misperception: An alcohol abuse prevention program. *Journal of Drug Education* **29**, 115–38.

Stenius K. and Babor T.F. (2009) The alcohol industry and public interest science. *Addiction* (online early access). DOI: 10.1111/j.360-0443.2009.02688.x.

Stenius K., Storbjörk J., and Romelsjö A. (2005) Decentralisation and integration of addiction treatment: Does it make any difference? A preliminary study in Stockholm county. Paper presented at the 31st Annual Alcohol Epidemiology Symposium of the Kettil Bruun Society for Social and Epidemiological Research on Alcohol (KBS), Riverside, California, June.

Stevenson M., Palamara P., Rooke M., Richardson K., Baker M., and Baumwol J. (2001) Drink and drug driving among university students: What's the skipper to do? *Australian and New Zealand Journal of Public Health* **2**, 511–13.

Stewart D.W. and Rice R. (1995) Non-traditional media and promotions in the marketing of alcoholic beverages. In: Martin S.E. and Mail P. (eds), *The effects of the mass media on the use and abuse of alcohol*, pp. 209–38. Bethesda, MD: US Department of Health and Human Services.

Stewart K. (1999) *Strategies to reduce underage alcohol use: Typology and brief overview.* Washington, DC: Office of Juvenile Justice and Delinquency Prevention.

Stewart L. (1993) *Police enforcement of liquor licensing laws: The U.K. experience.* Auckland, New Zealand: Alcohol and Public Health Research Unit; School of Medicine, University of Auckland.

Stewart L. and Casswell S. (1993) Media advocacy for alcohol policy support: Results from the New Zealand Community Action Project. *Health Promotion International* **8**, 167–75.

Stewart L., Casswell S., and Duignan P. (1993) Using evaluation resources in a community action project: Formative evaluation of public health input into the implementation of the New Zealand Sale of Liquor Act. *Contemporary Drug Problems* **20**, 681–704.

Stewart L., Casswell S., and Thomson A. (1997) Promoting public health in liquor licensing: Perceptions of the role of alcohol community workers. *Contemporary Drug Problems* **24**, 1–37.

Stockwell T. (1997) Regulation of the licensed drinking environment: A major opportunity for crime prevention. In: Homel R. (ed.), *Policing for prevention: Reducing crime, public intoxication and injury*, Vol. 7, pp. 7–33. Monsey, NY: Criminal Justice Press.

Stockwell T. (2001a) Editor's introduction to prevention of alcohol problems. In: Heather N., Peters T.J., and Stockwell T. (eds), *Handbook of alcohol dependence and alcohol-related problems*, pp. 680–3. Chichester, UK: Wiley.

Stockwell T. (2001b) Harm reduction, drinking patterns and the NHMRC Drinking Guidelines. *Drug and Alcohol Review* 20, 121–9.

Stockwell T. and Chikritzhs T. (2009) Do relaxed trading hours for bars and clubs mean more relaxed drinking?: A review of international research on the impacts of changes to permitted hours of drinking. *Crime Prevention and Community Safety: An International Journal* 11, 171–88.

Stockwell T. and Crosbie D. (2001) Supply and demand for alcohol in Australia: Relationships between industry structures, regulation and the marketplace. *International Journal of Drug Policy* 12, 139–52.

Stockwell T. and Gruenewald P.J. (2004) Controls on the physical availability of alcohol. In: Heather N. and Stockwell T. (eds), *The essential handbook of treatment and prevention of alcohol problems*, pp. 213–33. Chichester, UK: Wiley.

Stockwell T., Lang E., and Rydon P. (1993) High risk drinking settings: The association of serving and promotional practices with harmful drinking. *Addiction* 88, 1519–26.

Stockwell, T., Hawks, D., Lang, E., and Rydon, P. (1996) Unravelling the preventive paradox for acute alcohol problems. *Drug and Alcohol Review* 15, 7–15.

Stockwell T., Gruenewald P., Toumbourou J., and Loxley W. (eds) (2005) *Preventing harmful substance use: The evidence base for policy and practice*. New York: Wiley.

Stockwell T., Zhao J., and Thomas G. (2009) Should alcohol policies aim to reduce total alcohol consumption?: New analyses of Canadian drinking patterns. *Addiction Research and Theory* 17, 135–51.

Stout E.M., Sloan F.A., Liang L., and Davies H.H. (2000) Reducing harmful alcohol-related behaviors: Effective regulatory methods. *Journal of Studies on Alcohol* 61, 402–12.

Stout R.L., Rose J.S., Speare M.C., Buka S.L., Laforge R.G., Campbell M.K., and Waters W.J. (1993) Sustaining interventions in communities: The Rhode Island community-based prevention trial. In: Greenfield T.K. and Zimmerman R. (eds), *Experiences with community action projects: New research in the prevention of alcohol and other drug problems*, pp. 253–61. Rockville, MD: US Department of Health and Human Services.

Suh I., Shaten B.J., Cutler J.A., and Kuller L.H. (1992) Alcohol-use and mortality from coronary heart-disease: The role of high-density lipoprotein cholesterol. *Annals of Internal Medicine* 116, 881–7.

Sulkunen P. (1997) Logics of prevention: Mundane speech and expert discourse on alcohol policy. In: Sulkunen P., Holmwood J., Radner H., and Schulze G. (eds), *Constructing the new consumer society*, pp. 256–76. New York: St Martin's Press.

Sulkunen P., Sutton C., Togerstedt C., and Warpenius K. (eds) (2000) *Broken spirits: Power and ideas in Nordic alcohol control*. NAD Publication No. 39. Helsinki: Nordic Council for Alcohol and Drug Research.

Sutton C. and Nylander J. (1999) Alcohol policy strategies and public health policy at an EU-level: The case of alcopops. *Nordisk alkohol- & narkotikatidskrift* [Nordic Studies on Alcohol and Drugs] 16 (English Suppl.), 74–91.

Sutton M. and Godfrey C. (1995) A grouped data regression approach to estimating economic and social influences on individual drinking behaviour. *Health Economics* **4**, 237–47.

Sweedler B. and Stewart K.G. (2009) Worldwide trends in alcohol and drug impaired driving. In: Verster J.C., Pandi-Perumal S.R., Ramaekers J.G., and de Gier J.J. (eds), *Drugs, driving, and traffic safety*, pp. 23–41. Basel: Birkhäuser.

Sweedler B.M. (2000) The worldwide decline in drinking and driving: Has it continued? In: *Proceedings of the 15th International Conference on Alcohol, Drugs and Traffic Safety.* Stockholm, Sweden: ICADTS. Available at: http://www.ntsb.gov/speeches/s000501.htm (accessed 13 July 2009).

Szabo G. (1997a) Alcohol and susceptibility to tuberculosis. *Alcohol Health and Research World* **21**, 39–41.

Szabo G. (1997b) Alcohol's contribution to compromised immunity. *Alcohol Health and Research World* **21**, 30–8.

Taylor B., Rehm J., Trinidad Caldera Aburto J., Bejarano J., Cayetano C., Kerr-Correa F., Piazza Ferrand M., Gmel G., Graham K., Greenfield T.K., Laranjiera R., Lima M.C., Magri R., Monteiro M.G., Medina Mora M.E., Munné M., Romero M.P., Tucci A.M., and Wilsnack S. (2007) *Alcohol, gender, culture and harms in the Americas: PAHO Multicentric Study Final Report.* Washington, DC: Pan American Health Organization.

Television New Zealand (2008) The twin powers. Sunday, 5 October.

Tesler T.E. and Malone R.E. (2008) Corporate philanthropy, lobbying, and public health policy. *American Journal of Public Health* **98**, 2123–32.

Thamarangsi T. (2008) Alcohol policy process in Thailand. Doctoral dissertation. Auckland: Massey University.

Thombs D.L., Dodd V., Pokorny S.B., Omli M.R., O'Mara R., Webb M.C., Lacaci D.M., and Werch C.E. (2008) Drink specials and the intoxication levels of patrons exiting college bars. *American Journal of Health Behavior* **32**, 411–19.

Thombs D.L., O'Mara R., Dodd V., Hou W., Merves M., Weiler R.M., Pokorny S.B., Goldberger B.A., Reingle J., and Werch C.E. (2009) A field study of bar-sponsored drink specials and their associations with patron intoxication. *Journal of Studies on Alcohol and Drugs* **70**, 206–14.

Thomson A., Bradley E., Casswell S., and Wyllie A. (1997) A qualitative investigation of the responses of in treatment and recovering heavy drinkers to alcohol advertising on New Zealand television. *Contemporary Drug Problems* **24**, 133–46.

Thorsen T. (1990) *Hundrede års alkoholmisbrug: Alkoholforbrug og alkoholproblemer i Danmark* (Hundred years of alcohol abuse: Alcohol consumption and alcohol related problems in Denmark). Copenhagen, Denmark: Alkohol- og Narkotikarådet.

Tigerstedt C. (1990) The European Community and alcohol policy. *Contemporary Drug Problems* **17**, 461–79.

Tigerstedt C. (2000) Discipline and public health. In: Sulkunen P., Sutton C., Tigerstedt C., and Warpenius K. (eds), *Broken spirits: Power and ideas in Nordic alcohol control*, pp. 93–112. NAD Publication No. 39. Helsinki: Nordic Council for Alcohol and Drug Research.

Timko C., Moos R.H., Finney J.W., and Lesar M.D. (2000) Long-term outcomes of alcohol use disorders: Comparing untreated individuals with those in Alcoholics Anonymous and formal treatment. *Journal of Studies on Alcohol* **61**, 529–38.

Timmerman M.A., Geller E.S., Glindemann K.E., and Fournier A.K. (2003) Do the designated drivers of college students stay sober? *Journal of Safety Research* **34**, 127–33.

Tin S.T., Ameratunga S., Robinson E., Crengle S., Schaaf D., and Watson P. (2008) Drink driving and the patterns and context of drinking among New Zealand adolescents. Acta Paediatrica 97, 1433–7.

Tippetts A.S., Voas R.B., Fell J.C., and Nichols J. (2005) A meta-analysis of.08 BAC laws in 19 jurisdictions in the United States. Accident Analysis and Prevention 37, 149–61.

Tobler N.S. (1992) Prevention programs can work: Research findings. Journal of Addictive Diseases 11, 1–28.

Tobler N.S., Roona M.R., Ochshorn P., Marshall D.G., Streke A.V., and Stackpole K.M. (2000) School-based adolescent drug prevention programs: 1998 meta-analysis. Journal of Primary Prevention 20, 275–336.

Toomey T.L., Williams C.L., Perry C.L., Murray D.M., Dudovitz B., and Veblen-Mortenson S. (1996) An alcohol primary prevention program for parents of 7th graders: The Amazing Alternatives! Home program. Journal of Child and Adolescent Substance Use 5, 35–53.

Toomey T.L., Kilian G.R., Gehan J.P., Perry C.L., Jones-Webb R., and Wagenaar A.C. (1998) Qualitative assessment of training programs for alcohol servers and establishment managers. Public Health Reports 113, 162–9.

Toomey T.L., Wagenaar A.C., Gehan J.P., Kilian G., and Perry C.L. (2001) Project ARM: Alcohol risk management to prevent sales to underage and intoxicated patrons. Health Education and Behavior 28, 186–99.

Toomey T.L., Erickson D.J., Lenk K.M., Kilian G.R., Perry C.L., and Wagenaar A.C. (2008) A randomized trial to evaluate a management training program to prevent illegal alcohol sales. Addiction 103, 405–13.

Treisman D. (2008) Pricing death: The political economy of Russia's alcohol crisis. Los Angeles, CA: UCLA, Political Science Department. Available at: http://www.sscnet.ucla.edu/polisci/faculty/treisman/Mortal.pdf (accessed 9 July 2009).

Treno A.J. and Holder H.D. (1997) Community mobilization, organizing, and media advocacy: A discussion of methodological issues. Evaluation Review 21, 166–90.

Treno A.J., Nephew T.M., Ponicki W.R., and Gruenewald P.J. (1993) Alcohol beverage price spectra: Opportunities for substitution. Alcoholism: Clinical and Experimental Research 17, 675–80.

Treno A.J., Breed L., Holder H.D., Roeper P., Thomas B.A., and Gruenewald P.J. (1996) Evaluation of media advocacy efforts within a community trail to reduce alcohol-involved injury: Preliminary newspaper results. Evaluation Review 20, 404–23.

Treno A.J., Gruenewald P.J., and Ponicki W.R. (1997) The contribution of drinking patterns to the relative risk of injury in six communities: a self-report based probability approach. Journal of Studies on Alcohol 58, 372–81.

Treno A.J., Alaniz M.L., and Gruenewald P.J. (2000) The use of drinking places by gender, age and ethnic groups: An analysis of routine drinking activities. Addiction 95, 537–51.

Treno A.J., Grube J., and Martin S.E. (2003) Alcohol availability as a predictor of youth drinking and driving: A hierarchical analysis of survey and archival data. Alcoholism: Clinical and Experimental Research 27, 835–40.

Treno A.J., Gruenewald P.J., Lee J.P., and Remer L.G. (2007a) The Sacramento neighborhood alcohol prevention project: Outcomes from a community prevention trial. Journal of Studies on Alcohol and Drugs 68, 197–207.

Treno A.J., Johnson F.W., Remer L.G., and Gruenewald P.J. (2007b) The impact of outlet densities on alcohol-related crashes: A spatial panel approach. Accident Analysis and Prevention 39, 894–901.

Treno A.J., Ponicki W.R., Remer L.G., and Gruenewald P.J. (2008) Alcohol outlets, youth drinking, and self-reported ease of access to alcohol: A constraints and opportunities approach. *Alcoholism: Clinical and Experimental Research* 32, 1372–9.

Trolldal B. (2005a) The privatization of wine sales in Quebec in 1978 and 1983 to 1984. *Alcoholism: Clinical and Experimental Research* 29, 410–16.

Trolldal B. (2005b) An investigation of the effect of privatization of retail sales of alcohol on consumption and traffic accidents in Alberta, Canada. *Addiction* 100, 662–71.

Trolldal B. (2005c) Availability and sales of alcohol in four Canadian provinces: A time-series analysis. *Contemporary Drug Problems* 32, 343–72.

Trolldal B. and Ponicki W.R. (2005) Alcohol price elasticities in control and license states in the United States, 1982–99. *Addiction* 100, 1158–65.

Truong K.D. and Sturm R. (2007) Alcohol outlets and problem drinking among adults in California. *Journal of Studies on Alcohol and Drugs* 68, 923–33.

Truong K.D. and Sturm R. (2009) Alcohol environments and disparities in exposure associated with adolescent drinking in California. *American Journal of Public Health* 99, 264–70.

Tumwesigye N.M. and Kasirye R. (2005) Gender and the major consequences of alcohol consumption in Uganda. In: Obot I.S. and Room R. (eds) *Alcohol, gender and drinking problems: Perspectives from low and middle income countries*, pp. 189–208. Geneva, Switzerland: World Health Organization.

Turner S.C. (1997) Effects of peer alcohol abuse education on college students' drinking behavior. *Dissertation Abstracts International* 57, 4276A.

Ugland T. (2002) *Policy re-categorization and integration: Europeanization of Nordic alcohol control policies.* Oslo: Arena.

Uhl A. (2007) How to camouflage ethical questions in addiction research. In: Fountain J. and Korf D (eds), *Drugs in society: European perspectives.* pp. 116–30. Oxford: Radcliffe.

United Breweries (2006–7) *UB Annual report*, Delhi.

Urbano-Márquez A. and Fernández-Solà J. (1996) Musculo-skeletal problems in alcohol abuse. In: Peters T.J. (ed.) *Alcohol misuse: A European perspective*, pp.123–44. Amsterdam, The Netherlands: Harwood Academic Publishers.

Usdan S., Moore C., Schumacher J., and Talbott L. (2005) Drinking locations prior to impaired driving among college students: Implications for prevention. *Journal of American College Health* 54, 69–75.

Valde K.S. and Fitch K.L. (2004) Desire and sacrifice: Seeking compliance in designated driver talk. *Western Journal of Communication* 68, 121–50.

Valencia-Martín J.L., Galán I., and Rodríguez-Artalejo F. (2008) The joint association of average volume of alcohol and binge drinking with hazardous driving behaviour and traffic crashes. *Addiction* 103, 749–57.

VandenBos G.R. (2007) *APA dictionary of psychology.* Washington, DC: American Psychological Association.

Van den Bulck J. and Beullens K. (2005) Television and music video exposure and adolescent alcohol use while going out. *Alcohol and Alcoholism* 40, 249–53.

Van Hoof J., Van Noordenburg M., and De Jong M. (2008) Happy hours and other alcohol discounts in cafes: Prevalence and effects on underage adolescents. *Journal of Public Health Policy* 29, 340–52.

Vartiainen E., Jousilahti P., Alfthan G., Sundvall J., Pietinen P., and Puska P. (2000) Cardiovascular risk factor changes in Finland, 1972–1997. *International Journal of Epidemiology* **29**, 49–56.

Victorian Government (2008) *Victoria's alcohol action plan, 2008–2013*. Melbourne: Victorian Government.

Vingilis E., McLeod A.I., Seeley J., Mann R., Beirness D., and Compton C. (2005) Road safety impact of extended drinking hours in Ontario. *Accident Analysis and Prevention* **37**, 549–56.

Vingilis E., McLeod A.I., Stoduto G., Seeley J., and Mann R.E. (2007) Impact of extended drinking hours in Ontario on motor-vehicle collision and non-motor-vehicle collision injuries. *Journal of Studies on Alcohol and Drugs* **68**, 905–11.

Viser V. (1999) Geist for sale: A neoconsciousness turn through advertising in contemporary consumer culture. *Dialectical Anthropology* **24**, 107–24.

Voas R.B. (2008) A new look at NHTSA's evaluation of the 1984 Charlottesville Sobriety Checkpoint Program: Implications for current checkpoint issues. *Traffic Injury Prevention* **9**, 22–30.

Voas R.B. and DeYoung D. J. (2002) Vehicle action: Effective policy for controlling drunk and other high-risk drivers? *Accident Analysis and Prevention* **34**, 263–70.

Voas R.B. and Marques P.R. (2003) Barriers to interlock implementation. *Traffic Injury Prevention* **4**, 183–7.

Voas R.B. and Tippetts A.S. (1999) *Relationship of alcohol safety laws to drinking drivers in fatal crashes*. Washington, DC: National Highway Traffic Safety Administration.

Voas R.B., Holder H.D., and Gruenewald P.J. (1997) The effect of drinking and driving interventions on alcohol-involved traffic crashes within a comprehensive community trial. *Addiction* **92** (Suppl.), 221–36S.

Voas R.B., Lange J.E., and Johnson M.B. (2002) Reducing high risk drinking by young Americans south of the border: The impact of a partial ban on sales of alcohol. *Journal of Studies on Alcohol* **63**, 286–92.

Voas R.B., Tippetts A.S., and Fell J.C. (2003) Assessing the effectiveness of minimum legal drinking age and zero tolerance laws in the United States. *Accident Analysis and Prevention* **35**, 579–87.

Voas R.B., Fell J., McKnight A., and Sweedler B. (2004) Controlling impaired driving through vehicle programs: An overview. *Traffic Injury Prevention* **5**, 292–8.

Voas R.B., Romano E., Tippetts A., and Furr-Holden C. (2006) Drinking status and fatal crashes: Which drinkers contribute most to the problem? *Journal of Studies on Alcohol* **67**, 722–9.

Wagenaar A.C. (1981) Effects of the raised legal drinking age on motor vehicle accidents in Michigan. *HSRI Research Review* **11**, 1–8.

Wagenaar A.C. (1986) Preventing highway crashes by raising the legal minimum age for drinking: The Michigan experience 6 years later. *Journal of Safety Research* **17**, 101–9.

Wagenaar A.C. (1993) Research affects public policy: The case of the legal drinking age in the United States. *Addiction* **88** (Suppl.), 75–81S.

Wagenaar A.C. and Holder H.D. (1991) Effects of alcoholic beverage server liability on traffic crash injuries. *Alcoholism: Clinical and Experimental Research* **15**, 942–7.

Wagenaar A.C. and Holder H.D. (1995) Changes in alcohol consumption resulting from the elimination of retail wine monopolies: Results from five US states. *Journal of Studies on Alcohol* **56**, 566–72.

Wagenaar A.C. and Langley J.D. (1995) Alcohol licensing system changes and alcohol consumption: Introduction of wine into New Zealand grocery stores. *Addiction* **90**, 773–83.

Wagenaar A.C. and Maldonado-Molina M. (2007) Effects of drivers' license suspension policies on alcohol-related crash involvement: Long-term follow-up in forty-six states. *Alcoholism: Clinical and Experimental Research* **31**, 1399–1406.

Wagenaar A.C. and Maybee R.G. (1986) Legal minimum drinking age in Texas: Effects of an increase from 18 to 19. *Journal of Safety Research* **17**, 165–78.

Wagenaar A.C. and Toomey T.L. (2002) Effects of minimum drinking age laws: Review and analyses of the literature from 1960 to 2000. *Journal of Studies on Alcohol* **63**, S206–25.

Wagenaar A.C. and Wolfson M. (1994) Enforcement of the legal minimum drinking age in the United States. *Journal of Public Health Policy* **15**, 37–53.

Wagenaar A.C. and Wolfson M. (1995) Deterring sales and provision of alcohol to minors: A study of enforcement in 295 counties in four states. *Public Health Reports* **110**, 419–27.

Wagenaar A.C., Finnegan J.R., Wolfson M., Anstine P.S., Williams C.L., and Perry C.L. (1993) Where and how adolescents obtain alcoholic beverages. *Public Health Reports* **108**, 459–64.

Wagenaar A.C., Toomey T.L., Murray D.M., Short B.J., Wolfson M., and Jones-Webb R. (1996) Sources of alcohol for underage drinkers. *Journal of Studies on Alcohol* **57**, 325–33.

Wagenaar A.C., Gehan J.P., Jones-Webb R., Wolfson M., Toomey T.L., Forster J.L., and Murray D.M. (1998) *Communities Mobilizing for Change on Alcohol: Experiences and outcomes from a randomized community trial.* Minneapolis, MN: University of Minnesota.

Wagenaar A.C., Murray D.M., and Toomey T.L. (2000a) Communities Mobilizing for Change on Alcohol (CMCA): Effects of a randomized trial on arrests and traffic crashes. *Addiction* **95**, 209–17.

Wagenaar A.C., Murray D.M., Gehan J.P., Wolfson M., Forster J.L., Toomey T.L., Perry C.L., and Jones-Webb R. (2000b) Communities mobilizing for change on alcohol: Outcomes from a randomized community trial. *Journal of Studies on Alcohol* **61**, 85–94.

Wagenaar A.C., O'Malley P.M., and LaFond C. (2001) Very low legal BAC limits for young drivers: Effects on drinking, driving, and driving-after-drinking behaviors in 30 states. *American Journal of Public Health* **91**, 801–4.

Wagenaar A.C., Maldonado-Molina M.M., Erickson D.J., Linan, M., Tobler A.L., and Komro K.A. (2007a) General deterrence effects of U.S. statutory DUI fine and jail penalties: Long-term follow-up in 32 states. *Accident Analysis and Prevention* **39**, 982–94.

Wagenaar A.C., Maldonado-Molina M.M., Linan, M., Tobler A.L., and Komro K.A. (2007b) Effects of legal BAC limits on fatal crash involvement: analyses of 28 states from 1976 through 2002. *Journal of Safety Research* **38**, 493–9.

Wagenaar A.C., Maldonado-Molina M.M., and Wagenaar B.H. (2009a) Effects of alcohol tax increases on alcohol-related disease mortality in Alaska: Time-series analyses from 1976 to 2004. *American Journal of Public Health* **99**, 1464–70.

Wagenaar A.C., Salois M.J., and Komro K.A. (2009b) Effects of beverage alcohol price and tax levels on drinking: A meta-analysis of 1003 estimates from 112 studies. *Addiction* **104**, 179–90.

Waiters E., Treno A., and Grube J. (2001) Alcohol advertising and youth: A focus-group analysis of what young people find appealing in alcohol advertising. *Contemporary Drug Problems* **28**, 695–718.

Wallack L. (1983) Mass media campaigns in a hostile environment: Advertising as anti-health education. *Journal of Alcohol and Drug Education* **28**, 51–63.

Wallack L. (1990) Social marketing and media advocacy: Two approaches to health promotion. *World Health Forum* **11**, 143–54.

Wallack L. and DeJong W. (1995) Mass media and public health: Moving the focus from the individual to the environment. In: Martin, S. (ed.), *The effects of the mass media on the use and abuse of alcohol*, pp. 253–68. Research Monograph No. 28. Bethesda, MD: National Institute on Alcohol Abuse and Alcoholism.

Wallack L. and Dorfman L. (1992) Television news, hegemony and health [letter]. *American Journal of Public Health* **82**, 125–6.

Wallin E. and Andréasson S. (2005) Effects of a community action program on problems related to alcohol consumption at licensed premises. In: Stockwell T., Gruenewald P., Toumbourou J., and Loxley W. (eds), *Preventing harmful substance use: The evidence base for policy and practice.* New York: Wiley.

Wallin E., Gripenberg J. and Andréasson S. (2002) Too drunk for a beer?: A study of overserving in Stockholm. *Addiction* **97**, 901–7.

Wallin E., Norström T., and Andréasson S. (2003) Alcohol prevention targeting licensed premises: A study of effects on violence. *Journal of Studies on Alcohol* **64**, 270–7.

Wallin E., Lindewald B., and Andréasson S. (2004) Institutionalization of a community action program targeting licensed premises in Stockholm, Sweden. *Evaluation Review* **28**, 396–419.

Wallin E., Gripenberg J., and Andréasson S. (2005) Overserving at licensed premises in Stockholm: Effects of a community action program. *Journal of Studies in Alcohol* **66**, 806–15.

Walsh D.C., Hingson R.W., Merrigan D.M., Levenson S.M., Cupples L.A., Heeren T., Coffman G.A., Becker C.A., Barker T.A., Hamilton S.K., McGuire T.G., and Kelly C.A. (1991) A randomized trial of treatment options for alcohol-abusing workers. *New England Journal of Medicine* **325**, 775–81.

Walsh G.W., Bondy S.J., and Rehm J. (1998) Review of Canadian low-risk drinking guidelines and their effectiveness. *Canadian Journal of Public Health* **89**, 241–7.

Walsh P. (2005) Diageo 2005 preliminary results. Presentation slides and speech transcript. Available at: http://www.diageo.com/NR/rdonlyres/4DA6C679-AC5E-4F90–8E93-AB213FFCD958/0/PaulWalshInterviewTranscript.pdf (accessed 2 November 2005).

Walters S.T., Vader A.M., and Harris T.R. (2007) A controlled trial of web-based feedback for heavy drinking college students. *Prevention Science* **8**, 83–8.

Warburton A.L. and Shepherd J.P. (2000) Effectiveness of toughened glassware in terms of reducing injury in bars: a randomized controlled trial. *Injury Prevention* **6**, 36–40.

Warburton A.L. and Shepherd J.P. (2006) Tackling alcohol related violence in city centres: Effect of emergency medicine and police intervention. *Emergency Medical Journal* **23**, 12–17.

Watson B. and Freeman J. (2007) Perceptions and experiences of random breath testing in queensland and the self-reported deterrent impact on drunk driving. *Traffic Injury Prevention* **8**, 11–19.

Watson B.C. and Nielson A.L. (2008) An evaluation of the 'Skipper' designated driver program: Preliminary results. Paper presented at the Australasian College of Road Safety Conference on High Risk Road Users, Brisbane, 18–19 September. Available at: http://www.acrs.org.au/srcfiles/Watson.pdf (accessed 13 July 2009).

Webb R. (2006) *Excise taxation: Developments since the mid-1990s.* Parliamentary Library Research Brief No. 15. Canberra, Australia: Parliament of Australia. Available at: http://www.aph.gov.au/library/pubs/rb/2005–06/06rb15.pdf (accessed 9 July 2009).

Wechsler H. (1996) Alcohol and the American college campus: A report from the Harvard School of Public Health. *Change* **28**, 20–25 and 60.

Wechsler H. and Nelson T.F. (2008) What we have learned from the Harvard School of Public Health College Alcohol Study: Focusing attention on college student alcohol consumption and the environmental conditions that promote it. *Journal of Studies on Alcohol and Drugs* **69**, 481–90.

Wechsler H., Nelson T.F., Lee J.E., Seibring M., Lewis C., and Keeling R.P. (2003) Perception and reality: A national evaluation of social norms marketing interventions to reduce college students' heavy alcohol use. *Journal of Studies on Alcohol* **64**, 484–94.

Wechsler H., Seibring M., Liu I.C., and Ahl L. (2004) Colleges respond to student binge drinking: Reducing student demand or limiting access. *Journal of American College Health* **52**, 159–68.

Weisner C. (2001) The provision of services for alcohol problems: A community perspective for understanding access. *Journal of Behavioral Health Services and Research* **28**, 130–42.

Weisner C., Conell C., Hunkeler E.M., Rice D., McLellan A.T., Hu T.W., Fireman B., and Moore C. (2000) Drinking patterns and problems of the "stably insured": A study of the membership of a health maintenance organization. *Journal of Studies on Alcohol* **61**, 121–9.

Weitzman E.R., Folkman A., Folkman K.L., and Wechsler H. (2003) The relationship of alcohol outlet density to heavy and frequent drinking and drinking-related problems among college students at eight universities. *Health and Place* **9**, 1–6.

Wells S. and Graham K. (1999) The frequency of third party involvement in incidents of barroom aggression. *Contemporary Drug Problems* **26**, 457–80.

Wells S., Graham K., and West P. (1998) 'The good, the bad, and the ugly': Responses by security staff to aggressive incidents in public drinking settings. *Journal of Drug Issues* **28**, 817–36.

Wells S., Graham K., and West P. (2000) Alcohol-related aggression in the general population. *Journal of Studies on Alcohol* **61**, 626–32.

Wells S., Graham K., and Purcell J. (2009) Policy implications of the widespread practice of 'pre-drinking' or 'pre-gaming' before going to public drinking establishments: Are current prevention strategies backfiring? *Addiction* **104**, 4–9.

Wells-Parker E. (2000) Assessment and screening of impaired driving offenders: An analysis of underlying hypotheses as a guide for development of validation strategies. In: Proceedings of the 15th International Conference on Alcohol, Drugs, and Traffic Safety, pp. 575–94. Stockholm: Ekom Press.

Wells-Parker E., Bangert-Drowns R., McMillen R., and Williams M. (1995) Final results from a meta-analysis of remedial interventions with drink/drive offenders. *Addiction* **90**, 907–26.

Werch C.E., Lepper J.M., Pappas D.M., and Castellon-Vogel E.A. (1994) Use of theoretical models in funded college drug prevention programs. *Journal of College Student Development* **35**, 359–63.

West S.L. and O'Neal K.K. (2004) Project D.A.R.E. outcome effectiveness revisited. *American Journal of Public Health* **94**, 1027–9.

Wheeler D.R., Rogers E.M., Tonigan J.S., and Woodall W.G. (2004) Effectiveness of customized Victim Impact Panels on first-time DWI offender inmates. *Accident Analysis and Prevention* **36**, 29–35.

Whetten-Goldstein K., Sloan F.A., Stout E.M., and Liang L. (2000) Civil liability, criminal law, and other policies and alcohol-related motor vehicle fatalities in the United States, 1984–1995. *Accident Analysis and Prevention* **32**, 723–33.

White D. and Pitts M. (1998) Educating young people about drugs: A systematic review. *Addiction* **93**, 1475–87.

White S. (1996) *Russia goes dry: Alcohol, state and society*. Cambridge, MA: Cambridge University Press.

Whitlock E.P., Polen M.R., Green C.A., Orlean T., and Klein J. (2004) Behavioral counseling interventions in primary care to reduce risky/harmful alcohol use by adults: A summary of the evidence for the US Preventive Services Task Force. *Annals of Internal Medicine* **140**, 557–68.

Wilks J., Vardanega A.T., and Callan V.J. (1992) Effect of television advertising of alcohol on alcohol consumption and intentions to drive. *Drug and Alcohol Review* **11**, 15–21.

Witheridge J. (ed.) (2003) Worldwide brewing alliance: Global social responsibility initiatives. London: British Beer and Pub Association.

Wiers R.W., van de Luitgaarden J., vand den Wildenberg E., and Smulders F.T.Y. (2005) Challenging implicit and explicit alcohol-related cognitions in young heavy drinkers. *Addiction* **100**, 806–19.

Wiggers J.H., Jauncey M., Considine R.J., Daly J., Kingsland M., Purss K., Burrows S., Nicholas C., and Waites R.J. (2004) Strategies and outcomes in translating alcohol harm reduction research into practice: The alcohol linking program. *Drug and Alcohol Review* **23**, 355–64.

Wilkinson C. and Room R. (2009) Warning labels on alcohol containers and advertisements: International experience and evidence on effects. *Drug and Alcohol Review*, in press.

Wilks J., Vardenega A., and Callan V. (1992) Effect of television advertising on alcohol consumption and intentions to drive. *Drug and Alcohol Review* **11**, 15–21.

Williams A.F. (2008) *Licensing age and teenage driver crashes: A review of the evidence*. Arlington, VA: Institute for Highway Safety.

Williams A.F., Ferguson S.A., and Cammisa M.X. (2000) *Self-reported drinking and driving practices and attitudes in four countries and perceptions of enforcement*. Arlington, VA: Insurance Institute for Highway Safety.

Williams A.F., McCartt A., and Ferguson S. (2007) Hardcore drinking drivers and other contributors to the alcohol-impaired driving problem: need for a comprehensive approach. *Traffic Injury Prevention* **8**, 1–10.

Williams C.L., Perry C.L., Dudovitz B., Veblen-Mortenson S., Anstine P.S., Komro K.A., and Toomey T.L. (1995) A home-based prevention program for sixth-grade alcohol use: Results from Project Northland. *Journal of Primary Prevention* **16**, 125–47.

Williams J., Chaloupka F.J., and Wechsler H. (2005) Are there differential effects of price and policy on college students' drinking intensity? *Contemporary Economic Policy* **23**, 78–80.

Willis C., Lybrand S., and Bellamy N. (2004) Alcohol ignition interlock programmes for reducing drink driving recidivism. *Cochrane Database of Systematic Reviews*, Issue 4. Art. No. CD004168. doi: 10.1002/14651858.CD004168.pub2.

Willis J. (2001) *Alcohol in East Africa, 1850–1999*. Durham: Durham University, History Department.

Wilsnack R.W., Wilsnack S.C., and Obot I.S. (2005) Why study gender, alcohol and culture? In: Obot I.S. and Room R. (eds), *Alcohol, gender and drinking problems: Perspectives from low and middle income countries*, pp. 1–24. Geneva: World Health Organization.

Windle M. (1996) Effect of parental drinking on adolescents. *Alcohol Health and Research World* 20, 181–4.

Wines M. (2000) An ailing Russia lives a tough life that's getting shorter. *New York Times*, 3 December.

Winlow S. (2001) *Badfellas: Crime, tradition and new masculinities*. Oxford: Berg.

Winlow S., Hobbs D., Lister S., and Hadfield P. (2001) Get ready to duck: Bouncers and the realities of ethnographic research on violent groups. *British Journal of Criminology* 41, 536–48.

Witheridge J. (ed.) (2003) Worldwide brewing alliance: Global social responsibility initiatives. London: British Beer and Pub Association. Available at: http://ec.europa.eu/health/ph_determinants/life_style/alcohol/Forum/docs/alcohol_lib6_en.pdf (accessed 24 August 2009).

Wood E., Shakeshaft A., Gilmour S., and Sanson-Fisher R. (2006) A systematic review of school-based studies involving alcohol and the community. *Australian and New Zealand Journal of Public Health* 30, 541–9.

Woodall W.G., Kunitz S.J., Zhao H., Wheeler D.R., Westerberg V., and Davis J. (2004) The prevention paradox, traffic safety, and driving-while-intoxicated treatment. *American Journal of Preventive Medicine* 27, 106–11.

World Bank Group (2000) *World Bank Group note on alcoholic beverages*. Washington, DC: World Bank Group.

World Advertising Research Center (2005) *World drink trends*, 2005 edn. Henley-on-Thames, UK: World Advertising Research Center.

World Health Organization (1992a) *International statistical classification of diseases and related health problems*, 10th revision (ICD-10). Tabular list. Geneva: WHO.

World Health Organization (1992b) *The ICD-10 classification of mental and behavioural disorders: Clinical descriptions and diagnostic guidelines*. Geneva: WHO.

World Health Organization (1993) *Programme on substance abuse: Assessing the standards of care in substance abuse treatment*. Geneva: WHO.

World Health Organization (1998) *The world health report 1998: Life in the 21st century: A vision for all*. Geneva: WHO.

World Health Organization (1999) *Global status report on alcohol*. Geneva: WHO.

World Health Organization (2000) *The world health report 2000—health systems: Improving performance*. Geneva: WHO.

World Health Organization (2001a) *The international classification of functioning, disability and health*. Geneva: WHO.

World Health Organization (2001b) *Global status report on alcohol*. Geneva: WHO.

World Health Organization (2002a) *The world mental health (WMH2000) initiative*. Geneva: WHO Assessment, Classification, and Epidemiology Group.

World Health Organization (2002b) *The world health report 2002: Reducing risks, promoting healthy life*. Geneva: WHO.

World Health Organization (2004a) Global status report on alcohol. Geneva: WHO. Available at: http://www.who.int/substance_abuse/publications/global_status_report_2004_overview.pdf (accessed 18 October 2009).

World Health Organization (2004b) *Global status report: Alcohol policy*. Geneva: WHO. Available at: http://www.who.int/substance_abuse/publications/en/Alcohol%20Policy%20 Report.pdf (accessed 6 July 2009).

World Health Organization (2009a) About WHO Framework Convention on Tobacco Control. Available at: http://www.who.int/fctc/about/en/index.html (accessed 6 July 2009).

World Health Organization (2009b) Parties to the WHO Framework Convention on Tobacco Control. Available at: http://www.who.int/fctc/signatories_parties/en/index.html (accessed 24 June 2009).

World Health Organization Expert Committee on Problems Related to Alcohol Consumption (2007) *WHO Expert Committee on problems related to alcohol consumption: Second report*. WHO Technical Report Series 944. Geneva: WHO.

World Trade Organization (2008) The 128 countries that had signed GATT by 1994. Available at: http://www.wto.org/english/thewto_e/gattmem_e.htm (accessed 27 October 2008).

World Trade Organization (2009) Members and observers. Available at: http://www.wto.org/ english/thewto_e/whatis_e/tif_e/org6_e.htm (accessed 24 June 2009).

Wortley R. (2001) A classification of techniques for controlling situational precipitators of crime. *Security* **14**, 63–82.

Wyllie A., Waa A., and Zhang J.F. (1996) *Alcohol and moderation advertising expenditure and exposure: 1996*. Auckland: University of Auckland.

Wyllie A., Zhang J.F., and Casswell S. (1998a) Positive responses to televised beer advertisements associated with drinking and problems reported by 18 to 29 year olds. *Addiction* **93**, 749–60.

Wyllie A., Zhang J.F., and Casswell S. (1998b) Responses to televised alcohol advertisements associated with drinking behaviour of 10–17-year-olds. *Addiction* **93**, 361–71.

Young D. (1993) Alcohol advertising bans and alcohol abuse: Comment. *Journal of Health Economics* **12**, 213–28.

Young D.J. and Bielinska-Kwapisz A. (2002) Alcohol taxes and beverage prices. *National Tax Journal* **55**, 57–88.

Young D.J. and Bielinska-Kwapisz A. (2006) Alcohol prices, consumption, and traffic fatalities. *Southern Economic Journal* **72**, 690–703.

Young D.J. and Likens T.W. (2000) Alcohol regulation and auto fatalities. *International Review of Law and Economics* **20**, 107–26.

Younger S.D. (1993) *Estimating tax incidence in Ghana: An exercise using household data*. Cornell Food and Nutrition Policy Program Working Papers No. 48. Ithaca, NY: Cornell University. Available at: http://www.cfnpp.cornell.edu/images/wp48.pdf (accessed 9 July 2009).

Younger S.D. and Sahn D.E. (1999) *Fiscal incidence in Africa: Microeconomic evidence*. Cornell Food and Nutrition Policy Program Working Papers No 91. Ithaca, NY: Cornell University. Available at: http://www.cfnpp.cornell.edu/images/wp91.pdf (accessed 9 July 2009).

Yu Q., Scribner R., Carlin B.P., Theall K., Simonsen N., Ghosh-Dastidar B., Cohen D.A., and Mason K. (2008) Multilevel spatio-temporal dual changepoint models for relating alcohol outlet destruction and changes in neighbourhood rates of assaultive violence. *Geospatial Health* **2**, 161–72.

Zador P.L. (1991) Alcohol-related relative risk of fatal driver injuries in relation to driver age and sex. *Journal of Studies on Alcohol* **52**, 302–10.

Zador P.L., Krawchuk S.A., and Voas R.B. (2000) Alcohol-related relative risk of driver fatalities and driver involvement in fatal crashes in relation to driver age and gender: An update using 1996 data. *Journal of Studies on Alcohol* **61**, 387–95.

Zakhari S. (1997) Alcohol and the cardiovascular system: Molecular mechanisms for beneficial and harmful action. *Alcohol Health and Research World* **21**, 21–9.

Zaridze D., Brennan P., Boreham J., Boroda A., Karpov R., Lazarev A., Konobeevekaya I., Igitov V. Terechova T., Boffetta P., and Peta R. (2009) Alcohol and cause-specific mortality in Russia: A retrospective case–control study of 49557 adult deaths. *Lancet* **373**, 2201–14.

Zhang J-F. (2004) Alcohol advertising in China. Presentation to Asia Pacific NGO Meeting on Alcohol Policy. Auckland, New Zealand, 24–25 September.

Zeigler D.W. (2006) International trade agreements challenge tobacco and alcohol control policies. *Drug and Alcohol Review* **25**, 567–79.

Zeigler D.W. (2009) The alcohol industry and trade agreements: A preliminary assessment. *Addiction* **104** (Suppl. 1), 13–36.

Zielenziger M. (2000) Year-ending parties pour drunks onto trains of Japan. *The Hartford Courant*, Hartford, CT, December 28.

Zimmerman R. (1997) *Social marketing strategies for campus prevention of alcohol and other drug problems*. Newton, MA: Higher Education Center for Alcohol and other Drug Prevention.

Zwarun L. (2006) Ten years and one master settlement agreement later: The nature and frequency of alcohol and tobacco promotion in televised sport, 2000 through 2002. *American Journal of Public Health* **96**, 1492–7.

Zwarun L. and Farrar K. (2005) Doing what they say, saying what they mean: Self-regulatory compliance and depictions of drinking in alcohol commercials in televised sports. *Mass Communication and Society* **8**, 347–71.

Zwarun L., Linz D., Metzger M., and Kunkel D. (2006) Effects of showing risk in beer commercials to young drinkers. *Journal of Broadcasting and Electronic Media* **50**, 52–77.

Zwerling C. and Jones M.P. (1999) Evaluation of the effectiveness of low blood alcohol concentration laws for younger drivers. *American Journal of Preventive Medicine* **16** (Suppl. 1), 76–80.

Glossary

Most of the definitions below were adapted from the following sources: Keller *et al.* (1982), Babor *et al.* (1994), VandenBos (2007), and Wikipedia.

Administrative licence revocation (ALR) Driver's licence is revoked administratively, without the need for a judicial process, in the event of a drink-driving arrest or conviction.

Affective education Programmes that address self-esteem, general social skills, values clarification, or similar factors assumed to underlie underage drinking.

Aggregate Population level; summary data representing a collection of individuals.

Alcohol dependence syndrome Term used in psychiatric diagnostic classifications to identify the co-occurrence of at least three of six alcohol-related symptoms associated with dependence on alcohol: increased tolerance, withdrawal signs; continued drinking despite harmful consequences; preoccupation with alcohol; impaired control over drinking; and alcohol craving.

Alcohol education programmes Programmes implemented in school settings with the aim of teaching students about the dangers of alcohol and ultimately preventing underage drinking.

Alcohol intoxication A more or less short-term state of functional impairment in psychological and psychomotor performance induced by the presence of alcohol in the body.

Alcoholism Term traditionally used to identify chronic excessive drinking by individuals who are physically dependent on alcohol. See 'alcohol dependence syndrome'.

Alcopops A form of alcoholic beverage characterized by carbonation, artificial colouring, sweetness, and other characteristics. More formal names for alcopops are 'premixed spirits', 'RTDs' (ready to drink beverages), 'flavoured alcoholic beverages', and 'designer drinks'. While there are earlier forms, such as 'long drinks' in Finland, alcopops emerged as an international category and a concern in the 1990s. With an alcohol content (~5%) that is often slightly higher than beer, the marketing of alcopops has been criticized because of its potential attractiveness to children and young adults.

Alternatives to drinking Programmes that provide minors with alternative activities (e.g. sports, meditation) presumed to be incompatible with underage drinking.

Aquavit Scandinavian forms of aqua vitae or vodka flavoured with caraway seed or other flavourings.

Arrack A distillate from the fermented product of local vegetation in many parts of the world, often variously flavoured. Palm toddy or other juices, rice, and molasses are chiefly used in the East Indies and in India; grapes and other fruit in the Balkans; dates and other produce in the Middle East.

BAC or BAL Blood alcohol content/concentration (BAC) is the concentration of alcohol in a person's blood. Blood alcohol level (BAL) is an equivalent term. The abbreviations are also used concerning breath alcohol concentration, as an indicator of blood alcohol. BAC is commonly used as a metric indicating intoxication for legal or medical purposes. It is usually measured in terms of mass per volume, either in percent (e.g., the legal limit for driving in the U.S. is .08%) or per-mille (the legal limit for driving in many European countries is 0.5 per mille, equivalent to .05%).

Binge drinking A pattern of heavy drinking that occurs over an extended period of time. In earlier population surveys, the period was usually defined as more than one day of drinking at a time. More recently the term has been applied to drinking by young adults and has been defined by the number of alcoholic drinks (usually five or six) consumed on a single occasion.

Bratt rationing system A form of liquor control (named after a Swedish physician) incorporated into Swedish law in 1917, designed to discourage misuse of spirits by establishing individual alcohol rations for adult citizens. The system was abolished in 1955.

Chibuku Indigenous alcoholic beverage of southern Africa; also known as opaque beer.

Chicha A fermented drink made in Latin America mostly from maize but also from a great variety of juices.

Cochrane Reviews Systematic reviews and meta-analyses of the scientific literature that explore the evidence for and against the effectiveness and appropriateness of medical treatments as well as social and psychological interventions. These reviews are designed to facilitate the choices that doctors, patients, policymakers and others face in health care and social policy decisions.

Confounding A distortion of results that occurs when the apparent effects of a variable of interest actually result entirely or in part from an extraneous variable that is associated with the factor under investigation.

Counter-advertising Actions involving the use of advertising-styled messages about the risks and negative consequences of drinking. Counter-advertising is used to balance the effects of alcohol advertising on alcohol consumption. Such measures can take the form of print or broadcast advertisements (e.g. public service announcements) as well as product warning labels.

Dependence See Alcohol dependence syndrome.

Disability-adjusted life-years (DALYs) A composite health summary measure that combines years of life lost to premature death with years of life lost due to disability.

Dram shop liability Legal statutes imposing liability upon the commercial drinking establishment or its representatives (e.g. servers) for injuries caused to or by intoxicated persons to whom they have sold alcoholic beverages.

Drinking patterns A sequence of drinking behaviours that includes the kind and amount of alcoholic beverage as well as the frequency, timing, and context of drinking occasions.

Empowerment model A strategy that attempts to solve problems by 'empowering' those most affected by a problem to use their knowledge, experience, and local resources instead of expert opinion or external resources.

Graduated driver licensing Process by which drivers' licenses are issued with limitations on driving privileges together with loss of licence if tested as higher than BAC limit.

Harm reduction/harm minimization Policies or programmes designed to reduce the harm resulting from the use of alcohol, without necessarily reducing alcohol use *per se*. Examples include programmes that offer free rides home to persons who are too intoxicated to drive their own cars.

Health belief model A theoretical model developed in the 1950s stating that the perception of a personal health behaviour threat is itself influenced by three factors: general health values, which include interest and concern about health; specific health beliefs about vulnerability to a particular health threat; and beliefs about the consequences of the health problem.

Hours and days of sale Days of the week and hours of the day in which it is legal to sell alcoholic beverages for consumption on- or off-premises.

International Statistical Classification of Diseases and Related Health Problems, 10th revision (ICD-10) The International Classification of Diseases is the standard diagnostic classification for epidemiological and health management purposes as well as clinical use. These include the analysis of the general health situation of population groups and monitoring of the incidence and prevalence of diseases and other health problems. It is used to classify diseases and other health problems recorded on vital records including death certificates and health records. ICD-10 was endorsed by the Forty-third World Health Assembly in May 1990 and came into use in World Health Organization Member States in 1994.

Licensing system A scheme for controlling the sale and distribution of alcoholic beverages by means of licenses granted by a national or local government authority to qualified persons. Licenses vary according to type of drink (beer, wine, distilled spirits) and place of sale (on- or off-premises, tavern, bar, supermarket) with the aim of restricting sales to certain times, places, customers, age groups, etc.

Liquor licensing See licensing system

Mandatory jail sentences A minimum prison sentence mandated by law for those convicted in a court of a drink-driving offence. Mandatory jail sentences apply to both first-time and repeat offenders. In its original design, mandatory sentencing attempted to determine the punishment for drink-driving offences rather than leave the punishment to the discretion of the judge.

Media literacy The process of evaluating messages in a wide variety of media by encouraging people to ask questions about what they watch, see, and read. In alcohol policy, media literacy education provides tools to help young people to critically analyse alcohol advertising and other marketing messages and thereby gain greater awareness of the potential for misrepresentation and manipulation.

Mediator An intervening or intermediate factor (e.g. intoxication) that occurs in a causal pathway from a risk factor (e.g. alcohol consumption) and a health (or social) problem (e.g. an accidental injury). It causes variation in the problem indicator, and variation within itself is caused by the risk factor.

Meta-analytic reviews (e.g. meta analysis) Statistical analyses in which data from several different studies are culled and reanalysed. The approach is particularly useful when there is a specific question to answer and at least a few relatively strong studies that come to different conclusions.

Natural experiment The investigation of change within and in relation to its naturally occurring context, as when a policy is implemented in one community but not in a comparable community.

Normative education Classroom lectures, discussions, and exercises designed to provide objective information (often obtained from school surveys) about the extent of alcohol use in the school-age population, which is thought to be overestimated by students. This information is thought to reduce the pressure to imitate or conform to the perceived norm.

Number of retail outlets The number of commercial drinking establishments selling alcoholic beverages for consumption on- or off-premises in a particular geographical area.

Ouzo A Greek brandy flavoured with oil of caraway.

Pattern of drinking See Drinking patterns.

Per se **laws** Laws that clearly define drink-driving with a BAC at or above a prescribed level for the whole population or for young drivers.

Pisco A brandy made in South America (Chilean liquor).

Prevention paradox The notion that the majority of the alcohol-related problems in a population are not associated with drinking by alcoholics but rather with drinking by a larger number of non-alcoholic 'social' drinkers.

Price elastic The percentage change in the amount of alcohol consumed (or quantity demanded) is greater than the percentage change in price.

Price elasticity of demand The term 'elasticity' is used by economists to describe the responsiveness of one variable to changes in another variable. Price elasticity of demand measures the responsiveness of demand for alcoholic beverages to changes in price. It involves comparing the proportional changes in price with the proportional changes in the quantity demanded. The relationship is expressed in the form of a ratio or coefficient.

Price inelastic The percentage change in price is greater than the percentage change in the amount of alcohol consumed (or quantity demanded).

Public service announcements Messages prepared by non-governmental organizations, health agencies, and media organizations for the purpose of providing important information for the benefit of a particular audience. When applied to alcohol, they usually deal with 'responsible drinking', the hazards of driving under the influence of alcohol, and related topics.

Pulque Indigenous alcoholic beverage of Mexico. It is made out of juice from the maguey cactus that goes through a fermentation process (similar to that of beer).

Quasi-experimental Lacking complete control over the scheduling of experimental stimuli that make true experiments possible. A quasi-experimental design does not include random assignment. The causal certainty of a quasi-experimental design is lower than that of a true experimental design.

Random breath testing Roadside checks of randomly selected drivers to assess BAC based on breath alcohol content. Also called 'compulsory breath testing' in some countries.

Randomized clinical trial A research design in which study participants are randomly allocated either to a group that will receive an experimental treatment or to one that will receive a comparison treatment or placebo. Randomization is done to eliminate error from self-selection or other kinds of systematic bias.

Randomized controlled experiment See Randomized clinical trial.

Randomized controlled study See Randomized clinical trial.

Rationing The sale of alcoholic beverages is limited to a certain amount per person (usually determined by government authorities). The most notable example of rationing as a way to discourage alcohol misuse is the Bratt system, a form of legal control over alcohol availability in Sweden between 1917 and 1955.

Resistance skills training Classroom exercises designed to provide the social and verbal skills necessary to refuse peer pressure to consume alcohol or drugs.

Responsible beverage service An education programme that trains managers of alcohol outlets and alcohol servers or sellers how to avoid illegally selling alcohol to intoxicated or underage patrons. Training includes educating servers regarding state, community, and establishment-level alcohol policies; describing potential consequences for failing to comply with such policies (e.g. criminal or civil liability, job loss); and development of the necessary skills to comply with these policies.

Responsible drinking Drinking of alcoholic beverages in moderation; drinking that does not lead to loss of health or other harm to the drinker or to others.

Shochu A low-priced Japanese spirit having an alcohol content of about 25%.

Sick-quitter effect The fact that many people abstain from alcohol because they are already sick, thereby making abstainers look less healthy as a group than moderate drinkers.

Sobriety checkpoints Places where roadside tests, designed to evaluate whether an individual is driving under the influence of alcohol, are administered.

Soju Traditional Korean liquor distilled from rice, barley, and sweet potatoes.

Sorghum A species of grass used to produce beer in southern Africa. African sorghum beer is a brownish-pink beverage with a fruity, sour taste. Alcohol content can vary between 1% and 8%.

Temperance See Temperance society.

Temperance society An organization originally devoted to the restriction or prohibition of alcoholic beverages by means of mutual pledging, education, political advocacy, charitable activities, and the establishment of treatment and prevention programmes.

Time-series analysis A statistical procedure that allows inferences to be drawn from two series of repeated measurements made on the same individuals or organization over time. Where the emphasis is on understanding causal relationships, the key question is how a change on one series correlates with a change on the other.

Total ban on sales A law or regulation making the sale of all or a specific type of alcoholic beverage illegal. Sometimes called alcohol prohibition.

Universal strategy A prevention strategy directed at the entire population, rather than at high-risk drinkers. Mass media campaigns often use this approach.

Viral marketing A technique aiming at reproducing 'word of mouth', usually on the Internet or by e-mail, for marketing purposes. Also called viral advertising, it refers to marketing techniques that use pre-existing social networks to increase brand awareness or to achieve other marketing objectives (such as product sales) through self-replicating viral processes passed on from one person to another. Viral promotions may take the form of video clips, interactive games, or text messages.

Warning labels Messages printed on alcoholic beverage containers warning drinkers about the harmful effects of alcohol on health.

World Health Organization (WHO) A United Nations agency established in 1948 to protect and promote the health of member states through public health measures and relevant policy research. In addition to the WHO's headquarters in Geneva, Switzerland, there are six regional offices. The WHO's Department of Mental Health and Substance Abuse is responsible for developing a Global Strategy to Reduce Harmful Use of Alcohol.

Zero tolerance The concept of compelling legal and judicial authorities, who might otherwise exercise their discretion in making subjective judgements regarding the severity of a given drink-driving offence, to impose a predetermined punishment regardless of individual culpability or 'extenuating circumstances'. Now also commonly used to refer to a requirement of no drinking (i.e. zero blood alcohol level), e.g. for novice or teenage drivers.

Index